"I have nothing but the utmost respect for Joy and her work. For many years she has helped me and my family with dieting and nutrition. She is forever searching for new ways to improve health and wellness. She is a star in my eyes."

—Tommy Mottola, music mogul, former chairman Sony Music Entertainment

"When it comes to questions about nutrition, Joy Bauer is your go-to source. She's got all the facts, with great tips for healthy eating and living with a totally sensible, and more importantly, realistic outlook on all of it. In my experience, this is the woman—and now the book—with the answers."

—Bobby Flay, chef/owner Mesa Grill, Bolo, Bar Americain, and Bobby Flay Steak, and author of *Grilling For Life*

"While reading *Joy Bauer's Food Cures*, I felt like I was visiting with Joy at her office. The book captures her real life persona . . . one of encouragement, humor, resiliency, support, genuine concern . . . and, above all, her ability to present realistic and practical options in achieving your personal goals and objectives!"

—Paul Carlucci, publisher, *New York Post*

"This is an easy-to-read, absolutely comprehensive, medically accurate guide to food as a body fuel. This book is a real contribution to the field—it explains the principles of nutrition, and lays out the practices of eating for health and well being. It is a gem."

—Orli R. Etingin, MD, professor of clinical medicine, Weill Cornell Medical College, New York Presbyterian Hospital

"Joy Bauer has somehow made the impossible, possible. She makes smart eating, weight loss and now, in this book, preventative and curative health a reality. Joy's simple and practical steps are easy to follow, even for those who feel challenged in this area. Our family knows firsthand that success is inevitable when you listen to Joy."

—Jessica Seinfeld, author and founder/president, Baby Buggy, Inc.

"Joy has written a superb, readable, and tremendously useful book that distills all her expertise into a volume I will use personally and give to all my patients. It's uniquely valuable."

—Marianne J. Legato, MD, founder and director of the Foundation for Gender-Specific Medicine, Inc.; professor of clinical medicine, Columbia University; and adjunct professor of medicine, Johns Hopkins

"Joy brings the same thoroughness and understanding of nutritional needs to this book as she does to our high-performance dancers. Her expertise makes her an integral part of our wellness team at New York City Ballet."

—Ken Tabachnick, general manager, New York City Ballet

"Wow! Joy has finally given us what we need. She has written a comprehensive, well-researched, easy-to-use nutritional guide for people who want to protect their vision from cataracts and macular degeneration."

—Paul T. Finger, MD, FACS, clinical professor of ophthalmology, New York University School of Medicine, and author of *The Macular Degeneration Network* (http://www.macular-degeneration.org)

"Joy Bauer has been the 'go-to' nutritionist in New York for many years. This easy-to-read book captures her warmth, her humor, her clinical wisdom, and her vast experience, and gives sensible advice about managing your diet and staying healthy. It is a most-welcome resource!"

—B. Timothy Walsh, MD, Ruane Professor of Psychiatry, College of Physicians & Surgeons, Columbia University; director, Eating Disorders Research Unit, New York Psychiatric Institute

"Reading *Food Cures* is like having an extended session with Joy herself. She offers intelligent, doable, and new solutions to the age-old question: What should I eat? Anyone who has ever held a menu, read a cookbook, or tried a diet will benefit from her wisdom."

—Lucy Danziger, editor-in-chief, *SELF* magazine

"Joy is exactly what you want in a nutritionist: compassionate, insightful, and incredibly knowledgeable about the latest diet research. Her new book, *Joy Bauer's Food Cures,* is just like having a much-coveted one-on-one session with Joy; and she offers smart, effective and, best of all, easy-to-implement advice for every goal—from weight loss to beautiful skin to improved digestion. This book is a must-read for anyone who wants a step-by-step action plan to better their diet and get results without starving or sacrificing taste, thanks to several delicious recipes."

—Caroline Schaefer, deputy editor, *Us Weekly*

"Joy's book serves up heaping portions of useful nutritional and general health information, coupled with lots of common sense advice and guidance. She spices it up with great anecdotes and recipes, written in a conversation style that makes this book a joy to read. I thought I'd just glance at the Weight Loss and Radiant Skin chapters, but each chapter was filled with so many goodies I could not put it down."

—Marsha Gordon, MD, clinical professor, dermatology, Mount Sinai School of Medicine

"*Joy Bauer's Food Cures* offers a welcome addition to my shelf of trusted books. It is a well researched guidebook for helping select the foods that will make and keep you healthy."

—Evelyn Attia, MD, associate director, The Eating Disorders Clinic, New York State Psychiatric Institute, and associate clinical professor of psychiatry, Columbia University College of Physicians & Surgeons

"Whether you are trying to lose weight, manage a chronic medical condition, or just feel better, nutrition expert Joy Bauer has detailed and targeted advice that will help. Grounded in the latest medical science, clearly explained and illustrated, and rounded out with dozens of user-friendly recipes, *Joy Bauer's Food Cures* is highly recommended not only for clinicians, but also for anyone pursuing a more healthful lifestyle."

—Michael J. Devlin, MD, associate professor of clinical psychiatry, Columbia University College of Physicians & Surgeons; and associate director, Eating Disorders Research Unit, New York State Psychiatric Institute

"*Joy Bauer's Food Cures* is an extraordinary detailing of profoundly easy nutrition programs that yield dramatic results. Joy doesn't just play with generalities, she boldly details the way specific foods relate to specific medical conditions and diseases. *Joy Bauer's Food Cures* is a fun and easy-to-read book that delivers the critical facts for everyone!"

—Carlon M. Colker, MD, FACN, chief executive officer and medical director, Peak Wellness, Inc.

"Joy Bauer's new book is well-written, easily read, and is a great guide for eating properly. Her style and 4-step outlines make it easy for anyone to understand and to follow the programs. It is a great recipe for all of us to learn."

—Phillip Bauman, MD, orthopaedic consultant for the New York City Ballet

"In a world crammed with crack-head nutritionists, Joy Bauer is a beacon of sanity. No joke—she saved my life."

—Dany Levy, founder and editor-in-chief of *DailyCandy*

"As Joy says, 'Eating is a piece of cake.' What she fails to mention is that it is only that easy if you have a clear, articulate, authentic, and authoritative guide like *Food Cures*. Joy makes eating and healthy living carefree and enjoyable. Dig in."

—Deanna Brown, general manager, Yahoo Health

"Joy Bauer is an amazing food coach! *Food Cures* will connect the dots between eating well, feeling healthy, and really enjoying your life."

—Vicki Wellington, associate publisher, *Domino* magazine

"The most comprehensive, easy-to-read book on life-changing nutrition, with the most up-to-date science. An extraordinary book, which will be a must-have for every one of my patients. Joy has changed how I eat, as well as how I treat."

—Dr. Lorenzo Gonzalez, MD, faculty at the University of Miami School of Medicine, department of physical therapy

"Fantastic! A comprehensive guide for anyone who wants to live better and feel better. With topics ranging from having beautiful skin and a great smile to handling migraines or celiac disease, it gives realistic advice for everyone. Plus, the recipes and shopping lists remove all guesswork and are simple enough for anyone to follow."

—Jeff Wellington, vice president, group publisher, *Parenting* Magazine

"Never before in history have we humans been able to shape our destiny—for good or for bad—to the degree we can today. With this liberating potential come responsibility and choice, what we do, how we live and, yes, what we eat. Joy Bauer has written a remarkable book. It outlines with clarity and caring professionalism a road map to better health. It is easy to read and amazingly easy to live by—all one needs is a touch of discipline—and that seasoning is under your control."

—Maurice Tempelsman, chairman of the board/director at Lazare Kaplan International, Inc.,

"It never ceases to amaze me that Joy continues to make it easy and clear for me to understand the world of nutrition. She simply knows how to keep it real."

—Laura Geller, renowned makeup artist, working mother, and educator

JOY BAUER'S

FOOD CURES

EASY 4-STEP NUTRITION PROGRAMS for IMPROVING YOUR BODY

This book is being published simultaneously by Rodale Inc. as *Food Cures*

© 2007 by Joy Bauer, MS, RD, CDN

Rodale books may be purchased for business or promotional use or for special sales. For information, please write to: Special Markets Department, Rodale, Inc., 733 Third Avenue, New York, NY 10017
Printed in the United States of America
Rodale Inc. makes every effort to use acid-free ∞, recycled paper ♻.

Book design by Joanna Williams

Library of Congress Cataloging-in-Publication Data
Bauer, Joy.
    Joy Bauer's food cures : easy 4-step nutrition programs for improving your body / Joy Bauer with Carol Svec.
        p.   cm.
    Includes bibliographical references and index.
    ISBN-13 978–1-59486–466–7   paperback
    ISBN-10 1–59486–466-7   paperback
    1. Diet therapy—Popular works.   I. Svec, Carol.   II. Title.
    RM217.B38   2007
    615.8′54—dc22   2007001050

Distributed to the book trade by Holtzbrinck Publishers
4   6   8   10   9   7   5   paperback

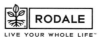

We inspire and enable people to improve their lives and the world around them
For more of our products visit **rodalestore.com** or call 800-848-4735

This book is dedicated to health and medical researchers everywhere.

Their brilliant, behind-the-scenes work allows me and other wellness educators to improve the health of millions of people.

ACKNOWLEDGMENTS

Many remarkable people were involved in the creation of this book. I'm especially grateful to the world-class physicians who continuously trust and support my work, and to my extraordinary clients—their successes have made this book possible by teaching me the things readers need and want to know.

Tremendous thanks to Carol Svec—appreciation is an understatement. You were my pillar of strength during this entire process and actually made hard work enjoyable. This book is a direct result of your extraordinary talent and professionalism. You're a brilliant writer, and it's a sheer honor to work with you and call you my friend.

Sincere thanks to *Dystel and Goderich Literary Management*. Jane Dystel, your wisdom, ongoing support, and direction mean the world. And many thanks to Miriam Goderich for your overall guidance and expertise.

Special thanks have to go out to two extraordinary experts and colleagues: Erica Ilton, the director of nutrition research for this project. This book substantially benefited from your genius research and exceptional input. And Jennifer Iserloh, a phenomenal chef with a passion for health. Your scrumptious recipe contributions and incredible commitment were a true blessing. Seriously, you are both angels.

Thanks to the entire crew at Rodale, Inc. Your enthusiasm, support, and dedication are greatly appreciated. Special thanks to Heather Jackson and Tami Booth Corwin for recruiting me, and to Gail and Jim Citrin for helping to ignite the fire. Many thanks also to Liz Perl, Nancy Hancock, Lois Hazel, Cindy Ratzlaff, Mary Lengle, Chris Rhoads, and Joanna Williams. Tremendous thanks to my two fabulous editors: Lisa Considine, for your valuable suggestions in writing, editing, and structuring the book . . . and Amy Super, who pulled everything together at the end.

I feel particularly grateful to Steven Rubenstein for your friendship, support, and ongoing kindness. And special thanks to Alice McGillion, Rachel Nagler, and Lori Ferme of Rubenstein Public Relations for helping to spread the word of good health!

Deep appreciation to Shaquille O'Neal—for making me a part of your dream team and mission to get kids healthy.

Lori Schulweis, I am so appreciative of your friendship and for all that you've done.

Many thanks to Jim Bell (for your kindness and ongoing support), Amy Rosenblum (for your confidence, friendship and expert tutelage—I'm forever indebted), Marc Victor (for your warm generosity), Rainy Farrell (for believing in me, and going way out on a limb), Elena Nachmanoff (for taking my calls!), and Jackie Levin (for giving my book a shot). Heartfelt thanks to all of you for regularly inviting me on your show and enabling me to improve the health of America. You make the studio feel like my home away from home. Also, thank goodness for Laura Bonanni and Barbara Kelly, Bianca Henry, Kristin Costa, Edward Helbig, and Deb Winson. And many thanks to Paul, Cindy and the hardworking prop department at *Today*.

Thanks to Kim Gerbasi and Emily Raiber—you gave me a shot and I'm forever grateful.

Much appreciation to my friends at Yahoo! . . . Deanna Brown, Rachel Friedlander, Harold Goings, and Maggie Nemser.

Sincere thanks to Jessica Seinfeld. Your passion for health makes it an honor to collaborate and call you a friend. Thanks, too, to the fabulous Pam Fink, for my "Charmed Life." Clearly, your Good Charma jewelry works!

I owe thank yous to so many people, all of whom play an important part in my life: Peter Martins, Ken Tabachnick, and the rest of the gang at *New York City Ballet* . . . and Mira-bai Holland at the 92nd Street Y . . . the crew at *SELF* magazine, especially Lucy Danziger, Carla Levy, and Donna Fennessy . . . my attorney, Richard Heller, for invaluable input and legal advice . . . Jon and Bonnie Ackerman, for expertise on teeth and cooking . . . and last (but never least) Judy Lieberman, for the outstanding gazpacho recipe.

Special thanks to Janice Johnston, Lois Perelson-Gross, Dany Levy, and Geralyn Coopersmith for your genuine support and friendship. And many thanks to Cindy Cinicolo, Louisa Guigli and Martha Rios.

For your ongoing advice, opinions, and positive energy, I send heartfelt thanks to the dedicated registered dietitians/nutritionists at *Joy Bauer Nutrition* who help keep New Yorkers healthy: Lisa Mandelbaum, Jennifer Medina, Laura Pumillo, Maria Baldo, Erica Ilton, Elyssa Hurlbut, Nicole DiLorenzo, Suzanne Magnotta, Rebecca Appleman, Amy Horwitz, and Ilana Derman. And many thanks to my interns for all your hard work and commitment; Barbara Ackerman-Kravitz, Ilyse Bernikow Schapiro, Janice Wen, and Rachel Dower.

Hugs to everyone in my wonderful families: the Beal family; (Debra, Steve, Ben, Noah, Becca, Harvey, and Jenny), the Schloss family (Ellen, Artie, Pam, Dan, Charlie, Glenn, Elena, and Otis), the Bauer family (Carol, Vic, Jason, Mia, Harley, and Jimmy), the Malachowsky family (Mary and Nat), and the Cohen/Shapiro family (Nancy, Jon and Camrin). And special thanks to Lisi Epstein, Kael Goodman, and Shannon Green.

I must give special mention to "the room" on the third floor in Stockbridge where I spent most of my summer, and to the Berkshire Co-Op in Great Barrington for providing me with a table and cup of coffee whenever my house was too filled with chaos to write.

Thanks, too, to Bill Svec, for keeping my coauthor sane and happy while she was working on deadline.

Infinite, deep, and ever-lasting thanks to my mom and dad. You are my lifelines and my touchstones. Your support means the world and I'm forever grateful for your encouragement, advice, cashews, and wine.

I can't say enough about my husband Ian, and my three children, Jesse, Cole, and Ayden Jane—I owe you big time! You all astonish me with your patience, understanding, support, flexibility, and forgiveness. You picked up the pieces when I was preoccupied, and you picked me up with your good humor and loving spirits. Just when I thought I saw the full magnitude of your generosity, you surprised me again and again. You are everything valuable in the world . . . my heart . . . my bliss . . . my home . . . my loves.

CONTENTS

PART SIX—SMOOTH SAILING

PART ONE

WELCOME TO MY OFFICE

CHAPTER 1

WELCOME TO MY OFFICE

My motto is this: Life is hard . . . food should be easy.

But for many people, knowing what to eat, when to eat, and how much to eat is a puzzle they have lost all hope of ever solving.

Anyone who has ever tried to make a commitment to healthy eating knows the obstacles: The dizzying number of choices in grocery stores and restaurants . . . the crazy, always-on-the-go schedules of nearly every member of the family . . . the relentless hype and marketing surrounding fatty and sugary snack foods . . . and the powerful appetites fueled by habits, traditions, and humongous portion sizes. As if that wasn't enough pressure, add in the swirl of conflicting information about specific diets—high-carb versus low-carb, high-fat versus low-fat, calorie-counting versus no-counting, cabbage versus grapefruit versus eggs versus whatever.

Who wouldn't feel overwhelmed and frustrated? And when we're frustrated, we tend to fall back into old, unhealthy eating patterns. Have you ever gone on a diet to lose weight, but ended up gaining weight instead? Or did you lose weight only to put it back on again within a year or two? Has your doctor ever put you on a special diet to treat a health problem, but you soon abandoned it because it was just too complicated for real life? If so, you're not alone. These scenarios happen more often than you might think. No one consciously plans to eat her way into a larger dress size, or to make himself a candidate for triple bypass surgery. But dietary uncertainty can turn the best intentions sour, even when the stakes are high. When it comes to good nutrition, it is so easy to go from being totally motivated to feeling utterly defeated.

It doesn't have to be that way. Whatever else is going on in your life, food should be the least of your worries. Eating is a piece of cake.

Really.

HOW FOOD MAKES US NUTS

I understand why you might be skeptical. We have a strange love/hate relationship with food. We want to eat cupcakes, but be as slim as Jennifer Aniston. We fantasize about our ideal meal, but settle for a burger and fries from a drive-through window. We buy "skinny jeans" for the body we want to have, but then eat comfort foods because those jeans don't fit anything but our dreams. Love/hate—two sides of the same sneaky cookie.

Food does more than nourish us, so it makes sense that it can elicit complex feelings. Of course, its most important role is to nourish us—to give us the vitamins, minerals, energy, and nutrients necessary to keep us alive and healthy—but food is also about love and family traditions. It's how we celebrate and comfort and nurture—which is why food is at the center of weddings and funerals, and it's the first thing we think to bring when we hear a friend is sick. Food is about taking away the pain that comes from hunger, but it also has become about easing our boredom, stress, or depression. We tend to eat too much of almost everything whenever we get the chance. We eat in the car, at work, in front of the TV, or standing over the kitchen sink. We snack before meals, after meals, and sometimes in the middle of the night, sometimes without even waking up. Next to sex, eating is the activity most responsible for making us feel any number of emotions, including happiness, longing, pride, pleasure, shame, weakness, and power.

Food is like that great, big proverbial elephant in the room—which also follows you around all day. We try to ignore it, but every time we turn around, there it is. Yet despite the huge (mammoth!) role food plays in our lives, we don't really know how to talk about it, at least not in a way that helps us make the best choices when it comes time to eat.

I believe the reason some diets become wildly popular for a time is that they allow us to understand food and eating in a new way, and they give us a different language to use when trying to sort out our confusion. Think about it: During the past few years, we've all learned the language of "Carbs"—what carbs are, what low-carb eating looks like, the difference between net carbs and total carbs, bad carbs and good carbs, et cetera, et cetera. Before that, we studied the language of "Fats." And before fats, we all knew how to parse calories.

So it's not that people lack information about food and eating. In fact, most of us have more information than we know what to do with. Literally. Many of my clients have such sophisticated vocabularies that they sound like third-year nutrition students. The problem is that they don't know how to combine all the disparate pieces of the diet puzzle into a plan that they can use to achieve their individual, highly personal goals. They are eager—desperate, even—to gain control over food. But they can't do it with words alone!

That's where I come in.

THE POWER OF A STEP-WISE PROGRAM

In my 16 years as a nutritionist, I've helped thousands of people overcome their worst problems with eating. In the process, they have grown stronger and healthier. In many cases, they have added 10, 15, or even 20 years to their lives by controlling or even reversing disease processes.

How can food turn your life around? Let me tell you about 56-year-old Stephen, a high-powered lawyer who was all but ordered by his doctors to make an appointment with me. To say he was initially resistant to seeing a nutritionist would be an understatement. It was a hard sell, but in the end the encouragement (and begging and pleading) of his wife and children persuaded him to come to see me.

He was a nutritional wreck. At 5' 9" tall, Stephen was significantly overweight at 250 pounds. His body mass index (BMI) was 37, officially classifying him as obese. His lab values were high across the board: High cholesterol and triglycerides put him at high risk of heart disease, and high fasting glucose levels meant Stephen was officially diagnosed with type 2 diabetes.

To try to get control over these risk factors, Stephen's doctors put him on three powerhouse medications—a blood pressure drug, a statin to lower his cholesterol, and Glucophage to lower his blood sugar. And then I got a hold of him.

I gave him a food plan to help him lose weight, lower blood sugar, and lower his cholesterol . . . and when he had an episode of gout, I gave him tips on how to treat that, too. Once he overcame his initial reluctance, Stephen approached his new eating program with the same intensity he used to succeed in every other aspect of his life. He made a spreadsheet to track his weight loss and his lab numbers, he used his eating plan like a script: he memorized and followed it religiously. He consulted me whenever circumstances made it more than likely he would need to deviate from it—to make sure he wouldn't do too much harm. He ate cake at his birthday party, he socialized with friends, and he enjoyed holiday celebrations—but all within the guidelines of his food program.

At the end of a year, Stephen had lost more than 60 pounds, bringing him down to under 190. His critical blood measurements—triglycerides, cholesterol, and fasting glucose—all dropped to within normal ranges. He continued to take the statin, but he was able to stop taking the Glucophage and the blood pressure medication. As of this writing, Stephen has maintained his weight loss and health benefits for three years. His doctor told him that because of the nutritional changes, Stephen has probably *added at least ten healthy years to his life.*

As amazing as this story sounds, Stephen's results are not unusual, and well within anyone's reach. No matter what your personal health goals are, I have a terrific food plan for you. I'll even help you figure out exactly what your goals should be.

My goal is to make reading this book as much as possible like a one-on-one consultation with me in my New York office. I'll tell you everything you need to know to lose weight, look gorgeous, improve your mood and memory, boost your bone density, and stay healthy. I'll even give you a script to follow—a focused four-step program that spells out everything you need to know to think *and eat* just like a nutritionist. In short, I'll provide everything you need for success.

STEP INSIDE MY OFFICE

Let's start at the beginning, with the absolute basics. One of the main questions I'm asked over and over is what defines *good nutrition*. In general, it means eating the right foods in the right combinations throughout the day to optimize your energy and overall health.

Of course, the people who come to see me lead different lives and strive to achieve a wide range of goals. So for some, good nutrition means focusing on increasing energy. I've worked with professional and student athletes, dancers, actors, and business executives who need to maintain a consistent level of performance. For other people who have a strong family history of disease, good nutrition means minimizing their risk of heart disease, diabetes, Alzheimer's disease, migraine headaches, arthritis, osteoporosis, or cancer. For others, it means finding a way to lose the weight they might have been struggling with for years.

A while ago, a man I'll call Bruce called me up and told me that one of his friends had lost a ton of weight after he became my client, and now he looked phenomenal. His buddy said that I worked miracles. Bruce was calling because he had a weight problem, but he was a busy person. He knew all the tricks, had been on all the diets, had gained and lost 100 pounds more times than he could count, and didn't want to bother with an appointment if I couldn't guarantee success. "Tell me," he said, "are you the person who is absolutely going to help me prevail, once and for all?"

He didn't mince words! But he just asked outright what everyone really wants to know—can my programs work, immediately, quickly, and forever? The short answer to that question is *Yes, dramatic and long-lasting results are absolutely possible . . . but the chance of success depends entirely on you.* I don't want to give anyone false promises, not in my office and not in this book. I'm only as good as my clients' follow-through, so if you're after the kind of transformation that your friends (like Bruce's) will call miraculous, I'm here to help. I can show you how to evaluate your needs, give you a dynamite eating plan, and guide you through some of the most common nutritional pitfalls. We are a team—I'm your food coach, but ultimately you're the one who'll be doing the heavy lifting.

A FEW WORDS ABOUT COMMITMENT

In the end, no matter what spurs you to seek help, three things are necessary for you to meet your goals:

1) The right coach. Well, you've got me, so cross this one off your list. I have a great track record for success with my clients.

2) Rock-solid nutrition and health information. Cross this one off the list, too, because that's what this book is all about.

3) Your personal commitment to stay in it for the long haul. This one is up to you!

Personal commitment is a big deal. None of this will work for very long if you're only following a food program because you're going on vacation, or because someone else is on your back about losing weight. You have to be doing this for you. You have to want results and be willing to work for them no matter what obstacles get in your way. After the September 11 attacks on the World Trade Center and the Pentagon, I heard lots of stories about how people ran for comfort foods and the liquor cabinet and gave themselves permission to overeat and drink . . . for weeks. My belief is that it's incredibly important—especially in times of crisis—to eat right and stay on top of your health.

Think about it: Whenever you say "I'm overwhelmed, I've got too many things on my plate"—or "I'm depressed . . . or too busy . . . or too anxious"—what do you do? If you're like most people, you give up on good nutrition and eat foods that make you sick, contribute to your illness, or put on weight you spent months trying to shed. In the end, you're left feeling depressed, sluggish, and easily angered. How is that helpful?

That's why I really think that any time could be the right time to make food changes. Your commitment is what's important, the commitment to eating well the majority of the time—not perfect foods, but healthy foods. It is a commitment you'll need to honor when you're home, when you're out, when you're shopping, and when you're socializing. It's a commitment to totally change your lifestyle.

PREPARE YOURSELF

Changing how you eat is never easy. The first step is to get in the right place mentally. If we're going to try to create a little nutritional magic, there are a few things you need to do to prepare for this adventure:

- **Limit your use of the word _diet_.** The word _diet_ seems to have horrible connotations. It is impossible to use the word _diet_ in a sentence without sounding sad or judgmental. Try it: "I really should go on a diet." "My doctor put me on a diet." "Boy, if anyone needs to diet, he does." The only time _diet_ doesn't sound like a prison sentence is when we talk happily about going off one. Try not to use the D-word; it will just demoralize you.

- **Repeat after me: "I can do this!"** The prospect of trying another weight-loss program can feel like staring into a black hole—no joy, no light, no end in sight. It's easy to feel defeated before you even begin, so some degree of nervousness is understandable. But a more appropriate response is enthusiasm and confidence. Trust me. I'm a professional. I've done this hundreds and hundreds of times before. No matter what your personal issues are, I've seen worse (and you'll read some of those stories in the chapters to come). I will give you all the secrets for success I've learned over the years.

- **Dare to make the leap.** Pop quiz: Which is more fun, wading into the shallow end of the pool or doing a cannonball off the diving board? When we were kids, all we wanted to do was jump into the deep end. We tend to lose that sense of courage and daring along the way. As adults, we need to find a way to get back that feeling of *one . . . two . . . three . . . let's go!* And we're talking about nutritional changes, so you can't hurt yourself by making a full, unrestrained leap. This is about your health—the only risk is if you don't do anything. So go ahead, take a deep breath, and jump in.

- **Think big.** As far as I'm concerned, small changes add up to small results. Grand changes equal grand, life-altering results. We're on this earth for such a short time that I don't believe we have the luxury to move slowly. And face it, it can be just as hard to make a small change as it is to go for the whole enchilada (so to speak). So, you might as well go for it. Make the big changes! The payoffs will be larger, and your gratification will come sooner.

- **When the going gets tough, remember that it's *just food*.** That probably sounds crazy coming from a nutritionist, but it's a critically important point to remember. Write it on a piece of paper and tape it up on your refrigerator: "It's just food." If you're in a restaurant trying to stick to your food plan, but salivating over the meal that the person next to you is eating, remember to ask yourself: Is it worth it? The food is only going to be there for 15 to 20 minutes at most, and then it is gone, a memory except for the effects it has on your health and your weight. Is it worth it? That's a question only you can answer. If, after careful and deliberate consideration, you answer yes, it is worth it, then go for it. We'll consider it your "meal off," like a little vacation day for your taste buds. But those meals off should be rare and special, just like real vacations.

- **Prepare to feel fabulous.** I won't try to fool you into thinking that there will ever come a time when you won't crave sweet, fatty foods, or that you will never want to go whole-hog at a buffet. We're all magnetically drawn to those foods that temporarily make us euphoric, and then drop us way down. Those yummy temptations are on every street corner, at every dinner party, and in all your friends' homes. They will always be there, every day for the rest of your life. But that said, the payoff in the form of improved quality of life is well worth the fight. You're going to want to continue to live through these struggles because you're going to feel so good when you meet your goals. When you give in to temptation and eat poorly, you end up feeling sluggish, lethargic, and unhealthy. What's the point?

So instead of giving in just to end up feeling bad, invest some energy and effort and feel fabulous. In the end, if you feel energetic and healthy, and you're more agile and comfortable, and you've added years and years onto your life, and you smile more often, and you're less moody, and you're more productive at home and at work, isn't it worth putting on the temptation blinders? Isn't it worth ducking the doughnuts? Isn't it worth enduring a little craving?

I say revel in your passion for life, not potato chips. And as your coach and nutritionist, I refuse to let you settle for anything less than success. You can do this, and I'm excited to help you.

CHAPTER 2

THINK LIKE A NUTRITIONIST

If you were visiting my office, I would ask you for two things. The first is a three-day food diary, essentially a snapshot of how food fits into your life. For three days, you would record everything you ate at every meal, every supplement or herb, every snack, every beverage. I would ask what brand of breakfast cereal you ate, how much pasta you had for dinner, how you prepared the vegetables, what type of spread you ate on your bread, the name of the restaurant where you ate lunch, what you added to your coffee, and what time of day you ate each meal or snack. Everything. This information would tell me exactly how much change would be needed to get your diet up to stellar quality.

Unfortunately, I don't have the personal luxury of reviewing your food habits . . . but you do. I highly recommend that you keep a modified food diary for yourself. Simply write down all the foods you eat for any three days of an average week. Don't worry about brands . . . but note what, when, and how much you eat and drink from the minute you wake up until you go to sleep. Everything counts—the quick snack from the vending machine, that "sliver" of cake from the office birthday party, the handful of French fries you grabbed off your son's dinner plate, the finger scoops of cookie dough you "tested" while baking for your family and yes, the two margaritas you sipped last night at happy hour. Everything you eat has consequences—good or bad—for your body, so record it all. This diary will provide us with a baseline, an indication of where your eating habits are now. We won't use it in the course of the book, but the diary is a terrific way to focus your mind on the details of eating (and of course, to help you notice patterns you'd like to change). Plus, a few weeks from now, when you've mastered a new way of eating, you'll be able to look back with pride when you see just how far you've come. It's often an incredible comparison, with a remarkable payoff.

The second thing I would ask for is your detailed medical history. My nutrition programs are designed to help you get control over your most pressing health problem first. Once you've mastered the first thing on the list, you'll be ready to tackle any other problems you might have. I recommend writing down all diseases, disorders, or diet-related concerns that affect your life. These can include being overweight, having a disease or disorder, or even having a history of medical tests that indicated a higher risk of disease. Beneath that, write down all diseases or disorders that run in your family, particularly those of your parents, grandparents, and siblings. When a biological family member has suffered with certain medical concerns, such as macular degeneration or breast cancer, this automatically puts you in a higher risk category. This list makes up your total universe of health issues. We're going to take them on, one at a time.

WHAT TO EXPECT FROM EACH CHAPTER

Each chapter of this book includes information about a particular health issue: how food, the environment, and other factors contribute to the issue; what foods to eat or avoid; which remedies might offer the best chance for curing or controlling symptoms; and other lifestyle changes you can make to feel better. Whenever possible, I include a story from my practice or personal experience, one which illustrates some particular aspect of how nutrition has helped change someone's life. (Although the basics of the stories are accurate, I have changed names and identifying information to protect my clients.)

The part I think you'll like best is my 4-Step Program. Each chapter has its own focused, customized program that summarizes all the advice offered in the rest of the chapter, and then goes full-force into specific food lists and meal plans. *Step 1: Start with the Basics* is a list of things you can do today, immediately, to take your first steps on the path to better health. *Step 2: Your Ultimate Grocery List* details foods that have been proven by scientific and clinical research to be beneficial, arranged in convenient grocery-aisle shopping lists. *Step 3: Going Above and Beyond* is a list of next steps, additional activities, supplements worth considering, or lifestyle changes that will improve your chances for success. *Step 4: Meal Plans* includes menus with the right mix of all the best foods—arranged into breakfast, lunch, dinner, and snack options—to help you accomplish your goals.

Common old-school wisdom says that you should eat breakfast as if you were royalty, lunch as if you were rich, and dinner as if you were flat broke. What this means is that breakfast really is the most important meal of the day, the time when you get to jump-start your day with energy and nutrition. Lunch is also important, because it gives you strength and stamina to make it through the toughest part of the day. Dinner is much less important because it comes at the end of the day, when you really don't need much fuel to carry you to bedtime. So ideally, you should eat the most calories at breakfast, nearly as many calories at lunch, and very few calories at dinner. Although I'm a health expert, I'm also a realist. I understand that the world doesn't work this way, so I've structured my meal plans to reflect the way people *really* eat. In each meal plan in every chapter, breakfast options are only 300 to 400 calories, lunch options are 400 to 500 calories, and dinner options are 500 to 600 calories.

Each chapter also contains at least two nutrition-rich—and delicious!—recipes. At the end of the book are additional sections to help you make great nutritional choices, including my favorite types and brands of foods to look for when you shop, how to read a food label, and references to the scientific studies mentioned throughout the book in case you want more details.

So, now that you've had a basic tour, it's time to choose where you want to start . . .

HOW TO CHOOSE WHICH PROGRAM TO FOLLOW

I'm willing to bet that you already know which health issue you would like—or need—to tackle first. Wait . . . don't tell me . . . could it be *weight loss*?

Unwanted pounds are the primary concern for about 60 percent of my clients, either because of how that extra weight makes them feel or because it contributes to another health disorder, such as diabetes or heart disease. If weight is an issue for you, begin by reading Weight Loss (page 19). It explains the basic mechanisms of weight loss, and reveals some of the secrets used by models, dancers, athletes, and others who absolutely need to control their weight. After more than 15 years spent working with all types of people—CEOs and store clerks, A-list celebrities and struggling musicians, supermodels and prima ballerinas, Olympic gold medalists and couch potatoes, and plenty of regular folks—I know what works. There is no one-size-fits-all plan. However, overweight people share many common struggles, and I present tricks that work. I know they work because they've been tested over and over again by my clients who have successfully lost weight and kept it off. If weight is your primary medical problem, then follow Joy's 4-Step Program for Weight Loss (page 41), from beginning to end.

If you have other health issues in addition to weight, I recommend reading the weight-loss chapter first to learn how to determine daily caloric intake for weight loss, and so that you understand how to apply my general principles. Follow one week of my 4-Step Program for Weight Loss. Then, look in the table of contents for the chapter that addresses your next most pressing health problem, read that chapter, and follow that 4-Step Program. You won't lose out on weight loss because this whole book is full of weight-loss guidance. The meal plans I provide in *every* chapter are scaled for weight loss, with specific calorie ranges listed for each and every breakfast, lunch, dinner, and snack. If you follow the plans precisely, your three meals and one or two daily snacks will amount to only 1,400 to 1,900 calories, depending upon the specific optional foods you choose. That's well below the 2,000 to 5,000 calories most Americans eat every day. So whether you follow the program for beauty, mood, migraines, or celiac disease, you can get the results you want, eat fantastic foods, *and* lose weight.

If weight is not an issue for you, congratulations! Either you have been blessed with the kind of metabolism that would make most people envious, or you have worked hard to maintain your weight. If you are part of this lucky minority, use the same food lists and meal plans listed in each chapter, but let your hunger cues guide portion size. You've done a great job thus far, so keep doing what you've always done . . . but with your specific program foods.

No matter which chapter you choose to focus on, the information in the 4-Step Program is your roadmap to success. But like all maps, it is designed for general navigation instead of a single strict path. Feel free to make adjustments for your personal taste and circumstances, as long as you stay within the general guidelines. For example, I might recommend a dinner of grilled salmon with a sweet potato and a mixed green salad with tomatoes and walnuts. If salmon isn't your favorite, choose another fish from the options given on the grocery list. Or, if you are eating out and they don't have sweet potatoes, ask for a serving of brown rice or a baked white potato instead. If tomatoes aren't in season, choose any mixed side salad and you'll still be within the general meal plan guidelines. If you only have time to microwave a frozen dinner, choose one that includes a grilled fish, a whole grain, and a vegetable. Similarly, if you are at a diner for an omelet breakfast, the cook certainly won't use a nonstick cooking spray on the griddle. So order an egg white omelet, ask them to fill it with your choice of vegetables, and eat your whole-wheat toast dry to compensate (at least somewhat) for the butter or grease used to cook the omelet. In other words, I provide the ultimate combinations of foods in calorie-controlled portions. You provide the creativity to make them work in your life.

TOP TIPS FOR THINKING LIKE A NUTRITIONIST

Before you begin, let me offer some helpful hints that will help you succeed, even if you've never been able to stick with a diet before.

1. **Watch out for weekends.** It is easiest to stay with the program during the week, when your time is probably more structured. It is more difficult during more unstructured time, such as on weekends and vacations. If you understand this in advance, you can make a plan of attack—try to give more structure to your downtime until the eating program becomes second nature.

2. **Pre-plan meals as much as possible.** Don't wait until you're starving before looking in the pantry. Say it's 8:00 p.m. and all you have on hand are crackers and potato chips. Well, that scenario might make a chip-eater out of even the most dedicated healthy eater. Try to shop on the same days of the week, every week, so you always have the right foods on hand. If you plan your lunch and dinner in the morning when you're having breakfast, you'll be able to pick up any missing ingredients during the day.

3. **Use the meal plans as a starting place.** The chapter meal plans use the recommended foods in the kinds of portions and combinations that are nutritionally sound and promote weight maintenance (or weight loss, if that's your goal). They are valuable if you want to follow them to the letter, but they also work as examples. Feel free to substitute other foods from your chapter's Ultimate Grocery List.

4. **Purge your home of foods that are unhealthy**—specifically foods that you tend to crave and overeat. If they are not easily available, you will be less likely to eat them. Don't just keep them around "for the kids." Buy treats for the kids that you don't enjoy, so they can have their goodies and you won't be tempted. Maybe later on, when you are feeling stronger and maybe even euphoric from your success, you can bring the chocolate chip cookies back into your life . . . or the doughnuts, or the Doritos, or whatever your personal "gotta have 'em" foods are.

5. **Load up on vegetables.** Eat vegetables whenever you can, in almost any quantity. There is no greater source of vitamins, minerals, and disease-fighting phytochemicals than vegetables. Aim to eat three to eight servings of vegetables daily.

6. **Eat 2+ servings of fresh fruits daily.** Fruits are healthy, but they are higher in calories and sugar than vegetables. Aim to eat two to four servings of fresh fruit daily. Calorie-laden fruit juices are another story; you'll want to dramatically limit them.

7. **Choose whole grains over refined white.** White flour is whole wheat flour, but with the nutritious part taken out. White rice is the same as brown rice, but with the nutritious part taken out. Whenever possible, choose whole grains over processed white grains.

8. **Account for liquid calories.** High-calorie beverages can undo the best weight-loss efforts if you forget to add them into your daily calorie count. Fruit juice and whole milk are healthy, but they are full of calories. Sugary beverages, especially soft drinks, are full of calories and nothing else. Wine and other alcoholic beverages also contain more calories than most people think. You'll notice that some of my meal plans recommend smoothie recipes and occasional healthy beverages. They are good for you, but they also contain calories (which I list in the recipe). If you are aiming for weight loss, remember to include the calories you drink in your daily tally. To enjoy more healthy foods without gaining weight, choose no-cal options, such as water, unsweetened tea, and other unsweetened beverages.

9. **Be wary of alcohol.** Many people don't realize that beer, wine, and liquor contain a significant number of calories. Plus, drinking alcohol can lower your inhibitions, which may make it more difficult to stick with your nutritional diet plans. Think about it. How many people do you know who make their best decisions after a few drinks? Plus alcohol has many effects on physiology, good and bad. In some chapters, you'll be advised to avoid alcohol altogether, but most people can drink moderately

with no ill effects. Most health professionals define *moderate* as one glass daily for women, and two glasses per day for men. If you regularly drink more than that, I recommend cutting down for the sake of your overall health.

10. **Don't forget breakfast—eat within 90 minutes of waking.** You're fasting for as long as you sleep, and your body needs to energize for the day ahead. That's what breakfast is for. It is your best opportunity to start each day on the right nutritional track.

11. **Maintain the right mix of foods.** Try to eat a combination of high-quality proteins and carbohydrates at every meal. You'll be energized throughout the day and stay full longer. In addition, combining foods will help your body maintain optimal levels of brain and other chemicals. (My meal plans include high-quality carbs and proteins in all meals, with the exception of dinners in my Insomnia chapter, where carbs are the focus to help induce sleep.)

12. **Fill up on fiber.** Fiber is naturally found in high-quality carbohydrate, such as vegetables, fruits, and whole grains. Fiber helps fill you up, lower your cholesterol, regulate your system, stabilize blood sugars, and more. My meal plans are loaded with fiber, so you don't have to worry about counting grams.

13. **Eat 3+ servings of calcium-rich foods daily.** Calcium does more than just build strong bones (although it is good for that). Calcium is necessary for muscle function and blood pressure management, which means that we need it every day . . . and way beyond the first years of our lives. Calcium is found in abundant amounts in dairy foods, some leafy green vegetables, fortified juice, enriched soy milk, almonds, fortified cereals and other whole-grain products, and salmon or sardines (with bones in). If you're a woman, and can't get enough through food, consider supplements to build and preserve bone density (see page 239 for more information).

14. **Eat every four to five hours.** Eating regularly will help you maintain level blood sugar, which is important for many health issues in this book, and also for general well-being, focus, and energy.

15. **Incorporate daily exercise.** Exercise is part of nutrition. Yup, you read that right. It allows us to use nutrients efficiently, to keep our minds active, to strengthen our bones and muscles, and any number of other valuable functions.

16. **Curb your calories after 8:00 p.m.** If you must eat after dinner, enjoy a small snack of 200 calories or less. (Nearly all snacks listed in meal plans are 200 calories or less.) If you have a history of nighttime nibbling, find a way to shut out food as an option after you finish dinner. You might follow dinner with a cup of herbal tea—then close down the kitchen and floss and brush your teeth. Eventually, your body will recognize the tea as a sign that eating is over, and the urge to snack will subside.

17. **Be patient.** Although a few chapters contain nutrition changes that can work quickly, most of the fixes here work more slowly. Some changes have invisible results, such as changes in cholesterol, which may not be noticeable until you have blood work done. It is important to stick with any nutrition program for at least six weeks. Resist all temptation to stop early. You'll be proud of yourself, and thrilled with the results.

FINAL WORDS OF ADVICE

No one expects you to be perfect. We're all human, even nutritionists. We, too, have days when we indulge our food lusts—remind me to tell you about my personal love affair with frozen peanut M&Ms. But I make healthy foods my *habit,* and frozen candy an occasional treat. If you really want to think like a nutritionist, start by becoming mindful of your eating habits. The good ones are your keys for overall health, weight management, and quality of life. Think of the indulgences as just that—a luxury you can only occasionally afford.

I know you can do it. Remember, we're in this together. Are you ready? Go ahead, find your starting chapter, and dive in!

PART TWO

LOSING WEIGHT

CHAPTER 3

WEIGHT LOSS

If you are reading this chapter, then you've decided you want to lose weight. Good for you! I'm going to help you do it.

Unwanted pounds are the number one reason people come to see me. Some of my clients are hundreds of pounds overweight, others have been trying for years to drop just 10 pounds. Some people are referred by doctors because their weight puts them at high risk for certain disorders, while others want to fit into a wedding dress, or to return to their wedding weight in time for an anniversary or a big birthday. I advise actors and actresses who need to look a particular way for a role, athletes who need to boost their strength and energy, and fashion models who need to be thin but not emaciated. No matter what your personal reasons or motivations, I'm thrilled that you have made the commitment to a healthier, slimmer you. Whatever brought you here, welcome to the party!

Yes, you read that correctly . . . this is a party, not a dreary march down a dark and fruitless dieting path. A plan that has enjoyed as much success as this one is a cause for celebration. Just think: If you had made this commitment a year ago, you would already be 12 to 50 pounds lighter, a few sizes smaller, and feeling happier and healthier than ever. By this time next year, you could be that person. Better still, you'll feel great doing it. Yes, I know that weight loss is your overall goal, but the process of getting there is empowering. After just one week following my 4-Step Program for Weight Loss, most people feel more confident and in control. They sleep better and feel more alert during the day. And, yes, their clothes are more comfortable, even a little looser. After a month, my clients can't imagine going back to their old ways. After three months, friends start asking *them* for their weight loss secrets. Your commitment is the first essential step in this process and visible results aren't far behind.

WEIGHT-LOSS BASICS

Most of my clients know everything there is to know about the mechanics of weight loss. Chances are you do, too, so I'm not going to go into exhaustive detail—I'll just review enough of the basics so that you understand the reasons behind some of my recommendations. I also include client stories (all names have been changed!) and weight-loss lessons to help you avoid some potential traps.

HOW MUCH SHOULD YOU WEIGH?

Are you overweight?

The answer is not as straightforward as you might think. Sure, there are scales and charts and different scientific methods for calculating "fatness," but determining whether a particular person is overweight isn't as easy as saying whether a light is on or off. It's more like trying to judge whether a particular light is "bright." Sometimes there will be a general consensus that a particular light is, indeed, bright—most people agree halogen floodlights are bright. But there are times when reasonable people could disagree. A 60-watt bulb might look dim at noon, but at midnight—when it is the only source of light—the same bulb might appear bright. Contextual factors play a role in judging whether someone is carrying extra pounds too—ballerinas and sumo wrestlers, for instance, have very different definitions of overweight. Physicians and their patients may have different definitions, too. Like judging artwork or the taste of a meal, there is an aspect of weight that is less scientific and more subjective.

HEIGHT AND WEIGHT

Ever hear someone say, "I'm not fat . . . I'm just short for my weight"? That really is one way to look at it—when doctors decide who is or is not overweight, they rely on charts that provide a range of healthy weights based on height. It's important for them (and you!) to know if you are overweight because hundreds of scientific studies confirm that those extra pounds increase the risk of many types of diseases . . . and losing weight can reduce those risks. The first height-weight charts were constructed in the 1940s by a life insurance company as a shorthand way to determine which applicants would be most costly to insure; the greater the risk of an early death, the more likely the company would be to lose money on that particular policy. The company collected years of mortality statistics and created tables of "desirable" weights by height, which were used, in part, to educate the

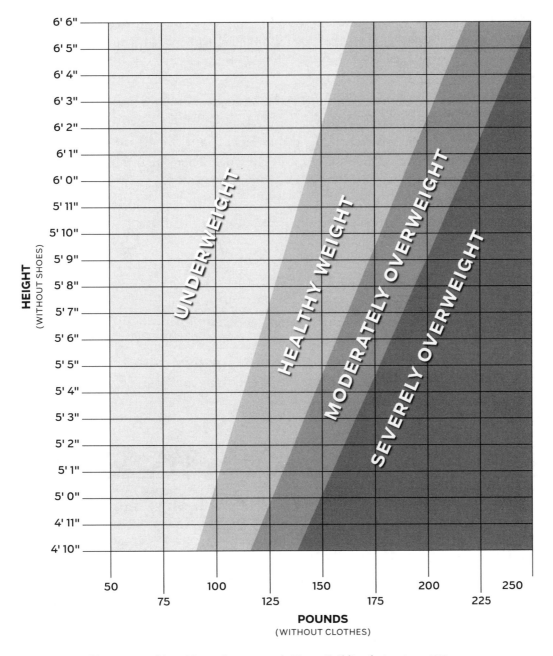

Source: Report of the Dietary Guidelines Advisory Committee on the Dietary Guidelines for Americans, 2000.

public about the health risks of weights that fell outside the desirable range. The charts have been revised and refined since then, but the concept is the same.

According to height-weight charts, people are considered overweight if they carry more weight than what is usually expected for someone their height. For example, a woman of 5'8" who weighs 155 pounds is at a healthy weight. However, 155 pounds puts a woman of 5'4" in the category of moderately overweight, and a woman of 5'0" in the category of severely overweight. Height and weight charts are a valid, if imperfect, way of defining overweight. Obviously some of your weight is muscle, bone, and other tissues that are essential to your physical functioning, and every inch of height adds healthy pounds to your total weight. Excess body fat, on the other hand, adds unhealthy pounds.

BODY MASS INDEX

In order to standardize the height-weight relationship to a simple numerical scale, scientists created the body mass index (BMI).

By using this chart instead of the height-weight chart, doctors use one number to determine whether you fall into a healthy weight range. There are five BMI categories:

- Underweight: BMI under 18.5
- Normal weight: BMI 18.5 to 24.9
- Overweight: BMI 25 to 29.9
- Obese: BMI 30 to 39.9
- Extreme obesity: BMI over 40

As with the height-weight measure, BMI is not perfect, but it's pretty darn good. It is a quick, inexpensive indicator that can be easily calculated during any physical examination. If you haven't already checked out where you fall on these charts, check now. Do the charts say you are overweight? If so, and you're not overly muscular (i.e., a body builder), chances are the charts are right.

Body Mass Index Table

	Normal						Overweight					Obese										Extreme Obesity														
BMI	19	20	21	22	23	24	25	26	27	28	29	30	31	32	33	34	35	36	37	38	39	40	41	42	43	44	45	46	47	48	49	50	51	52	53	54
Height (inches)															Body Weight (pounds)																					
58	91	96	100	105	110	115	119	124	129	134	138	143	148	153	158	162	167	172	177	181	186	191	196	201	205	210	215	220	224	229	234	239	244	248	253	258
59	94	99	104	109	114	119	124	128	133	138	143	148	153	158	163	168	173	178	183	188	193	198	203	208	212	217	222	227	232	237	242	247	252	257	262	267
60	97	102	107	112	118	123	128	133	138	143	148	153	158	163	168	174	179	184	189	194	199	204	209	215	220	225	230	235	240	245	250	255	261	266	271	276
61	100	106	111	116	122	127	132	137	143	148	153	158	164	169	174	180	185	190	195	201	206	211	217	222	227	232	238	243	248	254	259	264	269	275	280	285
62	104	109	115	120	126	131	136	142	147	153	158	164	169	175	180	186	191	196	202	207	213	218	224	229	235	240	246	251	256	262	267	273	278	284	289	295
63	107	113	118	124	130	135	141	146	152	158	163	169	175	180	186	191	197	203	208	214	220	225	231	237	242	248	254	259	265	270	278	282	287	293	299	304
64	110	116	122	128	134	140	145	151	157	163	169	174	180	186	192	197	204	209	215	221	227	232	238	244	250	256	262	267	273	279	285	291	296	302	308	314
65	114	120	126	132	138	144	150	156	162	168	174	180	186	192	198	204	210	216	222	228	234	240	246	252	258	264	270	276	282	288	294	300	306	312	318	324
66	118	124	130	136	142	148	155	161	167	173	179	186	192	198	204	210	216	223	229	235	241	247	253	260	266	272	278	284	291	297	303	309	315	322	328	334
67	121	127	134	140	146	153	159	166	172	178	185	191	198	204	211	217	223	230	236	242	249	255	261	268	274	280	287	293	299	306	312	319	325	331	338	344
68	125	131	138	144	151	158	164	171	177	184	190	197	203	210	216	223	230	236	243	249	256	262	269	276	282	289	295	302	308	315	322	328	335	341	348	354
69	128	135	142	149	155	162	169	176	182	189	196	203	209	216	223	230	236	243	250	257	263	270	277	284	291	297	304	311	318	324	331	338	345	351	358	365
70	132	139	146	153	160	167	174	181	188	195	202	209	216	222	229	236	243	250	257	264	271	278	285	292	299	306	313	320	327	334	341	348	355	362	369	376
71	136	143	150	157	165	172	179	186	193	200	208	215	222	229	236	243	250	257	265	272	279	286	293	301	308	315	322	329	338	343	351	358	365	372	379	386
72	140	147	154	162	169	177	184	191	199	206	213	221	228	235	242	250	258	265	272	279	287	294	302	309	316	324	331	338	346	353	361	368	375	383	390	397
73	144	151	159	166	174	182	189	197	204	212	219	227	235	242	250	257	265	272	280	288	295	302	310	318	325	333	340	348	355	363	371	378	386	393	401	408
74	148	155	163	171	179	186	194	202	210	218	225	233	241	249	256	264	272	280	287	295	303	311	319	326	334	342	350	358	365	373	381	389	396	404	412	420
75	152	160	168	176	184	192	200	208	216	224	232	240	248	256	264	272	279	287	295	303	311	319	327	335	343	351	359	367	375	383	391	399	407	415	423	431
76	156	164	172	180	189	197	205	213	221	230	238	246	254	263	271	279	287	295	304	312	320	328	336	344	353	361	369	377	385	394	402	410	418	426	435	443

Source: Adapted from *Clinical Guidelines on the Identification, Evaluation, and Treatment of Overweight and Obesity in Adults: The Evidence Report.*

WAIST/HIP RATIO

While young people with a high BMI are at an increased risk of disease and death, the relationship for older folks is less clear. As we age, our body composition changes and the predictive power of the BMI and height-weight charts weakens. Unhealthy pounds still matter, but BMI is not always an accurate measure of fatness among older people, especially those over age 75. Fortunately, the waist/hip ratio (WHR) succeeds where the BMI fails.

To calculate your WHR, measure your waist circumference with a flexible tape measure. (If you have a visible waist, measure around the narrowest part of your abdomen. Otherwise, take the measure at the level of your navel.) Record that number as your waist measurement. Then, measure around your hips—the widest part of your lower body, at or below the level of your pelvis. Record that number as your hip measurement. Now, take your waist measurement and divide by your hip measurement. That is your WHR. (For example, if your waist circumference is 30", and your hip measurement is 38": $30 \div 38 = 0.79$.) Higher WHRs indicate a greater proportion of weight carried as abdominal fat. In 2006, British researchers discovered that, for people older than 75, the greatest health risks are for men with a WHR greater than 0.99, and for women with a WHR greater than 0.90. For people younger than age 75, WHR also provides a measure of fatness that is related to an increased risk of cardiovascular disease, diabetes, and other disorders. For this younger group, the increased disease risk has a lower cut-off point: a WHR of 0.95 or greater for men, or 0.80 or greater for women.

PERSONAL EVALUATION

In addition to these mathematical formulations and charts, there is another expert you need to consult on the question of fatness—your own gut (pun intended). Do *you* think you are overweight?

Losing weight shouldn't be about pleasing other people or meeting some arbitrary social standard. Losing weight is about feeling great, both physically and emotionally. You know your body better than everyone else—your energy level, how well you're sleeping, whether your appetite is under control, and how your waist size has changed in the past year or two (or ten). You know whether you've been dragging or energetic and fit. And you know whether you are happy with the way you look and feel. That counts for a lot.

Weight loss requires hard work, faith in yourself, and a dream for your future. If it comes down to a battle between numbers on a BMI chart and emotions, emotions win every time. Your doctor can advise you, but he or she can't give you incentive. That part is all you. That's why I always encourage my clients to get in touch with their true motivations for wanting to lose weight, some personal reason, something to keep them going that has nothing to do with the numbers.

Take a moment now and think about your reasons for wanting to lose weight. You might be motivated by an milestone event you hope to enjoy with your family—like seeing your child graduate from college. It can be mundane, such as wanting to fit into a particular designer outfit. It can even be pure frustration with a weight issue that has stuck with you since childhood. Whatever your reasons, embrace them. They will carry you forward to success.

CALORIES COUNT

Calories are a measure of how much energy food provides. We need calories to do chores, run after the kids, make it through a full day of work, or go out with friends. All body processes use energy, too, including breathing, digesting, growing hair and fingernails, making hormones and enzymes . . . everything. Even the most inactive sofa sloth needs a certain number of calories to get through the day; active people need quite a bit more.

Here is the weight-loss formula: If you take in more energy (from food calories) than you use, the excess gets stored as body fat—most noticeably around your waist, hips, or thighs. If you use more energy than you take in, then your body gets the energy it needs by breaking down the stored fat, and you lose weight. That's it. That's what it takes to lose weight— use up more calories than you eat. Of course, you and I and everyone on the planet knows that it is *way more difficult* to do than it is to explain.

CALORIE CALCULATIONS

If your goal is to burn more calories than you take in, you need to know how many calories your body needs on an average day. There's a mathematical formula I use to make this estimate. And although this calculation can be incredibly helpful, it doesn't take into account genetics, your age, and muscular makeup—all of which play an important role in the amount of calories you burn each day. As we go along, I'll run through the numbers with our hypothetical 155-pound woman (height doesn't matter here).

1. Take your current weight (in pounds), and multiply by ten. That's the number of calories your body needs just to keep breathing and digesting and doing all that other maintenance work. This is called your *basal metabolic rate* (BMR).

    155 pounds × 10 = 1,550 calories (BMR)

2. Determine your *activity level:*
    - Average activity level: 0.30
      (Average activity is: desk job, little to no regular exercise)
    - More active than most: 0.40
      (More active is: engages in light, planned exercise or sports 1 to 3 times per week)
    - Very active: 0.50
      (Very active is: engages in moderate, planned exercise or sports 3 to 5 times per week)
    - Extremely active: 0.60
      (Extremely active is: engages in vigorous, planned exercise or sports 5 to 7 times per week)

    For our example, let's say the activity level is average:

    activity level = 0.30

3. Multiply your BMR by your activity level. This is your *activity factor.* (I'll talk more about this concept later!)

1,550 (BMR) × 0.30 (activity level) = 465 (activity factor)

4. Add your BMR and your activity factor to get your *maintenance calories*. You need about this many calories to make it through an average day. If you eat this exact number of calories, you will neither gain nor lose weight—you will maintain your current weight. *Important note:* When you lose weight, you'll have to recalculate your numbers.

1,550 (BMR) + 465 (activity factor) = 2,015 (maintenance calories)

So, for our 155-pound woman to maintain her weight, she should eat 2,015 calories a day. But, of course, you don't want to stay the same weight, do you? If you want to lose weight, you have to eat fewer calories than your maintenance calories. The greater the difference between your maintenance calories and the number of calories you eat daily, the faster you will lose weight. In our example, the maintenance calories are 2,015. Eating 1,800 calories per day will result in weight loss:

2,015 (maintenance calories) − 1,800 (actual calories) = 215 weight-loss calories

In order to lose a pound of fat, you need to accrue 3,500 weight-loss calories. In our example, the 215 weight-loss calories "spent" per day adds up to 78,475 weight-loss calories per year, which yields a projected weight loss of about 22 pounds in a year.

Reducing calories further to only 1,600 calories per day will result in faster weight loss:

2,015 (maintenance calories) − 1,600 (actual calories) = 415 weight-loss calories

These 415 weight-loss calories per day add up to 151,475 weight-loss calories per year, which yields a projected weight loss of about 43 pounds in a year. The greater the difference between your maintenance calories and your actual calories, the faster you will lose weight. *Important note:* Do not go lower than 1,000 actual calories per day. There is no advantage to ultra–low calorie dieting—your metabolism will slow, you'll be more likely to binge due to starvation, and you may develop some vitamin and mineral deficiencies from not eating healthfully.

Remember, you plug more than just the calories you eat into the equation—there's also your activity level. If you increase your maintenance calories by upping your activity level you'll also speed up weight loss. For example, if our hypothetical woman increases her activity to the 0.40 level, she will raise her maintenance calories to 2,170:

1,550 (BMR) × 0.40 (activity level) = 620 (activity factor)

1,550 (BMR) + 620 (activity factor) = 2,170 (maintenance calories)

Eating 1,800 calories per day will result in weight loss:

2,170 (maintenance calories) − 1,800 (actual calories) = 370 weight-loss calories

These 370 weight-loss calories per day add up to 135,050 weight loss calories per year, which yields a projected weight loss of about 39 pounds in a year.

But eating only 1,600 calories per day will result in faster weight loss:

2,170 (maintenance calories) − 1,600 (actual calories) = 570 weight-loss calories

These 570 weight-loss calories per day add up to 208,050 weight-loss calories per year, which yields a projected weight loss of about 59 pounds in a year.

Notice that even at the same calorie levels, weight loss is faster when you bump up the exercise and give your metabolism a boost. In the example, if our 155-pound woman ate 1,800 calories per day, she could lose 22 pounds in a year with an average activity level, but 39 pounds in a year by increasing her activity level just one notch above average.

BOOSTING METABOLISM

Clients—and just about everyone I meet who learns I'm a nutritionist—ask me this question all the time: How can I boost my metabolism?

Metabolism is simply the total of all body processes that burn calories—your basal metabolic rate plus your activity factor. When it comes to improving your metabolism, there's good news and bad news.

First the bad news: Most of what controls your metabolism isn't under your control. Some people are genetically blessed with a high-burning metabolism. They didn't ask for it, they were born with it. (So don't hate them for it, unless, of course, they rub it in!) On average, men have a metabolism that is 10 to 15 percent higher than women's, mainly because of their larger size and greater muscle mass. Whether you're a man or a woman, your metabolism naturally decreases with age. Scientists have estimated that metabolism slows about 5 percent per decade, beginning at age 40, as we lose muscle mass and increase body fat. Hypothyroidism (under-active thyroid) lowers metabolism and causes weight gain. Fortunately in this case, if a blood test confirms there's a problem, your doctor will prescribe medication that can boost it back up to baseline.

Now the good news: Your metabolism doesn't have to remain stagnant or take a nose-dive. You can burn more calories, lose more weight, just by changing the way you think about eating and moving.

FOOD FIXES FOR METABOLISM

Remember—our basal metabolic rate includes the energy we need for body processes, including digestion. About 10 percent of our calories are used to process the food we eat. As the calories are burned, our bodies generate heat. This phenomenon, known as the *thermic effect of food,* is influenced by how much, how often, and what we eat. In addition, food can directly affect metabolism by altering the way the body functions (which changes the amount of energy it needs). Here are my best recommendations for maximizing metabolism:

- **Eat at least 1,000 calories per day.** Although it is generally true that eating a low-calorie diet will help you take off weight, if you eat too few calories, your metabolism will get slower and slower as it tries to conserve energy. As your metabolism crashes, the weight you take off will most likely creep back on over time. Plus, you'll be more likely to binge on junk food if you reduce your calories by too much.
- **Eat every four to five hours.** A regular meal schedule helps keep your body working to digest and absorb foods. Between breakfast and bed, aim to eat a meal or snack every four to five hours. And try to eat breakfast within 90 minutes of rising. People who regularly eat a healthy breakfast are more likely to control

their weight. If you wait to eat until you're really ravenous, you're more likely to overeat later in the day. Also breakfast helps fire up your metabolism after a full night on a slow simmer.

- **Eat protein with every meal.** All foods contribute to the thermic effect, which means that all foods—carbohydrates, fats, and proteins—help to give metabolism a gentle nudge higher when we eat them. But protein has the greatest thermic effect of all. In addition, protein can increase metabolism by helping to maintain and build muscle mass. (For more information about good sources of protein, see page 28.)

FAQS

I'm tempted to try one of those metabolism-boosting supplements I see advertised on TV—do you recommend them?

If over-the-counter supplements worked, no one would be overweight. The supplements that are supposed to boost metabolism fall into two main categories—those that don't work, and those with stimulant ingredients that may cause a dangerous rise in heart rate and/or blood pressure. When the minor effect of the stimulants wears off, your metabolism soon returns to normal. As much as we wish otherwise, there is no quick fix for weight loss. Even prescription medications don't work as well as the scientists who developed them hoped. As of right now, your best bet is with healthy food choices in moderate portions, and metabolism-boosting exercise.

EXERCISE FIXES FOR METABOLISM

A big percentage of your maintenance calories—the amount you burn in the course of a day—comes from your activity level. If you go from having average activity levels to being extremely active, you can double the amount of calories burned (that's activity factor calories, not BMR calories). This is why *any* activity—every extra step you take—can help boost your metabolism. Part of my recommendation is to move as much as possible: climb the stairs instead of taking the escalator, park at the opposite end of the mall and walk to your favorite store, garden instead of watching TV . . . anything, as long as it is extra movement.

In addition, I strongly encourage everyone to exercise regularly. The optimal weight-loss exercise program consists of both aerobic exercise and strength training. Regular exercise can increase your activity factor and your metabolism. As you get older and your metabolism slows, you can rebalance your energy needs by increasing the duration or intensity of your workouts.

- **Aerobic exercise.** Aerobic exercises use energy and increase many different metabolic processes (such as your heart rate), all of which burn calories. All aerobic activities—including running, brisk walking, swimming, skating, skiing, and cycling—increase metabolism *while* you're exercising, and also keep your metabolism burning higher for hours afterward. I recommend doing some form of aerobic activity four or five days per week, for at least 30 minutes per day.
- **Strength training.** Exercises that work your muscles without necessarily raising heart rate are considered strength training. These include lifting weights, working with resistance bands, yoga, Pilates, circuit training, and calisthenics (including push-ups, chin-ups, and abdominal crunches). These activities directly increase your BMR by building muscle, so you will burn more calories every minute of every day. I recommend doing some form of strength training two or three days per week. Plan a strength training regimen that's realistic for both your schedule and personality. For some people that may mean 15 minutes of calisthenics in the privacy of your bedroom, and for others it may involve a more elaborate weight-training regimen at the gym.

HOW FOOD AFFECTS WEIGHT AND WEIGHT LOSS

I'm willing to bet you know exactly which foods are healthy choices, and which are guilty pleasures. At every meal and with every snack, you have an opportunity to decide which direction to go—you can make the energizing, slimming choice, or *fall back* on one of the choices that brought you to this chapter in the first place. Whenever you choose comforting, familiar junk food instead of healthy meals, that's a fall-back choice. Whenever you eat the wrong foods to reduce stress, that's a fall-back choice. If you ever sneak food, or find yourself thinking *I know it's bad but what the heck,* you're making a fall-back choice.

Don't you deserve more than the fall-back? Of course you do! Remember this important advice: The taste of food remains in your mouth for a very short time, but the calorie consequences remain LONG after. Before you go with a fall-back choice, consider how defeated you'll feel 30 minutes after finishing that fall-back food. Then consider how fabulous you'll feel 30 minutes after finishing a healthful nutrient-rich food. Don't make the wrong choice for short-term satisfaction. Instead, make the right choice for long-term results! You deserve better health. You deserve to lose inches from your waist and thighs. And you deserve foods that can help you lose weight and lower your risk of disease.

LEAN PROTEIN

As I already mentioned, eating protein can help raise metabolism because it has a high thermic effect, and because it can help maintain and increase your lean muscle mass. Protein also keeps you feeling satisfied longer, so you are less likely to snack on high-calorie fall-back foods between meals. In addition, when eaten as part of a well-rounded nutrition plan (which includes vegetables, high-quality carbohydrates, and healthy fats), protein helps to keep blood sugars at a nice, even level. That means that you'll generally be in a better mood, better able to handle stress, and less likely to reach for comfort foods to get through the day.

The key is to add *some* protein, but not to go overboard. Most Americans already eat far too much protein, and usually the wrong kind. The wrong kind contains large amounts of saturated or trans fats. I'm talking about hamburgers, hot dogs, salami, bologna, spareribs, full-fat dairy products (including whole and 2% milk, and full-fat cheese), fried foods, and poultry skin. The right kind, the kind you should choose instead, is *lean* protein, such as skinless chicken and turkey, low-fat or fat-free dairy products, and legumes. The meal plans in this chapter and throughout the book contain a healthy mix of proteins and other nutrients.

BEST FOODS FOR LEAN PROTEIN: *Turkey breast, chicken breast, seafood and fish, veal, pork tenderloin, lean ham, lean beef, egg whites, yogurt (fat-free, low-fat), milk (fat-free, 1% reduced-fat), enriched/fortified soy milk, cheese (fat-free, reduced-fat), beans (lima, black, navy, pinto, garbanzo), lentils, split peas, tofu, tempeh, soybeans.*

HIGH-QUALITY CARBOHYDRATES

Just as there are superior protein choices for weight loss and good health, there are good (and poor) carbohydrate choices. Carbs are necessary because your body breaks them down into glucose, the kind of simple sugar used by your cells for energy. When we eat low-quality carbs, we're essentially dumping glucose into our blood stream, which provides a quick rush of energy, followed eventually by a slump . . . which in turn causes us to eat more. It's a vicious cycle. A smart weight-loss plan limits or avoids low-quality carbs, including sugar and sugary foods, anything made with white flour, fruit juice, and soft drinks.

High-quality carbs, on the other hand, are rich in vitamins, minerals, and *fiber*. Fiber is the unsung hero of weight loss. There are two kinds of fiber, both abundant in whole grain foods, fruits, and vegetables. The first, *soluble fiber*, turns gooey when digested and stabilizes blood sugar, keeps you feeling full, and controls hunger. The second, *insoluble fiber*, is a volumizer—it adds bulk to food, so you can eat a lot more food without a lot of extra calories.

Fiber is critical to weight maintenance. Nutrition researchers at the University of Texas at Austin discovered that people who are not overweight eat 33 percent more fiber and 43 percent more complex carbohydrates than people who are overweight. This echoes the results of studies that have shown that people who eat high-fiber diets are less likely to be overweight than people who eat low-fiber diets. By including fiber-rich, high-quality carbohydrates with your meals, you'll feel energetic, full, and satisfied as you drop weight.

BEST FOODS FOR HIGH-QUALITY CARBOHYDRATES: *Vegetables, fruits, beans, peas, lentils, brown rice, wild rice, barley, oatmeal, whole grain cereals, whole grain breads, whole grain crackers, quinoa, amaranth, wheat berries, millet*

BEST FOODS FOR SOLUBLE FIBER: *Psyllium seeds (ground), oat bran, rice bran, oatmeal, barley, lentils, Brussels sprouts, peas, beans (kidney, lima, black, navy, pinto), apples, blackberries, pears, raisins, oranges, grapefruit, dates, figs, prunes, apricots, cantaloupe, strawberries, bananas, peaches, broccoli, carrots, cauliflower, cabbage, spinach, sweet potatoes, yams, white potatoes, tomatoes, avocado, raspberries, corn, almonds, ground flaxseed, sunflower seeds*

HEALTHY FATS: MONOUNSATURATED AND OMEGA-3

Along with protein and carbs, fats are an important component of a good nutrition program, but some fats are better than others. Unhealthy fats are saturated fats (found mainly in full-fat dairy products and fatty meats) and trans fats (found primarily in packaged baked goods). Healthy fats are omega-3 fatty acids (found mainly in fish oils and some nuts) and monounsaturated fats (found mainly in olive oil, canola oil, avocado, and some nuts).

Fats convey much of the flavor and texture that most people find—and here's the official term for it—*yummy*. It's natural to want to eat them. But fats contain more than twice the number of calories as the same weight of carbohydrates and proteins, so eating an ounce of a fatty food will put on more weight than an ounce of a nonfatty food. Studies have shown that people who are overweight tend to have diets that are high in fat. In fact, some intervention studies have shown that, over the long run, people who reduce the amount of fat in their diets (especially the bad fats) *and* increase the amount of fiber they eat lose up to three times more weight than people who followed other types of diets.

Still, it's not a good idea to eliminate all—or even most—fats. Fat can help satiate your appetite and stabilize blood sugar levels. Monounsaturated and omega-3 fats play an important role in maintaining good health, regardless of your body weight. People who eat monounsaturated fats (substituting them for unhealthy fats) lose weight, and so do people on very low-fat diets, but the good fats also help reduce the risk of heart disease by decreasing cholesterol and triglycerides.

BEST FOODS FOR MONOUNSATURATED FATS: *Olive oil, canola oil, avocado, macadamia nuts, hazelnuts, pecans, almonds, peanuts, cashews, Brazil nuts, pistachio nuts, pine nuts, peanut butter, olives*

BEST FOODS FOR OMEGA-3 FATTY ACIDS: *Wild salmon (fresh, canned), herring, mackerel (not king), sardines, anchovies, rainbow trout, Pacific oysters, omega-3–fortified eggs, flaxseed (ground, oil), walnuts, butternuts (white walnuts), seaweed, walnut oil, canola oil, soybeans*

JUICY FOODS

Some foods are mostly water. That's a good thing. These juicy foods help fill you up, much more than drinking plain water can. That's because plain water goes right through you—it's absorbed or eliminated very quickly. Water that's integrated into food hangs around your stomach, making you feel full longer. Fortunately, these high water-content foods are healthy fruits and vegetables. That doesn't mean they're calorie-free—you still need to count the calories. Still, my successful clients know that incorporating them into your meal and snack rotation is a big help in achieving your ideal weight.

BEST JUICY FOODS: *The following foods are at least 75 percent water (by weight): Apples, artichokes, asparagus, beets, bell peppers, blackberries, blueberries, broccoli, Brussels sprouts, cantaloupe, carrots, cauliflower, celery, cherries, cranberries, cucumbers, grapefruit, grapes, kale, kiwi, lemons, lettuce, limes, mangos, mushrooms, nectarines, olives, onions, oranges, papayas, peaches, pears, peas, pineapple, plums, potatoes, pumpkin, raspberries, rhubarb, spinach, squash, strawberries, tangerines, tomatoes, turnips, watermelon, yams*

FAQS

Is there a way I can lose belly fat first?

As much as you might like to lose weight specifically from your middle, or your thighs, or even your neck, weight loss doesn't work that way. Where fat settles depends on genetics. When you lose weight, your body will burn fat from all over your body—sometimes in your problem area, sometimes not. Keep to the program, exercise to strengthen and tighten your muscles, and eventually you'll have the lean shape you want.

THE PLAN: OVERVIEW

All the meal plans in this book (including the one in this chapter on page 45), have been calculated to provide 1,200 to 1,500 calories per day—from meals alone. All my meals break down like this: Each breakfast option provides 300 to 400 calories, each lunch option provides 400 to 500 calories, and each dinner option provides 500 to 600 calories. The additional calories you consume from snacks will be entirely up to you. You'll notice I provide snack options that are 100 calories or less, and snack options that are 100 to 200 calories. Depending on your daily caloric goal, pay close attention to the number and kind of snacks you consume.

If you want or need to lose weight, *and* have other medical concerns to address, I recommend following my 4-Step Plan for Weight Loss for the first full week—this will show you the basics of a low-calorie meal plan, jump-start your metabolism, and help you drop a few pounds fast. Then, if you have other health concerns, turn to that chapter and follow the specific recommendations there. As mentioned earlier, the meal plans in every chapter hold to the same calorie limits, so you can continue to lose weight while addressing other health issues. There are a three exceptions: If your primary concern is celiac disease, severe irritable bowel syndrome, or type 2 diabetes, read this chapter through to the end to understand the mechanics of weight loss, but don't follow the weight loss meal plan. Instead, turn to your appropriate chapter and begin that program immediately.

If weight loss is your primary concern, feel free to follow the 4-Step Plan for Weight Loss for as long as you like, or until you achieve your goal. The weight-loss meal plan contains custom-designed menus that are delicious and easy to follow. But if you prefer to create your own menus, use the following guidelines—they provide the basic building blocks for constructing healthy meals and snacks that will lead to weight loss while still allowing for personal flexibility. (Keep in mind that the meals listed in my custom-designed menus—in this and all other chapters—do not necessarily follow these guidelines. My calculations take into account many additional factors, but this is a good set of rules for simple meal planning.)

MAKE-YOUR-OWN WEIGHT-LOSS MEALS

■ At each meal, eat **1 SERVING of high-quality starchy carbohydrates,** for a total of three total servings per day. (During the first week, skip the dinner starch. It's an easy way to minimize calories during the meal when people are most inclined to overeat.)

> **One serving** *of high-quality starchy carbs can include your choice of the following: 1 slice whole wheat bread; 2 slices reduced-calorie bread; ½ cup brown or wild rice; ½ cup whole wheat pasta; 1 small whole wheat pita bread; ½ regular whole wheat pita bread; ½ medium baked white potato; ½ medium baked sweet potato; ¾ cup whole grain breakfast cereal (120 calories or less); ½ cup dry plain oatmeal; ½ whole grain English muffin; ½ cup peas; ½ cup corn; ½ cup kidney beans; ½ cup chickpeas (garbanzo beans); ½ cup acorn or butternut squash.*

■ At each meal, eat **1 SERVING of lean protein.**

> **One serving** *of lean protein can include your choice of the following: 3 to 5 ounces of lean meat, chicken, fish, seafood, or tofu; 1 cup fat-free milk; 1 cup fat-free yogurt; 1 cup reduced-fat cottage cheese; 1 or 2 ounces fat-free or reduced-fat cheese; 1 whole egg plus 3 egg whites.*

■ At each meal, eat no more than **1 SERVING of a fat.**

> **One serving** *of fat can include your choice of the following: 1 to 2 teaspoons olive oil; 1 tablespoon regular salad dressing; 2 to 4 tablespoons reduced-calorie salad dressing; 1 to 2 tablespoons nuts; 1 tablespoon peanut butter; 1 tablespoon regular cream cheese or 2 tablespoons light cream cheese; 1 tablespoon soft tub, trans fat–free margarine; 1 to 2 tablespoons guacamole; 1 to 2 tablespoons reduced-fat mayonnaise or 1 to 2 teaspoons of regular mayonnaise.*

■ Every day, you may eat **UNLIMITED SERVINGS of non-starchy vegetables** (all veggies are unlimited except corn, peas, and root vegetables).

■ Every day, eat **2 SERVINGS of fresh fruit.** These can be eaten at meals or as a snack.

> **One serving** *of fruit can include your choice of the following: 1 medium piece of fruit (apple, pear, peach, nectarine, orange, etc.); 1 small banana; ½ mango, papaya, or grapefruit; ¼ cantaloupe; 1 cup berries, grapes, or cut-up melon; ¾ cup fruit salad.*

■ Before lunch and dinner, drink **ONE 8-ounce GLASS of water.** During the first week on this program, make it two 8-ounce glasses before each of those meals.

■ Every day, feel free to eat **1 TREAT** (150 calories or less). This will help satisfy cravings, and lessen the feelings of deprivation. If you choose, you may skip the treat and enjoy an additional serving of any of the food categories: fruit, high-quality starchy carbohydrate, protein, or fat.

BEST LESSONS

To sum it all up, the ideal diet consists of moderate amounts of high-quality carbohydrates, lean protein, and healthy fats . . . all while reducing calories. I wish it could be sexier than that, but the information doesn't have to be exciting to work. My program definitely works.

But human nature can find loopholes in even the simplest program. Some of my favorite weight-loss secrets have come from finding solutions for the problems posed by my unique and wonderful clients. I'm sure you'll find some answers here, too.

Even very low-calorie foods can add up. Christina is principal ballet dancer with a national company who works diligently to perfect her craft and her body, putting in hours and hours at rehearsals every day. She came to see me because she had started gaining weight, despite counting every calorie. Her problem? Christina loved the "I Can't Believe It's Not Butter" spray. As the label says, a single serving of 5 sprays gives foods a buttery taste with zero calories. What Christina (and most people) didn't know was that each aerated spray serving has a little less than 1 calorie, and the label rounds down to zero. However, there are many, many servings per 8-ounce bottle, adding up to about 90 grams of fat and 820 calories. Because she thought the product had no calories, Christina went through an entire buttery bottle every day. When she broke the spray habit, the pounds dropped off. *The lesson: There are few foods you can eat in unlimited quantities. Even a so-called* zero-calorie *product can cause weight gain if you eat enough of it.*

There is no reason to be a Sally. In the movie *When Harry Met Sally,* there is a restaurant scene that shows Sally ordering a salad and pie a la mode. She wants her pie heated with ice cream on the side, strawberry not vanilla, but if there isn't strawberry then whipped cream, but only real whipped cream . . . if there isn't real whipped cream then the pie shouldn't be heated. As her list of special demands go on and on, we begin to understand that Sally is a high-maintenance kind of girl (adorably so in that Meg Ryan way!). Many of my high-profile clients are understandably afraid of being labeled high-maintenance or—even worse—a *diva.* They ask me the best way to stick to their meal plans while attending a dinner party or public function without acting like a Sally. Simple. I tell them to eat a single portion of whatever they are served (no matter what it is). They can even eat a dessert (or half a dessert) if it will put them and their hosts at ease. The key is to eat extra carefully the rest of the week. *The lesson: You can have a social life while trying to lose weight. Follow your meal plan as closely as possible when you are in control of cooking at home or ordering in a restaurant, but relax and allow yourself to be an easy dinner guest.*

Starvation diets backfire. Fashion model Rinna was convinced that if she lost just 10 more pounds she would be able to book more jobs, and resorted to starving herself when

FAQS

My husband and I both went on the same diet at the same time, but he's losing weight so much faster than me. How come?

Men generally burn more calories than women just by living and breathing. On average, men are taller, heavier, and have more lean muscle mass than women. It takes more energy (in the form of calories) to fuel all the body processes necessary to keep his larger body going than it does to keep your body going. Plus, lean muscle mass increases metabolism, so his testosterone-fed muscles give him an automatic weight-loss advantage. Increasing your muscle mass through resistance training will give you a boost, but his weight loss will always be easier than yours. Try not to make losing weight a competition. Instead, plan a celebration every time one of you loses 10 pounds—with the two of your losing at different rates, you'll be able to celebrate twice as often.

nothing else worked. By the time she came to see me, she was depressed and desperate—her self-imposed diet had worked for a little while, but then she regained every pound. Rinna skipped breakfast, exercised in the morning, skipped lunch, drank diet sodas all day long, chewed sugarless gum, and ate a calorie-controlled dinner. Then came what she called her all-night eating orgy—nonstop binging on the limited food items she kept in her apartment (things like dry cereal, oatmeal, and toast with peanut butter and jam). Her body craved food! She would wake up the next morning feeling bloated and sluggish, and then start the cycle all over again. We figured out that between the hours of 9:00 p.m. and midnight, she would eat about 1,800 calories—as much as many people eat all day! I encouraged her to start eating regular meals. She was terrified that she would gain even more weight, that she would eat all day and then eat all night, too! But eventually she trusted my experience and took the leap. She ate breakfast, lunch, an afternoon snack, dinner, and even a small snack before bed. After one week, she lost 4 pounds. All 10 pounds were gone after six weeks. *The lesson: You can feel good and look the way you want to, all while eating healthfully. Starvation is never a good choice, and it may even move you further from your goal.*

Limit or eliminate alcoholic beverages. Nearly every weekday, Scott—a brilliant CEO for a large, national company—meets with clients for lunch and dinner. These schmoozing fests often involve alcohol, sometimes two or three drinks each. Scott understands the use of alcohol as a social lubricant, but he has no particular craving for it himself. In fact, he would just as soon drink ice tea, but he wants clients to feel comfortable and typically matches them drink for drink. The problem, of course, is that alcohol is loaded with empty calories, and they contributed significantly to Scott's weight problem. Perhaps worse, the alcohol lowered Scott's usual inhibitions; his best laid plans to make healthy menu choices crumbled after a couple of drinks, and decadent, calorie-rich desserts often followed full meals. We did two things that helped Scott take control while still enabling him to court clients. First, I made him promise that his first drink of the meal would be club soda, and then he would alternate between club soda and his standard vodka. That way, if the client had three drinks, and Scott matched him order for order, Scott drank one vodka. He would not only save calories, but he would be sharper, less buzzed, more aware throughout the meeting. Second, he changed the way he ordered his drink. Scott enjoyed the flavor of vodka straight-up, with just a hint of extra flavor from a twist of lemon. We discovered that if he did without the lemon, he drank a little more slowly. The lemon twist made the drink go down easier. By removing the twist, his drinks lasted longer, so he ordered fewer of them. After just one week on his new routine, Scott lost 6 pounds. After four months, he had lost more than 30 pounds, and he was as gracious a host as ever. *The lesson: You can dilute the negative effects of alcohol on weight. Make each drink last as long as possible by removing your personal flavor "incentives." Also, always alternate alcoholic beverages with no-calorie drinks.*

It is possible to get too much of a good thing. Many of my most nutritionally knowledgeable clients are athletes. They know that their performances depend on good nutrition, so they do everything right. Emma is an Olympic medalist who was a nutrition fanatic. She ate whole grains, organic fruits and vegetables, fat-free dairy, and lean meats. She never ate sugar or bleached flour. And yet, she still needed to drop about 15 pounds to get to her optimal performance weight. It was a joy to see such stellar eating habits and I found it painful to nit-pick at her diet. It came down to nuts. She was a walnut and almond fanatic. Nuts are a healthy food choice, rich in healthy fats, vitamins, and minerals . . . but I don't recommend eating more than a small handful at one sitting. Emma ate a generous portion of nuts with breakfast, and as an afternoon snack. In all, she was eating about 1½ cups of nuts per day, or about 1,100 calories. Nuts are portable and bite-sized, which makes them easy to overeat. They are also high in calories. Emma cut back on the nuts, lost the weight she needed, and was back in award-winning form in just seven weeks. *The lesson: Go easy on foods (even healthy foods) that are easy to pop into your mouth—including grapes, olives, sunflower seeds, and dried fruit.*

Condiments are not always your friends. Many people forget that condiments contain calories. If you use them sparingly, they can add dimension and a little flavor to your meal. If you eat them in excess, they may be standing in the way of your weight-loss goal. One ounce of ketchup, for instance, contains about 40 calories (each tablespoon of ketchup provides 15 calories; barbecue sauce can often be higher). If you use more, the calories multiply. Other add-ons are worse: A tablespoon of mayonnaise contains about 100 calories; 1 tablespoon of French, bleu-cheese, or other creamy dressing has about 75 calories; a 1-ounce packet of tartar sauce can contain more than 150 calories. I have clients who have finally taken off those last 5 stubborn pounds when they learned that condiments aren't calorie-free. For intense taste with minimal calories, I recommend: tomato salsa (¼ cup has only 30 calories—much less than kethup); mustard (1 tablespoon has 9 to 15 calories, and you typically don't use that much); pickle relish (1 tablespoon has about 14 calories); reduced-sodium soy sauce (1 teaspoon has about 3 calories); and hot pepper sauce (1 teaspoon has about 1 calorie). *The lesson: Don't forget that condiments aren't just toppings—they are food. Use them wisely and sparingly.*

Beware of mindless eating—part one. Sarah never counted calories and never kept a food log because she thought she ate perfectly. She was frustrated that her weight never budged, despite being a busy mom who never seemed to sit down. I asked Sarah to pay close attention to every mouthful and she was surprised to discover that she actually did a lot of "tasting" while cooking, enough to add up to a significant number. We fixed that by having her chew sugarless gum whenever she prepared meals so she couldn't mindlessly enjoy these tasting portions before dinner. *The lesson: "Tasting" is eating. If you nosh your way through food preparations, keep your mouth otherwise occupied by chewing sugarless gum, sipping on hot tea, or singing along with your favorite CD.*

Beware of mindless eating—part two. Kimberly didn't overeat . . . she just picked off other people's plates. Because it was only a couple French fries from her son's portion or a cookie from her daughter's snack pack, Sarah didn't think those nibbles could account for the trouble she was having losing those few extra pounds. As an experiment, I asked her to carry a bunch of plastic zippered sandwich bags with her for a day. Every time she picked someone's food, she was to place it in a bag instead of eating it. Then, she brought that one day's worth of pickings to me. We were both surprised to discover that she was grazing through about 1,000 extra calories per day of *other people's food!* That's a full breakfast and dinner. *The lesson: Be picky about your pickings! If you plan for calories, you can enjoy them more. Be mindful.*

Choose your sweets for their staying power. Brenda is a writer who spends most of her days sitting in front of a computer. She kept a jar of hard candies on hand for whenever she got the urge for something sweet. Brenda inevitably crunched the candy instead of sucking it and ate one after the other, racking up calorie upon calorie. Each piece has less than 25 calories, but Brenda could easily eat six (about 140 calories) in just a few minutes. I had her swap her hard candy for Atomic FireBalls, which are very hot candies. They are hard as rocks, so Brenda couldn't just crunch them away. They give off two waves of "atomic" heat, so she never forgot that she had a candy in her mouth. After just one, Brenda was satisfied and didn't need any more "sweet" for the afternoon. Although each Atomic Fire-Ball has only 40 calories—more than a small sucking candy—Brenda still saved herself about 100 calories per day . . . and up to 10 pounds in a year! *The lesson: If you have a sweets habit that you can't break, look for a way around it by substituting similar treats that might last longer or give you fewer overall calories.*

Avoid the snack traps. Kevin, a television actor, had done a good job dropping most of the weight he had put on between seasons, but he had a snack habit that kept him from his weight-loss goal. His determination fell apart when faced with "snacky" foods—especially late in the afternoon. One serving would turn into two, which could turn into three or four before he would finally stop eating. For three weeks in a row, he vowed to me (and to himself) that he would stop after eating just one serving of pretzels, or one small bag of baked chips, or one granola bar. But vow or no vow, he ate two to three times more than he was allotted. They say that the camera adds 10 pounds, so he was justifiably worried that his extra weight would be magnified on the screen. I suggested that he switch from "snacky" foods to "real-food" snacks—calorie-controlled portions of foods that we typically eat at meals. For example, he now snacks on a two-serving container of fat-free cottage cheese, or 2 cups of hearty vegetable soup, or half a turkey sandwich on whole wheat bread with lettuce, tomato, and mustard. It worked like a charm! The key for Kevin was that the snacky nature of snack foods made him want to continue eating, while the food-like nature of my substitutes allowed him to feel satisfied sooner. Everyone has certain foods that are, well, let's say *problematic.* Foods that, once you start eating, trigger a need to keep eating. For Kevin, it was snacks. For other people, it is ice cream, or peanut butter, or even dry breakfast cereal. *The lesson: It is possible to break away from the never-ending snack, without going hungry. If you have a problem controlling snack portions, avoid your trigger. Try a different type of food that you don't usually associate with snacking.*

Slow difficult transitions. Long-standing habits can be difficult to break. Bill is a historian whose morning routine has long included a newspaper and two huge mugs of coffee. His weight loss plateaued when he was still about 15 pounds above his goal

JUMPING PAST A WEIGHT PLATEAU

The trickiest time during any weight-loss program is the plateau—that long stretch when the quick drop in pounds you saw at first tapers off, and every additional ounce feels hard-won. Frustration can turn to overeating, which leads to weight gain, which will move you off your plateau for sure—but in the wrong direction. Don't give up, and don't lose heart. There's hope:

- **Don't worry about the steady state.** If you're on a plateau, that means you've already lost weight. Enjoy it! Take a few days (or weeks, if necessary) to celebrate your new body. If you keep eating well and exercising, all plateaus end. Of course, it may be that you have reached your body's ideal weight, and striving for any new weight loss will be fighting against nature. If that's the case, acknowledge your great accomplishment and enjoy (and accept) the new body you have.

- **Exercise a little more.** As the weight comes off, metabolism slows down. The only way to rev it back up is by increasing the duration or intensity of your exercise. Just adding an extra ten minutes of aerobic exercise to your daily routine will help you burn an additional 50 to 100 calories per day, which could add up to an extra 10 pounds of weight gone by the end of the year!

- **Change your routine.** Maybe you and your body are becoming bored with the same old program. Vary your food choices, share recipes with a friend, try a new restaurant, modify your exercise routine. Sometimes little changes are just enough to get you out of a rut.

- **Look for sneaky foods.** Some foods that sound healthy (and some that actually ARE healthy) are weight-loss saboteurs. Granola and granola bars can be chock-full of calories, fat, and sugar. Dried fruit, yogurt-covered nuts or raisins, banana chips, trail mix, and so-called *natural* potato chips are all diet-busters. Eliminate the sneaky foods and see if that doesn't make a big difference.

- **Eliminate starchy carbohydrates with dinner.** Starchy carbohydrates are delicious, no doubt about it. But they also are relatively high in calories, easy to eat in large quantities, and some people even claim they're psychologically addictive. Of all healthy foods, people crave starches the most. So when you want to break a plateau, avoid all pasta, rice, bread, potatoes, corn, and peas for a week or two. Instead, choose dinners that consist of lean protein and non-starchy vegetables, such as broccoli, carrots, peppers, spinach, cauliflower, zucchini, and lettuce.

- **Close the kitchen after dinner.** Eliminate nighttime snacking and alcohol for a few weeks when you need a weight-loss boost. Clean the kitchen, put all dishes away, and move away from the pantry. Find a noncaloric way to train your body to understand that eating time is over—drink a cup of herbal tea (peppermint can be particularly soothing if you don't have heartburn), floss your teeth, and perhaps apply a tooth whitener . . . anything that keeps your mouth feeling clean and otherwise occupied.

FAQS

What about the vaccine against overweight I heard that scientists are working on—will that work for me?

Because overweight is such an overwhelming problem for so many people, scientists are always working on new angles for control. The media pick up on these stories, but the reports are often premature. In 2006, scientists at the Scripps Research Institute in La Jolla, California, developed a vaccine that slowed weight gain and decreased fat stores . . . *in rats*. The vaccine targeted a hormone called *ghrelin*, which is involved in regulating metabolism. Ghrelin promotes weight gain, so by creating a vaccine to combat ghrelin, the scientists were able to regulate weight gain in the laboratory animals. This is a potentially valuable discovery, but we are years—maybe even decades—away from seeing a practical tool for people based on this research.

Another hormone that has weight loss scientists salivating (so to speak) is leptin, which seems to help us feel full and satisfied. Research suggests that people who are extremely overweight may be resistant to leptin, and therefore are more likely to feel hungry, even after eating. If experts can find a way to increase leptin levels or sensitivity, it theoretically should be easier for people to lose weight. Research progresses slowly, so keep your eyes open for practical applications for leptin and ghrelin, but don't hold your breath.

weight, all due to his coffee habit. Bill liked his coffee very light and creamy, specifically with about ½ cup of half-and-half in each mug—1 cup of half-and-half per day. It was obviously the source of his extra weight. He fought this last change to his diet, but as it became clear his weight wasn't going to budge unless he broke this habit, he relented. It was a slow transition. Over the course of six months, Bill transitioned from half-and-half to whole milk . . . to 2% milk . . . to 1% reduced-fat milk . . . to fat-free milk. That saved him 232 calories every day, and enabled him to dropped 12 pounds. *The lesson: You don't have to make difficult changes all at once. Find intermediate steps that can make the process as painless as possible.*

Make evening hours less threatening. Busy people sometimes face the "feet-up" diet challenge—the minute they stop running around long enough to put their feet up, they binge. As a senior editor at a publishing company, Jillian doesn't have a spare private moment in her day. She is always in meetings or on the phone, planning for the next project or solving some problem with a current book. By the time she gets home—often after 9:00 p.m.—she would relax in front of the TV and eat. No matter what she had for dinner or when she finished, Jillian would create a buffet of high-calorie comfort foods—including cookies, cake, ice cream, dry cereal, and crackers. She woke up each morning with the best intentions for the evening, but by the time she reached home, exhausted from the day, her resolve went out the window. Jillian and I drew up a contract: Before starting her nighttime binge, she first had to eat three low-calorie foods that we agreed upon. So before she could spoon out the ice cream, Jillian committed to first eating two handfuls of baby carrots, one container of fat-free flavored yogurt, and one apple. After that, she could eat whatever she wanted. Of course, our strategy worked. She discovered that after she finished her three must-haves, she felt full and in control. Good-bye binges! Even though those snacks added an extra 250 calories to her daily food plan, they saved her from eating thousands of extra calories each night. *The lesson: If you can't stop yourself from eating at the end of the day (or whenever your particular challenging time is), front-load the binge with three healthy foods. If you vow to eat those three healthy snacks first, it gives your body time to feel satisfied while allowing your psyche the pleasure of eating.*

BONUS POINTS

- **Donate your "fat clothes."** Losing weight is a major accomplishment. As soon as an item of clothing is too big for you anymore, give it away. Don't keep it in your closet as part of your "just in case" wardrobe. It is easier to back-slide if you have bigger pants to slide into.

- **Keep a weight-loss journal.** Write down your food choices and portions, where you eat, why you eat, how much exercise you do, and anything else that allows you to see your healthy (and unhealthy) patterns. That way, you can spot areas for improvement and make adjustments as you go along. Use the journal to track your progress as you weigh yourself once or twice a week.

- **Consider the buddy system.** Some people do better if they have a friend, spouse, therapist, *someone* they can talk to about successes or setbacks. Ideally, this person is nonjudgmental and unconditionally supportive. If you thrive with a little help from your friends, go ahead and ask for their help and guidance.

- **Slow your eating.** Strive to make every mouthful a sensual experience. Taste your food. Savor the texture. Put your fork down between every two bites and sip water during your meal.

- **When you eat, focus.** This is not the time for multi-tasking. Make meal time (and snack time) all about the food. Avoid the mindlessness of eating while checking email, watching television, or other distracting activity.

- **Drink one or two glasses of water before meals.** Ten minutes before every meal, guzzle two glasses of water. This will help meet your daily fluid quota and remind you to follow through with smart food choices at the upcoming meal. Perhaps it will also fill you up and take the edge off your hunger, but most importantly, it will keep you thinking about your plan! Also, thirst can mimic the feelings of hunger—if you wait ten minutes after drinking water, you may find you don't want to eat at all.

- **Keep sugarless gum always on hand.** Sugarless gum can give you a hit of something sweet, keep your mouth busy (so you'll be less likely to snack), and clean your teeth when you can't brush. And, contrary to Internet rumors, sugarless gum won't stimulate your appetite.

- **Repackage snacks.** Before you dig into that mega-sized bag of pretzels, break it down. Divide the large bag into individual portions in snack-sized plastic zipper bags so that you'll be ready with appropriate servings when you need them. Also, seek out snacks that are in portion-controlled units—a Tootsie Pop, fat-free pudding cups, mini bags of microwave popcorn, or other individual snacks that are 100 calories or less per serving. Just remember to only eat one serving!

- **Shock your tongue.** Be liberal with spices—chile peppers, curry, hot salsa, wasabi. Hot and spicy flavors encourage slower eating. Hot (temperature-wise), low-calorie beverages can also help you feel satisfied and hydrated. When you're bored, it's possible to nurse a hot cup of skim latte, green or herbal tea, or diet hot cocoa for much longer than it would take to eat a snack.

- **Be patient with yourself.** There is a phenomenon well known among weight-loss experts—when people who are dieting slip up and overeat, they often decide that the entire effort is a bust and continue to overeat for days before they collect themselves. By then, all their hard work may have been undone. If you find yourself in this situation, be as kind and understanding with your own mistakes as you would be with a best friend who made a small slipup. All humans make mistakes—it is the nature of our species. Learn to forgive yourself.

- **Get enough sleep.** During sleep, our bodies rest and regenerate, so we can be strong and clear-headed the following day—clear-headed enough to make wise food choices. What's more, sleep deprivation causes an imbalance in certain hormones, including ghrelin (which causes weight gain) and leptin (which decreases appetite). When we don't get enough sleep, our levels of ghrelin go up (more weight gain) and levels of leptin go down (so we are hungrier). If it were up to me, I would write in a prescription for six to eight hours of sleep each night . . . but I can't, so it's up to you. Don't think of it as downtime, but as another important facet of your nutrition plan.

SUPPLEMENTS

While you are concentrating on the weight-loss part of your program, you may lose sight of your vitamin and mineral needs. As backup, I recommend:

1. **Multivitamin.** There's no need to go crazy with lots of different pills or megadoses. A single multivitamin that contains 100 percent DV of most vitamins and minerals is fine. If you are a man or a menopausal woman, choose a "senior formula" brand that doesn't contain iron.

2. **Calcium with vitamin D₃ and magnesium.** Many women trying to lose weight skimp on calcium-rich foods. To protect bone health, I recommend that *women only* take a calcium supplement daily. (There is some evidence that too much calcium may increase the risk of prostate cancer. Men should talk with their doctors before taking calcium supplements.) Take 500 to 600 milligrams of calcium twice a day, for a total of 1,000 to 1,200 milligrams daily. (You need to split the dose because the body can only absorb about 600 milligrams of calcium at a time.) Choose a brand that also contains vitamin D₃ (cholecalciferol, the most potent form of vitamin D) and magnesium. (The amount of vitamin D₃ and magnesium in each tablet will vary by brand. Aim to get a *daily total* of 400 to 800 IU vitamin D₃, and 400 milligrams magnesium.) Although *men* should not take calcium supplements, they may want to consider taking a total of 400 to 800 IU vitamin D₃ and 400 milligrams magnesium per day, including what they get from their multivitamin.

JOY'S 4-STEP PROGRAM
FOR WEIGHT LOSS

Follow this program if you want to lose weight.

STEP **1** ... **START WITH THE BASICS**

These are the first things you should do to start on a weight-loss program:

- Calculate your basal metabolic rate and your maintenance calories.

- Begin an exercise program that combines aerobic and strength training.

- Eat regularly—every four to five hours—to keep your metabolism up.

- Consider taking a multivitamin to ensure healthy levels of vitamins and minerals.

- Women may consider taking a calcium supplement; men and women may consider taking a supplement of vitamin D_3 and magnesium.

- Keep your pantry and refrigerator stocked with healthy foods from the grocery list below.

- Avoid or limit the worst weight offenders, including high-calorie drinks (including sugary soft drinks and fruit juices), low-quality carbs, and fatty proteins.

STEP 2 ... YOUR ULTIMATE GROCERY LIST

My weight-loss plan allows you to mix and match your meals based on nutrient categories. The foods on this list are all healthy. Combine them according to the meal plan guidelines (page 45).

FRUIT

ALL FRUITS, but especially:	Cantaloupe	Limes	Pears
Apples	Cherries	Mangos	Pineapple
Apricots	Cranberries	Nectarines	Plums
Bananas	Dates	Oranges	Prunes
Berries (blackberries, blueberries, raspberries, strawberries)	Figs	Oranges, mandarin, canned in light syrup (for meal plan)	Pumpkin puree
	Grapefruit		Raisins
	Grapes	Papaya	Tangerines
	Kiwi	Peaches	Watermelon
	Lemons		

VEGETABLES (NOT INCLUDING STARCHY VEGETABLES)

ALL VEGETABLES, but especially:	Cabbage	Kale	Rhubarb
Artichokes	Cauliflower	Lettuce (all varieties)	Seaweed
Asparagus	Celery	Mushrooms	Spinach
Beets	Collard greens	Okra	Swiss chard
Boysenberries	Cranberries	Onions (red, white)	Tomatoes and tomato paste
Broccoli	Cucumbers	Peppers (all varieties, hot and bell)	Turnips
Broccoli raab	Endive	Pumpkin; 100% canned pumpkin puree	Watercress
Brussels sprouts	Green beans		
	Honeydew		

LEAN PROTEIN

Beef, lean	Eggs (esp. omega-3–fortified)	(especially anchovies, herring, mackerel [not king], Pacific oysters, rainbow trout, sardines, wild salmon)	Tempeh
Cheese (fat-free, reduced-fat)	Flounder		Tofu
Cheese (for meal plan): reduced-fat Cheddar, goat, Parmesan, Romano, Swiss	Ham, lean		Tuna
	Milk (fat-free, 1% reduced-fat, enriched/fortified soy)		Turkey bacon, reduced-fat
		Seafood (for meal plan): smoked salmon, sushi	Turkey breast
Chicken breast	Mozzarella, reduced-fat		Turkey burgers, lean
Cottage cheese, reduced-fat	Pork tenderloin		Veal
	Seafood and fish	Shrimp	Veggie burgers
			Yogurt (fat-free, low-fat)

HIGH-QUALITY STARCHY CARBOHYDRATES (INCLUDING STARCHY VEGETABLES)

Amaranth	Corn (fresh or frozen kernels)	Pita, whole grain	Soybeans (edamame)
Barley		Potatoes, sweet	Squash
Beans (lima, lentils, black, kidney, navy, pinto, garbanzo)	Crackers, whole grain	Potatoes, white (with skin)	Tortilla (whole grain, spinach, tomato)
	Millet		
	Oat bran	Quinoa	Waffles, whole grain
Breads, whole grain, reduced-calorie	Oatmeal	Rice (brown, wild)	Wheat berries
	Peas, green	Rice bran	Yams
Carrots	Peas, split	Rice cakes	
Cereals, whole grain	Peas, sugar snap	Snow peas	

FOODS THAT COUNT TOWARD HEALTHY FATS

Almonds	Flaxseed (ground, oil)	Olives	Psyllium seeds (ground)
Avocado	Hazelnuts	Peanut butter	Soy nuts
Brazil nuts	Macadamia nuts	Peanuts	Sunflower seeds
Butternuts (white walnuts)	Oil, canola	Pecans	Walnuts
	Oil, olive	Pine nuts	
Cashews	Oil, walnut	Pistachio nuts	

MISCELLANEOUS

Applesauce, unsweetened	Honey	Paprika	Sour cream (fat-free, reduced-fat)
Broth, beef, low-sodium	Hot cocoa, diet	Pepper, ground	Soy sauce, reduced-sodium
	Hot sauce	Salad dressing, Caesar, reduced-calorie, or regular calorie	
Buttermilk, 1% reduced-fat	Hummus		Steak sauce
	Jam	Salad dressing, reduced-calorie	
Chili powder, sweet	Ketchup		Sugar
Cinnamon, ground	Margarine spread, soft tub, reduced-fat, trans fat–free	Salad dressing, vinaigrette, reduced-calorie	Sugar substitute
Cream cheese (fat-free, reduced-fat)			Thyme, dried
Croutons	Mayonnaise, reduced-fat	Salsa, jarred	Vinegar
Cumin, ground	Mustard, spicy	Salt	Vinegar, balsamic or red wine
Garlic	Mustard, Dijon	Salt substitute	Wheat germ
Garlic powder	Nonstick cooking spray	Soup, miso	Worcestershire sauce
Guacamole	Oil, sesame		

STEP3 ...GOING ABOVE AND BEYOND

To maximize weight-loss potential, here are some additional things you can try:

- Keep a weight-loss journal.

- Be aware of the foods that entice you to enter an eating danger zone. Keep them out of your pantry.

- Don't multitask while eating—focus and enjoy.

- Get enough sleep.

DON'T RUSH DINNER

Speed-eating through meals could be hurting your waistline. In an interesting experiment, women were invited to eat a pasta lunch on two different days. On one day, the women were given a small spoon and asked to take small bites, put the spoon down between bites, and chew each bite at least 15 times. On the second day, the women were given a large spoon and asked to eat as quickly as possible without stopping between bites. On both occasions, the women ate until they felt comfortably full. When researchers measured how many calories the women had eaten, they found that they ate 67 more calories when they ate quickly than when they ate slowly. Although this may not sound like much, calories add up. If you wolf down both lunch and dinner, it could mean an additional 134 calories per day, or 48,910 calories per year. That's the equivalent of 14 pounds. Once again, the tortoise beats the hare.

STEP4 ...MEAL PLANS

These sample menus include the foods and specific food combinations that will help you lose weight while feeling energized. Each meal is balanced with the right mix of high-quality carbs, protein, fat, and calories to help keep your blood sugars level and hunger at bay. Get ready to lose weight and feel *flabuloss*!

Some things you should know:

1. All 42 meals—*that's 14 options each for breakfast, lunch, and dinner (plus one bonus lunch, just because I couldn't decide which yummy option to eliminate!)*—are presented at the lower caloric range to accommodate people who have lower caloric needs. For example, although breakfast meals throughout the book range from 300 to 400 calories, breakfast options in this chapter are approximately 300 calories (lunch options are approximately 400 calories, and dinner options are approximately 500 calories). If you have higher caloric needs and/or find yourself too hungry at any one meal, I've also included instructions for adding 100 calories to each meal.

2. Don't feel you need to be limited to the meal plans. You can enjoy all the recipes in this book in your personal nutrition plan because I've provided caloric information on each. If you find that there are certain meals you love, by all means, repeat them. Although variety will ensure you get a wide variety of vitamins and minerals in your diet, it is okay to revisit the meals you enjoy the most. Also, if you sometimes eat frozen entrées, choose brands that fit within your calorie range for that meal. For example, a quick dinner might include a Lean Cuisine entrée and a pre-washed bag of salad with a reduced-calorie dressing. When eating out, keep your choices simple— grilled fish with steamed veggies and salad with dressing on the side. If you have some extra calories to play with, you may consider having a glass of wine with dinner or fresh berries for dessert.

3. Every day, choose *one* option for each of the three meals—breakfast, lunch, and dinner. Then, one or two times per day, choose from my variety of suggested snacks. Snacks are grouped according to their calorie amounts ("100 Calories or Less" and "100 to 200 Calories"). Your job is to strategically pick snacks that fit into your personal program. You may also enjoy up to one daily item on the Fun Foods list. Pay close attention to the number of snacks you choose (and their portions)—when you're trying to lose weight, everything counts. *Carefully note my recommendations for teaspoons and tablespoons. There are three teaspoons in a tablespoon—a mistake could get you three times the calories you counted on!*

4. For the first week, starch is omitted from dinner—all starch, even high-quality starch like sweet potatoes, brown rice, peas, and butternut squash. Instead, your dinner for the first seven days is comprised of lean protein and non-starchy vegetables like broccoli, peppers, cauliflower, salads, and more. I use this approach during the first week because many successful clients have found it incredibly effective . . . *I'm sure you*

will, too! If you miss eating starch with dinner, rest assured you'll be seeing them again—moderate amounts are incorporated during week two.

5. Beverage calories are *not* included. I encourage you to drink plenty of water with your meal, and two 8-ounce glasses of water *before* eating lunch and dinner (this will help keep you hydrated *and* thinking about our plan). If you'd prefer something other than water, stick with any preferred noncaloric beverages. Enjoy coffee and tea plain or with fat-free milk (and optional sugar substitute).

BREAKFAST OPTIONS

(Approximately 300 to 400 calories)

Each breakfast option is approximately 300 calories. If you'd like to increase to 400 calories, follow the instructions for adding 100 calories.

Fiesta Vegetable Omelet with Toast

In heated pan coated with nonstick cooking spray, sauté ½ cup chopped onion, ½ cup sliced mushrooms, and ½ cup chopped bell pepper (red, yellow or green) until soft. Beat 1 whole egg with 3 egg whites, pour over the sautéed vegetables, and add preferred seasonings. When bottom is cooked, gently flip. Fold omelet over and cook until egg mixture is firm. Serve with 1 toasted slice whole wheat bread (or 2 slices reduced-calorie bread), and top with 1 teaspoon reduced-fat, soft tub, trans fat–free margarine spread.

To add approximately 100 calories: Add ½ cantaloupe, 1 banana, or 1 cup berries.

Cold Cereal with Milk and Fruit

1 cup whole grain cereal (120 calories or less per ¾- to 1-cup serving and 3 grams or more fiber). Serve with 1 cup milk (fat-free, skim plus, 1% reduced-fat, or reduced-fat enriched/fortified soy milk) and ½ sliced banana (or 2 tablespoons raisins or ½ cup berries).

To add approximately 100 calories: Add 1 hard-boiled egg.

Strawberry-Banana Cottage Cheese with Almonds

1 cup fat-free or 1% reduced-fat cottage cheese mixed with ½ sliced banana, ½ cup chopped strawberries, and 1 tablespoon slivered almonds. For the cottage cheese, you can substitute 1 cup fat-free plain or flavored yogurt (180 calories or less).

To add approximately 100 calories: Add another tablespoon slivered almonds and 1 tablespoon wheat germ or ground flaxseed.

PB&J English Muffin

1 toasted whole grain English muffin, each half spread with 1 level teaspoon peanut butter and 1 teaspoon jam. Serve with ½ grapefruit (or 1 orange, peach, or plum).

To add approximately 100 calories: Use a total of 2 level teaspoons peanut butter and 2 teaspoons jam on each muffin half.

Scrambled Eggs with Turkey Bacon and Fruit

Beat 1 whole egg with 2 egg whites. Cook in heated pan coated with nonstick cooking spray, adding any preferred chopped vegetables (onion, red and green peppers, tomato). Enjoy with 2 strips reduced-fat turkey bacon and 1 orange (or ½ grapefruit or ¼ cantaloupe).

To add approximately 100 calories: Add 1 egg white (3 total) and 2 strips of turkey bacon (4 total).

Oatmeal with Berries and Nuts

½ cup dry oatmeal prepared with water, topped with 2 tablespoons chopped nuts (walnuts, pecans, soy nuts, slivered almonds) and ½ cup berries (sliced strawberries, blueberries, raspberries, and/or blackberries). Sweeten with optional sugar substitute.

To add approximately 100 calories: Enjoy a side serving of 6 ounces fat-free plain or flavored yogurt (100 calories or less).

Skinny Breakfast Burrito

Beat 1 egg with 2 egg whites. Scramble in heated pan coated with nonstick cooking spray. Mix cooked eggs with ¼ cup black beans and 2 tablespoons shredded fat-free or reduced-fat cheese. Wrap in 1 whole grain or spinach tortilla (100 calories or less). Add optional onion, bell pepper, salsa, and/or hot sauce.

To add approximately 100 calories: Add 2 tablespoons fat-free cheese and 2 tablespoons reduced-fat sour cream or guacamole.

Apple Slices with Peanut Butter

2 level tablespoons peanut butter spread over 1 sliced apple (or banana).

To add approximately 100 calories: Add 1 level tablespoon peanut butter (for a total of 3 level tablespoons).

Toast with Cream Cheese, Tomato, Onion, and Lox

2 toasted slices reduced-calorie whole wheat bread (45 calories or less per slice), each topped with 1 tablespoon fat-free or reduced-fat cream cheese, sliced tomato, onion, and 2 ounces smoked salmon.

To add approximately 100 calories: For the reduced-calorie bread, substitute 2 slices regular whole wheat bread, or instead add ¾ cup fruit salad.

Ham and Cheese Omelet with Toast

Beat 1 whole egg with 2 egg whites. Cook in heated pan coated with nonstick cooking spray. Add 2 ounces diced lean ham. When bottom is cooked, gently flip. Top with 2 tablespoons shredded fat-free cheese. Fold omelet over and cook until cheese is melted and egg mixture if firm. Season with preferred herbs. Enjoy with 1 slice whole wheat toast (or 2 slices reduced-calorie whole wheat toast) topped with 1 teaspoon reduced-fat, soft tub, trans fat–free margarine spread.

To add approximately 100 calories: Add an additional slice of whole wheat toast topped with 1 teaspoon reduced-fat, soft tub trans fat–free margarine, or ½ cantaloupe.

Whole Grain Waffles with Yogurt

2 frozen whole grain waffles, toasted and topped with 6 ounces fat-free flavored yogurt (100 calories or less) and 1 tablespoon wheat germ (or ground flaxseeds).

To add approximately 100 calories: Add 1 cup berries (or 2 tablespoons chopped walnuts, pecans, slivered almonds, peanuts, or soy nuts).

Rice Cakes with Cottage Cheese and Tomato

3 rice cakes topped with sliced tomato, onion, and 1 cup fat-free or 1% reduced-fat cottage cheese.

To add approximately 100 calories: Add ½ cantaloupe (or 1 apple, 1 banana, or ¾ mango).

Peanut Butter Pita and Yogurt

1 (70-calorie) whole grain pita bread (or 1 slice whole wheat bread) with 1 level tablespoon peanut butter. Enjoy with 1 cup fat-free plain or flavored yogurt (120 calories or less).

To add approximately 100 calories: Add 1 regular-size whole wheat pita bread (150 calories or less) and 1 extra teaspoon (not tablespoon) peanut butter.

Tomato-Cheddar Melt

2 slices reduced-calorie whole wheat bread, lightly toasted. Top each slice with sliced tomato, optional onion, and ¾-ounce slice reduced-fat Cheddar cheese. Bake in 350°F oven until cheese melts. Enjoy with 1 cup fresh berries (or 1 apple or 1 grapefruit).

To add approximately 100 calories: For the 2 slices reduced-calorie bread, substitute regular whole wheat bread (or add 6 ounces fat-free plain or flavored yogurt—100 calories or less).

LUNCH OPTIONS

(Approximately 400 to 500 calories)

Each lunch option is approximately 400 calories. If you'd like to increase to 500 calories, follow the instructions for adding 100 calories.

Ham and Cheese Sandwich

2 slices reduced-calorie whole wheat bread (45 calories or less per slice), toasted. On 1 slice, layer 1 tablespoon reduced-fat mayonnaise, optional spicy mustard, 4 ounces lean ham (or smoked turkey), and 1 ounce fat-free or reduced-fat cheese. Top with sliced tomato, onion, and remaining slice of bread. Enjoy with 1 cup baby carrots.

To add approximately 100 calories: For the reduced-calorie bread, substitute 2 slices regular whole wheat bread, or add a side serving of 6 ounces fat-free flavored yogurt, or 1 apple.

Caesar Salad with Grilled Chicken or Shrimp

Unlimited Romaine lettuce leaves topped with 4 ounces grilled chicken or cooked shrimp, 3 tablespoons grated Parmesan cheese, and optional anchovies (4 fillets). Toss with 4 tablespoons reduced-calorie Caesar dressing (40 calories or less per tablespoon) or 1 to 2 tablespoons regular Caesar dressing.

To add approximately 100 calories: Enjoy with 1 whole wheat pita (70 calories) or add ½ cup croutons to the salad.

Cottage Cheese with Cantaloupe and Almonds

½ cantaloupe filled with 1 cup fat-free or 1% reduced-fat cottage cheese, topped with 2 tablespoons slivered almonds (or chopped walnuts or sunflower seeds). For the cottage cheese, you can substitute 1 cup plain or flavored fat-free yogurt (180 calories or less).

To add approximately 100 calories: Add 2 tablespoons chopped nuts or seeds, for a total of 4 tablespoons.

Open-Faced Tuna Melt

Mash 3 ounces water-packed light tuna (or canned wild salmon or chicken breast) with 2 to 3 teaspoons reduced-fat mayonnaise, minced onion, and freshly ground black pepper. Spread on 2 slices reduced-calorie whole wheat toast (45 calories or less per slice). Top each open slice with thinly sliced tomato and small (¾-ounce) slice fat-free or reduced-fat cheese (any variety, including Cheddar, Swiss, or American). Bake in 350°F oven until cheese melts. Enjoy with crunchy celery and red, yellow, and green pepper sticks.

To add approximately 100 calories: Use the entire 5-ounce can of light tuna in water (or 5 ounces salmon or chicken breast) and add 2 to 4 tablespoons reduced-calorie dressing to your veggies for dipping.

Turkey Burger with Veggies

1 (5-ounce) lean turkey burger or veggie burger (250 calories or less) with lettuce, tomato, onion, and 2 tablespoons ketchup. Serve on ½ whole grain bun or in 1 (70-calorie) whole wheat pita pocket. Enjoy with 1 cup steamed vegetables (broccoli, cauliflower, spinach).

To add approximately 100 calories: Enjoy the burger on 1 whole bun, and top the steamed vegetables with 1 tablespoon grated Parmesan cheese (or 2 teaspoons reduced-fat, soft tub, trans fat–free margarine).

Mediterranean Pita and Yogurt

Spread 1 medium whole wheat pita (150 calories or less) with ⅓ cup hummus, then stuff it with shredded lettuce, thin slices tomato, onion, and cucumber. Enjoy with 6 ounces fat-free plain or flavored yogurt (100 calories or less).

To add approximately 100 calories: Add 5 sliced olives to the pita sandwich and enjoy the yogurt with 1 cup fresh berries.

Broccoli-Cheese Omelet with Salad

Sauté 1 cup broccoli florets in nonstick cooking spray until soft. Beat 1 whole egg with 3 egg whites and pour around broccoli. When bottom is cooked, gently flip. Top with 3 tablespoons shredded fat-free or reduced-fat cheese. Fold omelet over and cook until cheese melts and egg mixture is firm. Season with preferred herbs. Enjoy with mixed green salad tossed with 1 to 2 teaspoons olive oil and unlimited balsamic vinegar or fresh lemon juice (or 2 to 4 tablespoons reduced-calorie dressing).

To add approximately 100 calories: Add 1 slice whole grain bread or 70-calorie whole wheat pita bread.

Turkey, Cheese, and Avocado Sandwich

4 ounces sliced turkey breast (or grilled chicken or lean ham), 1 ounce reduced-fat Swiss cheese, 2 to 3 thin slices avocado, lettuce, tomato, and onion on 2 slices reduced-calorie whole wheat bread (45 calories or less per slice). Add optional mustard, and 2 teaspoons reduced-fat mayonnaise (or hummus). Enjoy with 1 cup cut-up bell peppers.

To add approximately 100 calories: For the reduced-calorie bread, substitute regular whole wheat bread. Or add 1 apple, 1 pear, or 1 cup berries.

Edamame with Wild Salmon Dijonnaise

1 cup boiled edamame (soybeans in the pod), lightly sprinkled with salt or salt substitute. Enjoy with 5 ounces canned wild salmon with bones, drained, mashed, and mixed with 1 tablespoon reduced-fat mayonnaise, 1 to 2 teaspoons Dijon mustard, minced onion, and black pepper to taste. Serve on large bed of leafy greens (lettuce, spinach, romaine) tossed with fresh lemon juice or 2 tablespoons reduced-calorie dressing.

*To add approximately 100 calories: Add 2 plain rice cakes or 1 small 70-calorie whole wheat
pita bread.*

Spinach Salad with Beets, Goat Cheese, and Walnuts

Large bed of spinach leaves topped with ½ cup sliced beets, ½ cup sugar snap peas,
2 ounces soft goat cheese (preferably reduced-fat), and 1 tablespoon lightly toasted,
chopped walnuts. Toss with 2 teaspoons olive oil and unlimited vinegar or fresh lemon
juice (or 2 to 4 tablespoons reduced-calorie dressing).

*To add approximately 100 calories: Add 2 tablespoons lightly toasted, chopped walnuts (or
½ cantaloupe, 1 cup grapes, 1 cup cherries, 1 apple, 1 pear, or 1 cup berries).*

Baked Potato with Broccoli and Cheese

1 medium baked potato topped with 1 cup steamed or boiled chopped broccoli and
1 ounce melted reduced-fat or fat-free cheese (or ½ cup 1% reduced-fat cottage cheese).
Serve with 2 tablespoons fat-free or reduced-fat sour cream and optional salsa.

*To add approximately 100 calories: Add 1 cup baby carrots and 2 tablespoons reduced-calorie
dressing.*

Grilled Chicken-Pepper Wrap

5 ounces grilled chicken and unlimited onion and bell peppers sautéed in nonstick
cooking spray or 1 teaspoon olive or canola oil. Wrap in a whole wheat, spinach, or
tomato tortilla (100 calories or less). Enjoy with 1 cup crunchy baby carrots and unlimited sliced cucumber.

*To add approximately 100 calories: Add 1 cup fresh grapes (or 1 cup cherries, 1 small banana,
½ cantaloupe, 1 apple, or 1 pear).*

Salad with the Works

Choose one 4-ounce serving from the following protein options: canned sardines,
canned light tuna in water, canned wild salmon, chicken breast, turkey breast, lean
ham, shrimp, lean roast beef, tofu, or a favorite fish. Place on top of a large bed of leafy
greens (lettuce, spinach, collard greens, endive) and mix with ½ chopped bell
pepper (red, yellow, green), 5 cherry tomatoes, and ¼ cup each sliced mushrooms,
chopped cucumbers, sliced beets, chopped red onion, and artichoke hearts. Add 2
tablespoons chickpeas (garbanzo beans) and 5 sliced olives. Toss with 2 teaspoons
olive oil and 2 tablespoons vinegar or fresh lemon juice (or 2 to 4 tablespoons reduced-
calorie dressing).

*To add approximately 100 calories: Add ¼ chopped avocado to the salad; or enjoy with 1 slice
whole grain bread or 1 whole wheat pita bread (70 calories), toasted and topped with
optional 1 teaspoon reduced-fat, soft tub, trans fat–free margarine.*

Veggie Tuna Salad with Pita

Veggie Tuna Salad (page 274; if you like, substitute canned chicken breast or wild salmon for the tuna) on a bed of romaine or spinach leaves. Serve with mini whole wheat pita bread (70 calories or less). Enjoy with 1 cup baby carrots with 2 tablespoons reduced-calorie vinaigrette dressing.

To add approximately 100 calories: For the 70-calorie mini pita bread, substitute a regular size version (150 calories or less).

Japanese Spread: Miso Soup with California Rolls

1 small miso soup with 1 six-piece California roll and side order of steamed vegetables. Serve with optional ginger, wasabi, and reduced-sodium soy sauce.

To add approximately 100 calories: Add 3 additional pieces California roll (½ order).

DINNER OPTIONS

(Approximately 500 to 600 calories)

Each dinner option is approximately 500 calories. If you'd like to increase to 600 calories, follow the instructions for additional 100 calories. For the first week, only select options listed in Week One (these menus do *not* include starch). During your second week (and weeks that follow), enjoy meal options listed in Week Two . . . or feel free to repeat the menus from week one.

Week One

Rosemary Chicken with Sautéed Spinach and Salad

5 ounces grilled or baked chicken breast with preferred seasonings (or Rosemary Chicken, page 347). Enjoy with 1 cup sautéed spinach (4 cups raw spinach leaves sautéed in 1 teaspoon olive oil, seasoned with minced garlic, and salt and pepper to taste). Serve with a side salad of chopped lettuce, cucumber, carrot, onion, and mushrooms, tossed with 1 tablespoon chopped walnuts, 1 teaspoon olive oil, and 1 to 2 tablespoons vinegar or fresh lemon juice (or 2 tablespoons reduced-calorie dressing).

To add approximately 100 calories: Add 3 ounces chicken breast (total 8 ounces).

Pork Tenderloin with Cauliflower Mashed "Potatoes"

5 ounces grilled, baked, or broiled lean pork tenderloin (or grilled chicken breast). Enjoy with 1 serving Cauliflower Mashed "Potatoes" (page 222), and a side salad of 2 cups chopped lettuce, ¼ cup each chopped pepper, onion, cucumber, mushrooms, and grated or chopped carrots. Toss with 1 to 2 teaspoons olive oil and 1 to 2 tablespoons vinegar or fresh lemon juice (or 2 to 4 tablespoons reduced-calorie salad dressing).

To add approximately 100 calories: Add 2 ounces of pork tenderloin (total 7 ounces).

Cheddar-Turkey Burger with Mixed Greens

5 ounces turkey burger (or lean hamburger or veggie burger; 250 calories or less), topped with sliced tomato, onion, 1 ounce reduced-fat Cheddar cheese and optional 2 tablespoons ketchup or salsa. Serve with unlimited leafy greens tossed with 2 to 4 tablespoons reduced-calorie vinaigrette (or 1 teaspoon olive oil and unlimited vinegar or fresh lemon juice).

To add approximately 100 calories: Add ¼ avocado, thinly sliced (or 2 heaping tablespoons guacamole).

Sirloin Steak with Mozzarella and Tomato Salad

5 ounces grilled sirloin steak (trimmed of all fat) with optional 2 tablespoons steak sauce or ketchup. Enjoy with mozzarella and tomato salad (½ sliced red tomato and 1 ounce reduced-fat mozzarella cheese; line alternate slices of tomato and cheese on plate, and drizzle with 2 tablespoon reduced-calorie balsamic vinaigrette). Serve with 12 steamed or grilled asparagus spears.

To add approximately 100 calories: Add 2 ounces steak (total of 7 ounces).

Sweet Salmon over Arugula with Broccoli

Mix 1 tablespoon reduced-sodium soy sauce and 1 tablespoon honey. Drizzle over 1 (6-ounce) wild salmon fillet and grill or broil 10 to 15 minutes, basting every few minutes. Serve over a large mound of baby arugula leaves tossed with 1 tablespoon lightly toasted, slivered almonds and 2 tablespoons reduced-calorie dressing. Enjoy with 1 cup steamed broccoli. For the salmon, you may substitute any preferred grilled or baked fish.

To add approximately 100 calories: Add 2 ounces salmon or other fish (8 ounces total).

Tofu Salad with Snow Peas, Almonds, and Mandarin Oranges

Toss 6 to 8 ounces extra-firm tofu, cubed and chilled, with 2 to 3 cups baby spinach leaves, 1 cup steamed and chilled snow peas, ½ chopped tomato, and ½ cup mandarin oranges (canned in light syrup). Drizzle with 1 teaspoon sesame oil and 1 tablespoon reduced-sodium soy sauce and top with 1 to 2 tablespoons slivered almonds. For the tofu, you may substitute grilled chicken breast or shrimp.

To add approximately 100 calories: Add 2 to 3 slices turkey or soy bacon, on the side or crumbled into the salad. (Or add ¼ cup of your favorite reduced-fat cheese to the salad.)

Orange Pepper Beef Stir-Fry with Cucumber Slices

1 serving Orange Pepper Beef Stir-Fry (page 101). Enjoy with 1 sliced cucumber.

To add approximately 100 calories: Skip the cucumber and add a mixed vegetable salad of lettuce, tomato, cucumber, onion, pepper, carrots, and mushrooms. Toss with 1 teaspoon olive oil and 1 to 2 tablespoons vinegar or fresh lemon juice (or 2 tablespoons reduced-calorie dressing).

Week Two (Starch Added)

Grilled Fish with Brussels Sprouts and Sweet Potato

1 (6-ounce) fish fillet (wild salmon, flounder, sole, tilapia, or trout), grilled with 1 teaspoon olive oil and lemon juice and preferred seasonings. Enjoy with 1 cup steamed Brussels sprouts (or cauliflower, sugar snap peas, or summer zucchini), topped with 1 tablespoon reduced-fat, soft tub, trans fat–free margarine and ½ plain baked sweet potato.

To add approximately 100 calories: Enjoy 1 whole sweet potato.

Southwestern Meat Loaf with Cauliflower Mashed "Potatoes"

1 serving Southwestern Turkey Meat Loaf (page 60). Enjoy with 2 servings Cauliflower Mashed "Potatoes" (page 222) or 2 cups steamed cauliflower or broccoli topped with 2 to 4 tablespoons grated Parmesan or Romano cheese. Serve with 1 cup crunchy baby carrots.

To add approximately 100 calories: Add ½ serving meat loaf.

Sweet and Sour Tofu-Veggie Stir-Fry with Brown Rice

1 serving Sweet and Sour Tofu-Veggie Stir-Fry (page 251) with ¾ cup cooked brown rice (or ½ medium baked or sweet potato topped with 1 tablespoon reduced-fat, soft tub, trans fat–free margarine or 2 tablespoons fat-free or reduced-fat sour cream).

To add approximately 100 calories: Add ½ cup cooked brown rice (1¼ cups total); or enjoy the whole potato.

Turkey Tacos with Lettuce, Tomato, and Cheese

3 servings Turkey Tacos (page 250) with optional salsa and hot sauce.

To add approximately 100 calories: Add 1 cup baby carrots dipped in 1 heaping tablespoon guacamole.

Chinese Takeout

1 order steamed seafood, tofu, or chicken and vegetable entrée (such as steamed chicken and broccoli); request garlic, black bean, or ginger sauce on the side. Enjoy with 1 cup brown rice. Pile your plate with the steamed entrée and flavor with 1 tablespoon side sauce and unlimited reduced-sodium soy sauce.

To add approximately 100 calories: Add 2 steamed vegetable dumplings or an additional ½ cup brown rice.

Skinny Shepherd's Pie

1 serving Skinny Shepherd's Pie (page 58). Enjoy with a side salad of chopped lettuce, cucumber, tomato, mushrooms, and onion tossed with 1 teaspoon olive oil and 1 to 2 tablespoons vinegar or fresh lemon juice (or 2 tablespoons reduced-calorie dressing).

To add approximately 100 calories: Add ½ cup chickpeas (garbanzo beans) to the side salad (or 2 tablespoons chickpeas and 1 tablespoon chopped nuts).

Turkey Chili with Cheese

1 serving (2 cups) Turkey Chili (page 367) topped with 1 ounce shredded fat-free or reduced-fat Cheddar cheese and 2 tablespoons fat-free or reduced-fat sour cream. Serve with mixed green salad of bell peppers, carrots, onion, and mushrooms tossed with 1 teaspoon olive oil and unlimited balsamic vinegar or fresh lemon juice.

To add approximately 100 calories: Add ¾ cup chili (total 2¾ cups).

SNACK OPTIONS

100 calories or less

- *Best Vegetables:* 1 cup raw or cooked bell peppers (red, green, yellow), broccoli, broccoli raab, chile peppers, kale, cauliflower, Brussels sprouts, cabbage, tomato, mushrooms, green beans, okra, carrots, lettuce and leafy greens (mustard greens, turnip greens, endive, or escarole), spinach, collard greens, Swiss chard, watercress, asparagus, okra, artichokes, beets, cauliflower, or seaweed

- *Best Fruits:* 1 apple, orange, pear, nectarine, tangerine, kiwi, or peach; 2 plums or clementines; ½ papaya, ½ mango, ½ banana, or ½ grapefruit; ¼ cantaloupe; 1 cup blueberries, boysenberries, blackberries, raspberries, sliced strawberries, cranberries, cherries, grapes, watermelon, pineapple, or honeydew; 4 apricots or prunes; 2 dates or figs; 20 whole strawberries; 2 tablespoons raisins

- 10 almonds

- 1 cup fat-free milk

- 1 diet hot cocoa (100 calories or less)

- 1 small skim café latte or cappuccino (decaffeinated, if caffeine makes you jittery or if you have PMS)

- 1 reduced-fat string cheese (or 1 ounce fat-free or reduced-fat cheese)

- ½ cup fat-free or 1% reduced-fat cottage cheese (with optional cinnamon)

- 1 hard-boiled egg (or 3 to 4 cooked egg whites)

- ½ cup natural, unsweetened applesauce

- 4 level tablespoons fat-free cream cheese (or 2 level tablespoons light cream cheese) with celery sticks

56   LOSING WEIGHT

- 6 ounces fat-free, plain or flavored yogurt (100 calories or less)
- 1 level tablespoon peanut butter with celery sticks

100 to 200 calories

- 10 almonds plus 1 serving fruit (from fruit list)
- 10 almonds plus 1 reduced-fat string cheese (or 1 ounce fat-free or reduced-fat cheese)
- 2 rice cakes, each topped with sliced tomato and a small slice fat-free cheese
- 1 cup edamame (boiled soybeans in the pod)
- Whole nuts: 1 ounce (about ¼ cup) almonds, soy nuts, cashews, toasted pecans, walnuts, or peanuts
- ¼ cup pistachio nuts or sunflower seeds in the shell
- ½ cup 1% reduced-fat cottage cheese mixed with ½ cup berries (or 2 tablespoons ground flaxseed or wheat germ)
- 70-calorie whole wheat pita bread with 1 level tablespoon peanut butter (or 2 tablespoons hummus)
- 1 cup fat-free, plain or flavored yogurt (120 calories or less) mixed with 2 tablespoons wheat germ
- 1 cup baby carrots or pepper sticks with 2 heaping tablespoons hummus or guacamole
- 1 sliced apple with 1 level tablespoon peanut butter
- Frozen banana: Slice peeled banana into several ½" wheels; place in a small plastic bag and freeze.
- Strawberry-Banana Fruit Smoothie: In a blender, mix 1 cup fat-free milk, 1 cup frozen strawberries, and ½ frozen banana.
- Vanilla Pumpkin Yogurt Pudding: Mix 1 cup vanilla fat-free, flavored yogurt with ½ cup canned 100% pure pumpkin puree.
- 1 baked apple with 1 to 2 teaspoons sugar and cinnamon
- 1 Banana Almond Muffin (page 414)
- 1 Berries and Jam Muffin (page 415)
- 1 Carrot 'n' Oat Muffin (page 416)

FUN FOODS (150 CALORIES OR LESS)

In addition to your healthy snack options, here's a list of calorie-controlled fun foods. Pick one item from this list each day . . . or, know that they're available and save for those occasional cravings. All items are 150 calories or less. If you have a personal favorite that's not on my list, simply portion out 150 calories worth and enjoy. It's very important that you always remember to count these calories towards your snacks.

- 1 ounce dark chocolate

- ½ cup fat-free pudding

- ½ cup low-fat ice cream, frozen yogurt, or sorbet (150 calories or less)

- 1 low-fat ice cream pop (150 calories or less)

- 4 to 5 cups light popcorn (150 calories or less)

- 2 standard cookies (150 calories or less)

- 1 fun-size candy bar (150 calories or less)

- 100-calorie snack pack (any variety)

- 1 ounce baked chips

- 1 ounce vegetable chips

- 1 ounce pretzels

- 1 small bag soy crisps (150 calories or less)

- 10 strawberries with 2 heaping tablespoons reduced-fat whipped topping

- 1 glass wine (white or red)

- 1 bottle light beer

- 1 serving Warm Dark Chocolate Sauce with Fresh Fruit (page 81)

SKINNY SHEPHERD'S PIE

When most people think of shepherd's pie, they imagine splurging on a calorie-heavy meal in an English pub—with a favorite cold ale, of course! Now you can enjoy the delicious taste without any guilt—really. And if you need the cold ale—go for a light beer.

Makes 4 servings

1	tablespoon olive oil
1	cup finely chopped onion
2	cloves garlic, minced
1¼	pounds lean ground turkey
2	tablespoons low-sodium tomato paste
1	tablespoon Worcestershire sauce
½	teaspoon garlic powder
½	teaspoon dried thyme
¼	teaspoon paprika
1	cup fat-free low-sodium beef broth
	Salt
	Ground black pepper
2	to 3 large sweet potatoes (about 1½ pounds), cubed and boiled (or softened in the microwave)
½	cup 1% reduced-fat buttermilk or reduced-fat sour cream
2	egg whites
2	tablespoons shredded reduced-fat Cheddar or Swiss cheese
1	tablespoon grated reduced-fat Parmesan cheese

1. Preheat the oven to 350°F. Coat a 6- to 8-cup ceramic or glass gratin dish with cooking spray.
2. In a large skillet, heat the olive oil over medium-high heat. Add the onion and garlic and cook, stirring, until softened and translucent, 4 to 5 minutes. Add the turkey, and increase the heat to high. Cook, stirring, until the turkey is browned, 3 to 4 minutes longer.

3. Stir in the tomato paste, Worcestershire sauce, garlic powder, thyme, and paprika. Cook, stirring, 2 minutes. Add the broth and cook 2 to 3 minutes, until the turkey is cooked through and a light sauce forms. Season to taste with salt and pepper. Set aside.

4. In a large bowl, mash the sweet potatoes with the buttermilk or sour cream until smooth. Season to taste with salt and pepper. In a large metal bowl, beat the egg whites with a pinch of salt on high speed until stiff but not lumpy, 4 to 6 minutes. They should cling firmly to the side of the bowl when tilted. With a spatula, gently fold the egg whites, one-third at a time, into the sweet-potato mixture, until all the egg whites are just incorporated and not deflated.

5. Spread the meat mixture into the prepared casserole dish, and top with the sweet-potato mixture. Sprinkle with the Cheddar or Swiss cheese and the Parmesan cheese. Bake, uncovered, until the potato topping is puffed and browned around the edges, 30 to 35 minutes. Serve immediately.

PER SERVING
403 calories, 41 g protein, 44 g carbohydrate, 7 g fat (2 g saturated), 61 mg cholesterol, 368 mg sodium, 6 g fiber

SOUTHWESTERN TURKEY MEAT LOAF

My recipe has less than half the calories of traditional meat loaf. If you'd like to kick up the heat, add a few hits of hot sauce to the meat mixture or serve with super spicy salsa (like we do in my house). Thanks to the extra bonus of soluble fiber from added oatmeal and corn, your waistline and blood sugar BOTH benefit!

Makes 4 servings

1	pound lean ground turkey
1	cup instant oatmeal
3/4	cup fat-free milk
2	egg whites
1	small red onion, minced
1/2	small green bell pepper, minced
1/2	cup fresh corn kernels or thawed frozen corn kernels
2	cloves garlic, minced
1/2	teaspoon sweet chili powder
1/4	teaspoon ground cumin
	Salt
	Ground black pepper
5	tablespoons jarred salsa, plus more for serving

1. Preheat the oven to 350°F. Coat a 1-quart loaf pan with cooking spray or line with aluminum foil.
2. In a large bowl, combine the turkey, oatmeal, milk, egg whites, onion, green pepper, corn, garlic, chili powder, and cumin. Season with salt and pepper. Press the turkey mixture into the prepared pan and cover with aluminum foil.
3. Bake 40 to 45 minutes. Remove foil and cover with the salsa. Bake, uncovered, 5 to 10 minutes longer, until the center is no longer pink. Serve immediately with additional salsa on the side.

PER SERVING
254 calories, 34 g protein, 23 g carbohydrate, 3 g fat (1 g saturated), 46 mg cholesterol, 193 mg sodium, 3 g fiber

PART THREE

LOOKING GREAT

CHAPTER 4

BEAUTIFUL SKIN

Everybody wants beautiful, healthy skin—especially women, many of whom are concerned (dare I say obsessed?) with signs of aging. Though I doubt it's high on the list of things people name when they're asked what first attracted them to another person, we all want that luminous glow from within. I know because people approach me all the time with questions about skin health—not just in my office, but at cocktail parties, on the street, during interviews, and even backstage during my television appearances.

Their interest is perfectly logical. Skin is, quite literally, the face we show to the world. It is our shell, the most exposed part of us. It is our first line of physiological defense as well as exquisitely sensitive to touch and temperature. It reflects our state of health, capable of turning yellow from liver toxins, red from a rush of blood, blue from a lack of oxygen, or grey from cell death.

But all this versatility and responsibility goes largely unappreciated. Most of us care mainly about the superficial beauty of skin. There's nothing wrong with that. Beautiful skin is healthy skin. If battling acne or wrinkles makes you want to eat healthier . . . if the search for clear, smooth skin leads you to exercise more . . . I can't see anything wrong with that! What's good for your skin is good for the rest of you too.

WHAT AFFECTS SKIN HEALTH?

In the search for more beautiful skin, the two main concerns are acne and wrinkles. Acne happens when hair follicles (sometimes called pores) become blocked with natural oils. If the pore is open to the air, the clog will appear as a blackhead. But if oil is trapped below the surface of the skin, it provides a nice little breeding ground for bacteria, leading to pimples—skin eruptions that can look red and inflamed. Because hormones affect how much oil your skin produces, acne is more likely to flare up during times of hormonal upheaval, including adolescence, pregnancy, and premenstrual weeks, as well as times of stress.

Wrinkles are a fact of life. As we age, collagen and elastin, the substances that keep skin firm and elastic, gradually decrease. Fat pads in the face also thin out. Without this underlying structure, skin sags, creases form, and—ugh!—we have wrinkles.

How quickly your skin shows signs of aging is largely determined by genetics, but the process accelerates if your skin is somehow damaged. Skin damage occurs as a result of *oxidation,* a chemical process in which unstable molecules called *free radicals* steal electrons from healthy cells. On the skin, oxidative stress can appear as wrinkling, thickening, discoloration, and decreased elasticity. The most damaging oxidative factors are smoking and sun exposure, and the extent of the damage depends on how long and how much you smoke, how much time you spent in the sun, and how many severe sunburns you've had.

Cigarette smoke fills your body with free radicals. Every lungful sends free radicals coursing through your blood stream, where they can damage every organ in the body, including your skin. Smoking also impairs blood flow to the skin, starving the cells of nutrition and oxygen. It also damages the underlying collagen and elastin, and keeps your skin from its natural renewal process. These problems evolve slowly, so the damage to skin can take up to ten years to appear. Unfortunately, those effects are irreversible. To prevent skin damage from cigarette smoke, including wrinkles, don't smoke and don't spend extensive amounts of time in smoky rooms.

Sunlight, as pleasant as it is, is a form of radiation. Ultraviolet (UV) radiation, to be more specific. UV radiation not only causes free radical damage, it can cause cells to mutate. With enough mutations, cells can turn cancerous. So excess sun exposure is a triple threat: sunburn in the short run, wrinkles in the long run, and the possibility of skin cancer to boot.

HOW FOOD AFFECTS SKIN

Skin is built from the inside out. Day to day and year to year, skin draws its healthy glow from good nutrition. Even though acne and wrinkles have different causes, and occur at different times in our lives, nutrition can help minimize or prevent both these problems and enhance your skin's natural beauty.

ANTIOXIDANTS

The best defense against the free radical damage of *oxidation* is a diet rich in anti*oxidant* vitamins and minerals. Research suggests that certain antioxidants—vitamin C, vitamin E, selenium, and vitamin A (in the form of beta carotene)—nourish and protect skin to extend its youthful appearance.

Topical preparations of these antioxidants—applied to the skin in a cream or ointment—have been shown to help protect the skin against radiation from the sun, and may even help *reverse* some of the damage that may already have occurred. They may even help prevent skin tumors. Some—such as the vitamin A prescription medications tretinoin (Retin-A, Renova) and isotretinoin (Accutane)—have become popular as treatments for acne and wrinkles.

Antioxidant-rich foods also can help:

Vitamin C, naturally found in the skin, is involved in collagen production and protects cells from free radical damage. Scientific studies found that when lab animals ate vitamin C–fortified food, their skin was better able to fight off oxidative damage. Because vitamin C is destroyed by exposure to sunlight, spending even a short time in the sun can leave skin depleted. It is important to replenish your skin's vitamin C stores by eating plenty of vitamin C–rich fruits and vegetables.

> **BEST FOODS FOR VITAMIN C:** *Guava, bell peppers (yellow, red, green), orange juice, hot chile peppers, oranges, grapefruit juice, strawberries, pineapple, kohlrabi, papaya, lemons, broccoli, kale, Brussels sprouts, kidney beans, kiwi, cantaloupe, cauliflower, red cabbage, mangos, grapefruit (pink, red), white potato (with skin), mustard greens, cherry tomatoes, sugar snap peas, snow peas, clementines, rutabagas, turnip greens, tomatoes, raspberries, Chinese cabbage, blackberries, green tomatoes, cabbage, watermelon, tangerines, lemon juice, okra, lychees, summer squash, persimmons*

Vitamin E helps protect cell membranes and guard against UV radiation damage. Some research suggests that vitamin E may work in combination with vitamin C to provide an extra boost of antiaging skin protection. However, because recent studies have raised some questions about the safety of vitamin E supplements, these nutrients should come from your diet, not from potent pills. I recommend you stick with food sources (and the small amount found in a multivitamin).

> **BEST FOODS FOR VITAMIN E:** *Wheat germ oil, fortified whole grain cereals, sunflower seeds, almonds, hazelnuts, peanut butter, wheat germ, avocado, pine nuts, tomato paste, flaxseed oil, red bell pepper, canola oil, kiwi, peanuts, olive oil, mangos, turnip greens, Brazil nuts, asparagus, peaches, papaya, radicchio, collard greens, broccoli, Swiss chard, spinach*

Selenium is an antioxidant mineral that helps safeguard the skin from sun damage and delays aging by protecting skin quality and elasticity. Dietary selenium has been shown to reduce sun damage, and even to prevent some skin cancers in animals. Be sure to get your selenium from food, though, and not from supplements. The Nutritional Prevention of Cancer Trial found that people with a high risk of nonmelanoma skin cancers who took selenium supplements actually had a 25 percent increased risk of squamous cell carcinomas.

BEST FOODS FOR SELENIUM: *Brazil nuts, tuna (canned light), crab, oysters, tilapia, whole wheat pasta, lean beef, cod, shrimp, whole wheat breads (including crackers, buns), turkey, wheat germ, brown rice, chicken breast, cottage cheese (fat-free, 1% reduced-fat), mushrooms, eggs*

Beta carotene, another antioxidant critical for skin health, is converted to vitamin A in the body. Beta carotene/vitamin A is involved in the growth and repair of body tissues, and may protect against sun damage. In extremely high doses, straight vitamin A from supplements can be toxic, so I never recommend them. However, ample beta carotene from food is entirely safe.

BEST FOODS FOR BETA CAROTENE: *Sweet potatoes, carrots, kale, butternut squash, turnip greens, pumpkin, mustard greens, cantaloupe, red bell pepper, apricots, Chinese cabbage, spinach, lettuce (romaine, green leaf, red leaf, butterhead), collard greens, Swiss chard, watercress, grapefruit, watermelon, cherries, mangos, red ripe tomatoes, guava, asparagus, red cabbage*

ZINC

Your skin contains about 6 percent of all the zinc in your body. This mineral is necessary for protecting cell membranes and helping to maintain the collagen that keeps skin firm. People with severe zinc deficiencies can develop redness, pustules, scaling, and lesions. (There's a pretty picture.) In addition, there are microscopic changes in the structure of skin cells themselves. On top of that, zinc is critically involved in skin renewal—which means that if you want to keep your skin fresh and as youthful as possible, be sure to include zinc-rich foods in your menu.

BEST FOODS FOR ZINC: *Oysters, lean beef, crab, ostrich, pork tenderloin, peanut butter, wheat germ, turkey, veal, pumpkin seeds, chicken, chickpeas (garbanzo beans), fat-free yogurt, fortified whole grain cereals, pine nuts, cashews, sunflower seeds, lima beans, lentils, pecans, cheese (fat-free, reduced-fat), fat-free milk, almonds, walnuts, peanuts, black-eyed peas, green peas*

OMEGA-3 FATTY ACIDS

Healthy fats known as omega-3 fatty acids help maintain cell membranes so that they are effective barriers—allowing water and nutrients in, and keeping toxins out. Omega-3s also seem to be able to protect skin against sun damage. In a study of skin cancer in sunny, skin-scorching southeastern Arizona, people who ate diets rich in fish oils and other omega-3 fats had a 29 percent lower risk of squamous cell skin cancer than those who got very little omega-3s from food. Not too shabby—grill some fish, prevent some cancer.

BEST FOODS FOR OMEGA-3 FATTY ACIDS: *Wild salmon (fresh, canned), herring, mackerel (not king), sardines, anchovies, rainbow trout, pacific oysters, omega-3–fortified eggs, flaxseed (ground, oil), walnuts, butternuts (white walnuts), seaweed, walnut oil, canola oil, soybeans*

WATER

It is so basic, but I can't emphasize enough how important water is for skin's health and beauty. Water helps your body flush away toxins, allows the smooth flow of nutrients into cells, and keeps organs functioning their best. Plus, cells that are well-hydrated are plump and full, which means that your skin will look firmer and clearer (but not "fat"). Recommendations vary, but current thinking says that you should let your thirst guide how much water you drink every day.

Although liquids are the main source of water, many foods have such high water content that they contribute to overall hydration. The following foods are at least 75 percent water (by weight):

Fruits: apples, blackberries, blueberries, cantaloupe, cherries, cranberries, grapefruit, grapes, kiwi, lemon, limes, mangos, nectarines, oranges, papaya, peaches, pears, pineapple, plums, raspberries, strawberries, tangerines, watermelon

Vegetables: artichokes, asparagus, beets, broccoli, Brussels sprouts, carrots, cauliflower, celery, cucumbers, kale, lettuce, mushrooms, onions, peas, potatoes, pumpkin, peppers (red, yellow, green), rhubarb, spinach, squash, tomatoes, turnips, yams

TEA

Another good option for hydration is tea. Teas contain natural compounds known as *polyphenols,* which have antioxidant properties. In animal studies, polyphenols helped prevent sun-related skin cancers and improve immune functioning. In people, topical polyphenols seem to help increase collagen production and decrease growth of skin cancer cells.

FAQS

I tried everything for my acne, and my doctor wants to put me on Accutane (isotretinoin). Do you have an opinion about this medication?

This powerful medication is a godsend to many of my acne-prone clients and friends (even celebrities!). It can improve skin significantly by drying up the oil-producing sebaceous glands. As you might imagine, it dries more than those glands, namely your skin and lips—and pretty badly. You'll want to be diligent about drinking plenty of water, and using skin cream and lip balm to conserve as much moisture as possible. Accutane also can increase the body's production of cholesterol, so the medication may temporarily raise your cholesterol levels. If you go on this medication, be sure to have your blood cholesterol measured regularly. If it starts going up, you should take steps to lower your cholesterol, even if you are young (see page 129 for more on cholesterol). There are some important warnings about using Accutane, so be sure to discuss this medication thoroughly with your doctor. For example, Accutane can cause birth defects, so it cannot be taken by women who are pregnant or considering getting pregnant. Also, some people become depressed or anxious while taking this medication (or soon after stopping), sometimes fatally depressed. If you have a history of depression, or if you find yourself feeling depressed or anxious while taking Accutane, see your doctor immediately.

Although there are no definitive studies about the effects of *drinking* tea for skin health, tea—green or black, caffeinated or decaffeinated—is always a better choice than sugary drinks, soft drinks, or fruit juice.

BONUS POINTS

- **Use sunscreen.** Whenever you are going to be spending more than a few minutes outside, protect your skin from some of the sun's damaging rays by applying sunscreen to all exposed areas of your body. Look for formulas designed to filter both UVA and UVB radiation, with a skin protection factor (SPF) of at least 15. The SPF is an indication of how long you will be protected, based on your skin type. The higher the number, the more time you can spend outside without burning. Use sunscreen with an SPF of at least 30 if you want longer protection, or if you tend to burn easily. Every day, apply moisturizer with SPF to guard your skin even during casual sun exposure.

- **Avoid sugary foods, refined-flour baked goods, and soda.** Some researchers have theorized that low-quality carbohydrates raise insulin levels, which, over time, may increase levels of certain acne-causing hormones. These foods also cause inflammation in skin cells and throughout the body, causing premature aging and wrinkles.

- **Consider a topical antioxidant.** Most drug store and cosmetic brand preparations don't contain enough of these antioxidants to make a difference to your skin's health. The more potent—and potential irritating—preparations aren't for everybody. Some are only available by prescription, so if you want to try antioxidant skin cream, talk with your dermatologist.

SUPPLEMENTS

To improve skin health, I strongly recommend getting all your nutrients from food sources. However, if you would also like to consider supplements, I recommend:

1. **Multivitamin.** Taking a multivitamin will assure that you get the minimal amount of vitamins and minerals necessary for good skin health, even on days when you might not eat as well as you should. Choose a brand that contains 100% DV for vitamin A (optimally 100%—or at least 50%—coming from beta carotene and/or mixed carotenoids), vitamin C, vitamin E, and zinc and which provides about 55 micrograms selenium.

2. **Omega-3s.** If you find it difficult to get all the omega-3 fatty acids you need from foods, try fish oil supplements. I recommend taking 650 milligrams of omega-3 fatty acids. There are two sub-types of omega-3s, called DHA (docosahexaenoic acid) and EPA (eicosapentaenoic acid). When buying fish oil supplements, choose brands that contain at least 220 milligrams each of both DHA and EPA. The remaining 200+ milligrams

can come from either DHA or EPA. Check labels for these details.

To prevent rancidity, always store bottles of fish oil supplements in the fridge. To lessen the chance of fishy burps or aftertaste, choose an enteric-coated variety, which is digested in the intestines instead of the stomach so it is less likely to repeat on you. Avoid getting omega-3 fats from cod liver oil because it may contain too much vitamin A. *Important note:* Because fish oil acts as a blood thinner, it should not be taken by people who have hemophilia, or who are already taking blood thinning medications or aspirin. People with diabetes should talk with their doctors before trying fish oil supplements because they may affect blood sugar.

FAQS

Can dairy foods cause acne breakouts?

It is entirely possible, although not necessarily for the reason you think. Cows are given iodine-fortified feed to help fight infection, and some of it naturally finds its way into the cows' milk. Iodine can cause acne in some people. Some experts believe that the amount of iodine found in milk—although low—is enough to cause skin problems for some sensitive people. In addition, the current prevailing thought is that dairy-acne connection may be caused by the hormones in milk. Apparently dairy cows are allowed to become pregnant while they are lactating, and the pregnancy hormones go into the milk. If you want to test your personal reaction, I recommend eliminating all dairy foods from your diet for one month. These include milk, yogurt, all cheeses, sour cream, and ice cream. (No matter what your age, be sure to get enough daily calcium from non-dairy sources or take 1,000 milligrams of calcium supplements daily to make up for what you're missing.) If you see no difference, then dairy is not a problem for you. If your acne improves, add dairy back into your diet—two servings a day for four or five days. If your acne comes back, then dairy is a definite acne-booster for you.

JOY'S 4-STEP PROGRAM
FOR BEAUTIFUL SKIN

Follow this program if you want healthier skin, now and in the future.

STEP 1 ... START WITH THE BASICS

These are the first things you should do to improve the state of your skin, today and tomorrow:

- See your doctor if you have any unusual skin growths, moles or freckles that have grown or gotten darker, or a scaly patch or scab that won't heal. These may be early signs of skin cancer. If caught early, most cancers can be stopped before they turn deadly.

- If you smoke, quit.

- Stay out of the sun as much as possible. If you do go outdoors, wear sunscreen to protect your skin . . . but don't depend on it to keep you entirely safe. Even the best sunscreen, applied liberally and often, allows some radiation through.

- Drink plenty of water.

STEP2 ... YOUR ULTIMATE GROCERY LIST

This list contains foods with high levels of nutrients that will help your skin look the best it can, plus foods included in meal plans and recipes. You don't have to purchase every item . . . but integrate as many of these foods as possible into your diet.

FRUIT

Apricots	Clementines	Lychees	Pineapple
Berries (blackberries, raspberries, strawberries)	Grapefruit and juice (pink, red)	Mangos	Tangerines
		Oranges and juice	Watermelon
	Guava	Papaya	
Cantaloupe	Kiwi	Peaches	
Cherries	Lemons and juice	Persimmons	

VEGETABLES

Artichokes	Cucumbers	Potatoes, sweet	green tomatoes,
Asparagus	Kale	Potatoes, white	red ripe tomatoes,
Avocado	Kohlrabi	Pumpkin	cherry tomatoes,
Beans (garbanzo, kidney, lima)	Leeks	Radicchio	tomato paste)
	Lentils	Rhubarb	Tomatoes, canned,
Beets	Lettuce (romaine, green leaf, red leaf, butterhead)	Rutabagas	whole peeled
Broccoli		Scallions	(for meal plan)
Brussels sprouts		Seaweed	Turnips
Cabbage (including Chinese and red)	Mushrooms	Snow peas	Turnip greens
	Mustard greens	Soybeans (edamame)	Watercress
Carrots	Okra	Spinach	Yams
Cauliflower	Onions	Squash, winter (especially butternut)	
Celery	Peas (green, sugar snap)		
Chickpeas (garbanzo beans)	Peas, black-eyed	Squash, summer	
	Peppers, (hot; yellow/ red/green)	Swiss chard	
Collard greens		Tomatoes (especially	

SEAFOOD

Anchovies	Mackerel (not king)	Salmon, wild (with bones)	Tilapia
Cod			Trout, rainbow
Crab	Oysters (especially Pacific)	Sardines	Tuna (canned light)
Herring		Shrimp	

LEAN MEATS/EGGS/SOY FOODS

Beef, lean	Eggs, omega-3–fortified	Pork tenderloin	Veal
Chicken	Ostrich	Turkey	

NUTS AND SEEDS (PREFERABLY UNSALTED)

Almond butter
Almonds
Brazil nuts
Butternuts (white
   walnuts)
Cashews
Flaxseed, ground
Hazelnuts
Peanut butter
Peanuts
Pecans
Pine nuts
Pumpkin seeds
Sunflower seeds
Walnuts

WHOLE GRAINS

Bread, whole grain
   (including crackers,
   buns)
Cereal, fortified whole
   grain
Pasta, whole wheat
Rice, brown
Wheat germ

DAIRY

Cheese (fat-free,
   reduced-fat)
Cheese, Parmesan
Cottage cheese (fat-free,
   reduced-fat)
Milk, fat-free
Milk, evaporated fat-
   free (for meal plan)
Sour cream, fat-free
Yogurt, fat-free
Yogurt, Greek
   non-fat (for meal
   plan)

MISCELLANEOUS

Basil
Broth, low-sodium
   (chicken, vegetable)
Caesar dressing,
   reduced-calorie
Cinnamon, ground
Cocoa powder
Coffee, instant
Cornstarch
Dill, fresh
Garlic
Honey
Ketchup
Leeks
Margarine spread, soft
   tub, trans fat–free
Mayonnaise, reduced-fat
Mustard, Dijon
Nonstick cooking spray
Oil, canola
Oil, flaxseed
Oil, olive
Oil, walnut
Oil, wheat germ
Oregano
Pepper, black
Salt
Scallions
Soup, butternut squash
   (low-fat)
Spice mix, Cajun
Sugar, granulated
   (or sugar substitute)
Tea (green, black;
   caffeinated,
   decaffeinated)
Thyme, dried
Vanilla extract
Vinegar, balsamic or
   red wine
Vinegar, white

STEP3 ...GOING ABOVE AND BEYOND

If you want to do everything you can to improve your skin, here are some additional things you might try:

- Consider taking a daily multivitamin.

- If you don't eat at least two servings of a fatty fish every week, consider taking fish oil supplements.

ACNE AND FRIED FOOD

You'll notice that I didn't warn you to avoid fried, greasy, oily foods in my discussion about acne. That's because eating grease doesn't cause skin problems. *However,* if you eat French fries, potato chips, or other oily foods and then scratch your nose or rub your chin, you spread that grease to your skin. That kind of topical oil can block pores and cause acne. In fact, any time you touch your face you risk transferring dirt and bacteria that can cloud your complexion. Make a point of washing your hands with soap before laying a finger on your face.

STEP4...MEAL PLANS

These sample menus include foods that have been shown to improve skin health, specifically foods high in vitamins C and E, beta carotene, selenium, zinc, and omega-3 fatty acids.

Every day, choose *one* option for each of the three meals—breakfast, lunch, and dinner. Then, one or two times per day, choose from among my suggested snacks. Approximate calories have been provided to help adjust for your personal weight management goals. If you find yourself hungry (and if weight is not an issue), feel free to increase the portion sizes for meals and snacks. Beverage calories are *not* included. For the best skin, water and green tea are your best bets for beverage selections.

BREAKFAST OPTIONS

(Approximately 300 to 400 calories)

Yogurt with Almonds and Berries

8 ounces fat-free plain or flavored yogurt (or Greek yogurt), mixed with 1 cup berries and topped with 1 to 2 tablespoons slivered almonds (or pumpkin seeds or chopped walnuts) and 2 tablespoons wheat germ.

Southwest Omelet with Whole Grain Toast

Coat a small skillet with nonstick cooking spray or 1 teaspoon canola oil. Sauté ½ cup each sliced onion and sliced red or yellow pepper until soft. Beat 1 whole egg with two egg whites and pour over sautéed vegetables. Add ½ cup chopped tomato, season with a pinch of salt and ground black pepper, and cook until bottom becomes firm. Gently flip over and cook until egg mixture becomes firm. Fold omelet over and serve. Enjoy with 1 slice whole grain bread, toasted (with optional 1 teaspoon soft tub, trans fat–free margarine spread).

Oatmeal with Chopped Walnuts and Fruit

½ cup dry instant oatmeal prepared with ½ cup water and ½ cup fat-free milk or enriched/fortified soy milk (sweeten with optional 1 teaspoon white or brown sugar, honey, jam, or artificial sweetener). Top with 1 tablespoon chopped walnuts (or almonds or sunflower seeds) and ½ cup berries (or ½ mango or 1 orange).

Peanut Butter Toast

2 slices whole grain bread, toasted; each slice topped with 1 level tablespoon peanut butter (or almond butter).

Cottage Cheese with Apricots and Pecans

1 cup fat-free or 1% reduced-fat cottage cheese topped with 4 diced whole apricots (or 1 cup berries or ½ chopped mango) and 2 tablespoons chopped pecans or slivered almonds (if you like, sprinkle with ½ teaspoon cinnamon).

LUNCH OPTIONS

(Approximately 400 to 500 calories)

Butternut Squash Soup with Salad and Fish

2 servings (3 cups) Butternut Squash Soup (page 80) or 2 to 3 cups of any prepared low-fat soup without cream. Serve with unlimited leafy greens topped with 3 ounces canned sardines (or wild salmon, light tuna, or grilled chicken) and drizzled with fresh lemon juice or vinegar.

Vegetarian Chili and Sweet Potato

2 cups vegetarian chili (or Turkey Chili, page 367, substituting kidney beans for black beans). Serve with ½ medium baked sweet or white potato (with optional 1 teaspoon soft tub, trans fat–free margarine spread, or 1 tablespoon fat-free sour cream).

Open-Faced Tuna Melt

Mash 6 ounces canned water-packed light tuna (or canned chicken breast or wild salmon) with 1 tablespoon reduced-fat mayonnaise, minced onion, and freshly ground black pepper (or use Veggie Tuna Salad, page 274); spread on 2 slices whole grain bread, toasted; top each open slice with thinly sliced tomato and 1 small (¾-ounce) slice fat-free or reduced-fat cheese (any variety, such as Cheddar, Swiss, or American). Bake in a 350°F oven until the cheese melts. Enjoy with red/yellow/green pepper sticks.

Turkey Burger with Sautéed Mushrooms and Broccoli

1 cooked 5-ounce turkey burger (or lean hamburger or veggie burger), topped with sliced tomato, sautéed mushrooms, and optional 1 tablespoon ketchup, on a standard size hamburger bun (preferably whole grain). For ½ the bun, you may substitute 1 small slice reduced-fat cheese. Serve with 1 cup steamed broccoli or sugar snap peas.

Caesar Salad with Grilled Chicken or Shrimp

Unlimited Romaine lettuce leaves, 4 ounces grilled chicken or cooked shrimp, 1 ounce grated Parmesan cheese (4 to 5 level tablespoons), and optional anchovies (4 fillets). Toss with ¼ cup reduced-calorie Caesar dressing (40 calories or less per tablespoon), or 2 tablespoons regular Caesar dressing.

DINNER OPTIONS

(Approximately 500 to 600 calories)

Beef Stir-Fry with Brown Rice and Steamed Broccoli

5 ounces lean beef (round, sirloin, or flank), trimmed and stir-fried in 2 teaspoons canola oil with ½ cup sliced bell peppers, ½ cup sugar snap peas, and 2 chopped scallions (plus optional minced garlic, salt, and black pepper to taste). Enjoy with ½ cup cooked brown rice and 1 cup steamed broccoli (or spinach, kale, or Swiss chard).

Wild Salmon with Mustard, Lemon, Dill, and Potato

1 poached 5-ounce wild salmon fillet topped with 1 tablespoon Dijon mustard and 1½ teaspoon dried dill, and drizzled with juice from ½ lemon (or 1 serving Easy! 3-Step Microwave Salmon, page 345). Enjoy with ½ medium baked sweet or white potato (with optional 1 tablespoon soft tub, trans fat–free margarine spread) and 1 cup steamed asparagus (or spinach, broccoli, kale, Swiss chard, or sugar snap peas).

Rosemary Chicken with Butternut Squash Soup and Cauliflower

5 ounces skinless chicken breast sautéed in 2 teaspoons canola or olive oil and minced garlic and seasoned with preferred herbs (or 1 serving Rosemary Chicken, page 347). Enjoy with 2 servings (3 cups) Butternut Squash Soup (page 80) and 1 cup steamed cauliflower (or broccoli, spinach, kale or Swiss chard).

Whole Wheat Pasta with Turkey Meatballs

1 serving Turkey Meatballs in Red Pepper–Tomato Sauce (page 79). Enjoy with ½ cup cooked whole wheat pasta (or ½ plain medium baked sweet or white potato).

Grilled Oysters with Cajun Fish and Brussels Sprouts

1 serving Grilled Rockefeller Oysters (page 186) with 6 ounces fish (tilapia, black cod, shrimp, wild salmon, or trout) rubbed with Cajun spice and baked or grilled. Enjoy with leafy green salad tossed with 1 teaspoon olive oil and fresh lemon juice or balsamic vinegar (or 2 tablespoons reduced-calorie dressing) and 1 cup steamed Brussels sprouts (or broccoli, Swiss chard, or spinach).

SNACK OPTIONS

100 calories or less

- *Best Vegetables:* 1 cup raw or cooked spinach, kale, red/yellow/green peppers, broccoli, cauliflower, asparagus, carrots, collard greens, sugar snap peas, kohlrabi, mushrooms, rutabagas, summer squash, Swiss chard, tomatoes, turnip greens, watercress, seaweed, okra, Brussels sprouts, mustard greens, cabbage

■ *Best Fruits:* 1 guava, peach, orange, persimmon, kiwi, clementine, or tangerine; 4 apricots; 6 lychees; 1 cup blueberries, blackberries, raspberries, cherries, watermelon, or pineapple; 20 strawberries; ½ mango, cantaloupe, papaya, or grapefruit

■ 2 level teaspoons peanut butter or almond butter with celery sticks

■ ½ cup fat-free or 1% reduced-fat cottage cheese with red, yellow, and/or green pepper sticks

100 to 200 calories

■ 1 serving (1½ cups) Butternut Squash Soup (page 80)

■ 1 serving Warm Dark Chocolate Sauce with Fresh Fruit (page 81)

■ 1 ounce raw almonds, cashews, toasted pecans, walnuts, or peanuts (about ¼ cup)

■ ¼ cup sunflower seeds in the shell

■ 1 slice whole grain bread (or 70-calorie pita bread) topped with 1 level tablespoon peanut butter or almond butter

■ Red, yellow, and/or green pepper sticks and baby carrots dipped in ¼ cup hummus (any store-bought brand)

■ 1 cup fat-free plain or flavored yogurt mixed with ½ cup blackberries, raspberries, or sliced strawberries plus 1 tablespoon wheat germ

■ ½ mango or small cantaloupe with ½ cup fat-free or 1% reduced-fat cottage cheese

TURKEY MEATBALLS
IN RED PEPPER–TOMATO SAUCE

I call these Beautiful Meatballs. By mixing wheat germ, egg whites, and plain yogurt into lean ground turkey meat, I'm able to boost the vitamin E, selenium, and zinc. Together with bell pepper–tomato sauce—rich in vitamin C and beta carotene—it's a perfect meal for a healthy complexion.

Makes 4 servings, 2 cups each (approximately 5 meatballs)

½	cup wheat germ
2	egg whites
2	cloves garlic, minced
2	small onions, minced
½	cup plain fat-free yogurt
¼	cup packed fresh basil leaves, chopped
1	pound lean ground turkey
	Salt and freshly ground pepper
1	can (28 ounces) whole peeled tomatoes
1	cup water
2	tablespoons olive oil
1	small red bell pepper, minced
1	sprig of fresh thyme or 1 teaspoon dried thyme
1	teaspoon dried oregano

1. In a large bowl, mix the wheat germ, egg whites, half the garlic, half the onions, the yogurt, and basil. Add the turkey. Season with salt and pepper and mix well. (The mixture will be sticky.) Cover and place in the freezer 20 minutes, for easier handling.
2. Meanwhile, in a blender or food processor, purée the tomatoes with the water.
3. In a large nonstick skillet, heat 1 tablespoon olive oil over medium-high heat. Sauté the remaining onion and garlic until translucent, 3 to 4 minutes. Add the red pepper, and cook 5 to 6 minutes longer, until the pepper softens slightly. Add the thyme, oregano, and puréed tomatoes, and bring to a low simmer.
4. Roll the turkey mixture into about 20 meatballs, 2 inches in diameter. Coat a nonstick skillet with nonstick cooking spray. Add the remaining 1 tablespoon olive oil and heat over high heat. In batches, add the meatballs and sauté until they are browned on all sides, 6 to 7 minutes total.
5. Carefully transfer the meatballs to the tomato sauce as they finish cooking. Simmer, partially covered, about 20 minutes longer, until the meatballs are cooked through. Season with additional salt and pepper. Serve immediately.

PER SERVING
390 calories, 33 g protein, 25 g carbohydrate, 19 g fat (4 g saturated), 176 mg cholesterol, 536 mg sodium, 6 g fiber; plus 54 mg vitamin C (90% DV), 326 mcg beta carotene: 3 mg zinc (20% DV)

BUTTERNUT SQUASH SOUP

This is, by far, one of my favorite, low-calorie comfort soups. It's easy to make, and 1½ cups provide a BLAST of vitamin C and beta carotene for radiant skin!

Makes 4 servings, 1½ cups each

1	tablespoon olive oil
2	large leeks, trimmed and chopped
⅛	teaspoon ground cinnamon
⅛	teaspoon freshly grated nutmeg
1½	pounds butternut squash, peeled and cubed (about 4 cups)
2	large carrots, peeled and grated
3	cups fat-free, low-sodium chicken or vegetable broth
	Salt
	Freshly ground black pepper

1. Spray a large stockpot with nonstick cooking spray. Add the oil and heat over medium-high heat. Add the leeks and sauté until translucent and soft, 6 to 7 minutes. Add the cinnamon and nutmeg, and cook an additional minute to release the flavor of the spices. Add the squash, carrots, and broth, and bring to a boil.

2. Reduce to a simmer and cook 20 to 25 minutes longer, until the vegetables are tender. Purée the soup with an immersion blender or in a food processor or blender. Season with salt and pepper and serve immediately.

PER SERVING
158 calories, 5 g protein, 30g carbohydrate, 4 g fat (0 g saturated), 0 mg cholesterol, 452 mg sodium, 5 g fiber; plus 43 mg Vitamin C (73% DV): 10,160 mcg beta carotene

WARM DARK CHOCOLATE SAUCE WITH FRESH FRUIT

Here's the most wonderful news: Research published in the *Journal of Nutrition* (June, 2006) suggests that consuming flavanol-rich cocoa may improve your skin. If you dip fresh fruit into my guilt-free dark chocolate sauce, you'll get the added benefits of vitamin C. If you're diabetic, or would like to lower the calories even further, substitute Splenda for the sugar.

Makes 6 servings, ¼ cup sauce each with fruit

1	tablespoon cornstarch
1	can (12 ounces) fat-free evaporated milk
½	cup unsweetened cocoa powder
½	cup granulated sugar or Splenda Sugar Blend for Baking
½	teaspoon instant coffee
½	teaspoon vanilla extract
⅛	teaspoon salt
1	cup whole strawberries
1	cup fresh pineapple chunks

In a medium saucepan, whisk the cornstarch into the evaporated milk. Place over low heat and stir in the cocoa powder, sugar or Splenda, coffee, vanilla, and salt. Cook, whisking constantly, until thoroughly combined and the liquid starts to thicken, 5 to 6 minutes. Serve immediately with strawberries and pineapple.

PER SERVING (USING SUGAR)
153 calories, 6 g protein, 33 g carbohydrate, 1g fat (0 g saturated), 0 mg cholesterol, 133 mg sodium, 3 g fiber; plus 24 mg vitamin C (40% DV)

CHAPTER 5

HEALTHY HAIR

Unless you are balding, chances are you take hair for granted. A little shampoo and conditioner, a bit of styling product, and a good hair day is in your future . . . right? Not necessarily. Like all other body tissues, the state of your hair is related to your overall health and individual physical characteristics.

Hair starts its lifespan in small, sack-like structures in the skin known as *follicles*. Each follicle produces a single hair shaft composed of a hard protein called *keratin* arranged in long, tightly bound strands. New growth begins in the follicle, and pushes outward so that the oldest part of the hair is furthest from the scalp.

Each hair has a distinct growth cycle—active growth, maturation, and rest. During the resting phase, the follicle relaxes its hold on the shaft, so hair can easily fall or be pulled out. Every hair on your head goes through the growth cycle, but not at the same time. At any given moment, about 15 percent of all the hairs on your head are resting, and therefore capable of shedding . . . in your hairbrush, in the shower, on the bathroom floor. This is totally normal, and is not a harbinger of baldness. Between my two daughters and myself, our shower drain needs cleaning about every two weeks—that's about all the "resting" hair it can take before it's thoroughly clogged. Trust me, none of us is even close to bald. But if you have been experiencing unusual hair loss or problems with dryness, splitting, or breakage, or if you simply want to have more beautiful locks, nutrition can help.

WHAT AFFECTS HAIR HEALTH?

It is estimated that we each lose about 100 hairs a day. The actual number you'll lose on any given day depends on how abundant and healthy your follicles are, as well as medications you're taking, and many other factors, some of which are beyond your control. For example, the recommendations in this chapter won't reverse thinning hair due to male pattern baldness or aging—typical male baldness is genetic. As we age, our hair spends more time in the resting phase, which means that we'll shed more hair than usual, and it won't grow back as quickly. For more general hair problems, here are some factors that you should be aware of:

HORMONAL SHIFTS

Both male and female hormones affect hair growth. Male hormones known as *androgens*—a category that includes testosterone—stimulate hair growth on the face and body, and create fuller, thicker hair on the head. In women, ovaries and adrenal glands naturally produce androgens, but very small amounts. If a woman suddenly starts growing facial hair, she should see her doctor—it could be a sign of a hormone-related health problem.

For some men with a genetic susceptibility to baldness, normal testosterone levels are converted to a more potent form of testosterone (dihydrotestosterone, or DHT), which binds to cells in the follicle. DHT alters the growth/shed cycle and eventually kills the follicle. These men find themselves becoming bald in their 20s, a few years after their testosterone levels peak. Because the follicle itself shrinks and dies, this type of baldness is irreversible. Some prescription medications may short-circuit the balding process if caught early enough, though the medications need to be continued for life.

In both men and women, levels of androgens decrease after about age 40, which leads to thinner, slower-growing, less luxurious hair as we get older.

In contrast to androgens, the female hormone estrogen slows hair growth, and creates a finer, thinner shaft of hair, which is why women are, on average, naturally less hairy than men. After menopause, levels of estrogen fall off dramatically, causing some genetically susceptible women to lose significant amounts of hair. Experts believe that female balding follows a processes much like male balding—without enough estrogen to off-set the tiny amounts of androgens in their bodies, they also can have androgen-related hair loss. But male and female hair loss aren't identical. While men tend to bald in a distinct pattern that includes a receding hairline and hair loss at the crown, women tend to lose hair evenly, leaving them with a sparse head of hair instead of a totally bald scalp. Hormone replacement therapy, which restores levels of estrogen, stops hair loss in some women, but not all.

The "other" female hormone, progesterone, has almost no direct action on hair.

However, when levels of estrogen and progesterone are both high, such as during pregnancy, the combination works to synchronize the hair growth cycles, so more hair is in the growth stage at the same time. In the second and third trimester of pregnancy, the percent of hair in the resting phase falls by one-third to about 10 percent. For those few months, pregnant women have the fullest, richest head of hair they'll have in their entire lives. About three months after delivery, the percent of shedding hairs goes back up to 15 percent. As all those synchronized hairs enter the resting phase together, it can look like you're suddenly losing all your hair. Don't panic! Once the hair starts to regrow, it returns to its usual growth/rest cycle.

STRESS

Stress is one of the most common causes of unusual hair loss. Severe emotional reaction to the death of someone close, an accident, or other traumatic event can send hair follicles into the resting phase prematurely. Three months later, when those resting follicles release the hair shaft, large amounts of hair can seem to fall out simultaneously, and for no discernable reason since several months have passed since the event that triggered this whole episode. Again, getting through this is simply a matter of waiting it out. Your hair should begin to regrow almost immediately.

LACK OF PROTEIN

Hair is made of protein. All basic nutrients contribute to keeping us whole and healthy, but protein provides the building blocks that allow us to repair, replace, or grow bones, skin, muscles, and hair. Although we tend to think of dietary protein as coming from steak, fish, chicken, and other meats, it is also found in eggs, legumes, milk, whole grains, and some vegetables. People who don't get enough protein in their diets, such as those with anorexia nervosa or who follow any extreme weight-loss diet, will slow the rate of new hair growth. As hair is naturally shed, it won't grow back as quickly. With enough hair loss, the scalp will start to show through.

Starvation also depletes the body of other nutrients important for hair growth and quality. And over the long term, starvation and extreme weight loss will lead to a reduction in hormone production, which can also lead to thinning hair.

FAQS

My doctor tested my iron level in the office, and it came up a little on the low side, but still normal. My thyroid, blood sugar, and all other blood tests turned out normal. Is there anything else I should test that might explain my hair loss?

Since your iron tested low-normal, make sure you eat lots of iron-rich protein (coupled with vitamin C, if you're vegetarian) for the next several weeks. This will help bring your iron levels back into the mid-normal range. You might also want to go back to your doctor and ask for a more extensive test for iron levels. There are actually three main tests for iron: 1) serum iron, which measures the amount of iron in blood; 2) ferritin, which is a measure of the amount of iron stored in the body; and 3) TIBC—Total Iron Binding Capacity—which is a measure of how much iron could be/should be in the body. Many doctors will only test serum iron, but unless you have severe anemia, serum iron can appear normal even if ferritin and TIBC are low. The other two tests are more sensitive. Low ferritin means low iron stores, which means that you may need more iron. High TIBC means that your body has a big gap between how much iron the body has and how much it can use. It indicates pre-anemia. Talk with your doctor about these additional tests. Your iron levels may yet be the problem. You may be a candidate for a supplemental dose, but don't try self-diagnosing this problem—never take iron pills unless a medical professional confirms you need them.

FAQS

I was losing a lot of hair, had no energy, gained weight, and felt miserable. Finally I was diagnosed with low thyroid hormone (hypothyroid). I've been on Synthroid for a couple of weeks, and I'm feeling better, but my hair still hasn't come back. What's up?

There's a good chance your hair will come back; you just have to give it more time. Your body needs a chance to recover from illness, and your follicles need a few months to recover from the resting phase. If your hair hasn't started to regrow within six months after your blood levels of thyroid hormone have returned to normal, talk with your doctor to see if there might be another reason for your continuing problem.

MEDICATIONS AND SUPPLEMENTS

Many medications can lead to hair loss. Most people understand that chemotherapy treatments for cancer can lead to widespread balding, but many other medications may cause less extensive hair loss. These include anticoagulants (such as warfarin), antidepressants, oral contraceptives, and medications for blood pressure, gout, or arthritis. In addition, very high doses of vitamin A and selenium are toxic, and can cause hair loss. This type of toxicity happens only if you take high-dose supplements. Don't take individual supplements for vitamin A or selenium. If you take a multivitamin supplement, it shouldn't contain more than 100% DV for vitamin A (5,000 IU) or selenium (70 micrograms). Better yet, make sure your multivitamin provides 50 to 100% of its vitamin A in the precursor form of beta carotene and/or mixed carotenoids. Most health experts agree there is no known chance of Vitamin A toxicity when you're getting your standard supplemental dose for vitamin A from carotenoids. Once you stop taking the medication or supplements, hair will usually begin to grow back within a few months.

THYROID GLAND MALFUNCTION AND OTHER DISORDERS

Thyroid hormones affect metabolism of all cells, including cells in hair follicles. Too much thyroid hormone (*hyper*thyroid) or too little thyroid hormone (*hypo*thyroid) can result in thin, brittle hair or hair loss.

With uncontrolled diabetes, body cells (including cells in hair follicles) starve because glucose can't get in; and in systemic lupus erythematosus, the body attacks its own collagen, including the collagen in hair follicles. These disorders and many others—including celiac disease, rheumatoid arthritis, ulcerative colitis, and Crohn's disease—may cause hair loss or damage by altering cell metabolism or structure. Once the underlying disease is treated, hair growth should return to normal. The lesson is that all cases of unexplained hair loss should be investigated by a physician to rule out the possibility of serious disease.

HOW FOOD AFFECTS HAIR

Hair is a great marker of overall health. Good hair depends on the body's ability to construct a proper hair shaft, as well as the health of the skin and follicles. Good nutrition assures the best possible environment for building strong, lustrous hair. But this is not a quick fix. Changing your diet now will affect only new growth, not the part of the hair that is already visible. You could get a completely fresh start if you shaved your head today, and start eating a perfect, hair-improving diet tomorrow. Your new head of hair would positively radiate with health. But there's really no need. Take my word for it: Starting a hair-healthy diet today will mean a more gorgeous head of hair within six months to a year, depending on how fast your hair grows. Hair growth rates vary between about ¼" and 1½" per month (depending on personal differences). On average, a person can expect to have about 6 inches of new growth every year, so it will take about that long to notice the effects of your nutritional changes.

B VITAMINS: FOLATE, B$_6$, B$_{12}$

These vitamins are involved in the creation of red blood cells, which carry oxygen and nutrients to all body cells, including those of the scalp, follicles, and growing hair. Without enough B vitamins, the cells can starve, causing shedding, slow growth, or weak hair that is prone to breaking.

BEST FOODS FOR VITAMIN B$_6$: *Fortified whole grain breakfast cereals, chickpeas (garbanzo beans), wild salmon (fresh, canned), lean beef, pork tenderloin, chicken breast, white potatoes (with skin), oatmeal, bananas, pistachio nuts, lentils, tomato paste, barley, rice (brown, wild), peppers, sweet potatoes, winter squash (acorn), broccoli, broccoli raab, carrots, Brussels sprouts, peanut butter, eggs, shrimp, tofu, apricots, watermelon, avocado, strawberries, whole grain bread*

BEST FOODS FOR VITAMIN B$_{12}$: *Shellfish (clams, oysters, crab), wild salmon (fresh, canned), fortified whole grain cereal, enriched/fortified soy milk, trout (rainbow, wild), tuna (canned light), lean beef, veggie burgers, cottage cheese (fat-free, 1% reduced-fat), yogurt (fat-free, low-fat), milk (fat-free, 1% reduced-fat), eggs, cheese (fat-free, reduced-fat)*

BEST FOODS FOR FOLATE: *Fortified whole grain cereals, lentils, black-eyed peas, soybeans, oatmeal, turnip greens, spinach, mustard greens, green peas, artichokes, okra, beets, parsnips, broccoli, broccoli raab, sunflower seeds, wheat germ, oranges and juice, Brussels sprouts, papaya, seaweed, berries (boysenberries, blackberries, strawberries), beans (black, pinto, kidney, garbanzo, navy), cauliflower, Chinese cabbage, corn, whole grain bread, pasta (preferably whole wheat)*

BIOTIN

People ask me about biotin for hair health all the time. Usually, they've heard about it on a shampoo commercial or read a magazine article that recommended biotin supplements. Biotin is a B vitamin essential for hair growth and overall scalp health. Because our bodies make their own biotin in the intestines, and it is plentiful in many common foods, deficiency is very rare. In those few cases where people are very ill and don't have use of their intestines, biotin deficiency causes hair loss. So yes, biotin is important for hair health, but you don't need to take supplements. Just eat a balanced diet that includes some high-biotin foods.

> **BEST FOODS FOR BIOTIN:** *Liver, eggs, peanuts (and peanut butter), almonds, wheat bran, walnuts, Swiss chard, whole wheat bread, wild salmon (fresh, canned), cheese (fat-free, reduced-fat), cauliflower, avocado, raspberries*

IRON-RICH PROTEIN

Iron helps red blood cells carry oxygen. With iron deficiency, a condition known as *anemia,* cells can't get enough oxygen to function properly. The result can be devastating to the whole body, causing weakness and fatigue . . . and maybe even hair loss. One large-scale study found that premenopausal women who had severe hair loss were more likely to have low iron reserves (as measured by a test for a form of iron called *ferritin*) than women with sufficient reserves of iron. Women of childbearing age are more likely to experience iron deficiency because they lose a significant amount of iron from the blood shed during menstruation. Women with heavier periods will lose more iron than those with lighter flow.

For most people, foods can provide all the iron necessary for good health and strong hair. I recommend iron-rich *protein* for two reasons. First, protein is necessary for all cell growth, including hair cells. Hair gets its structure from hardened proteins called *keratin.* Without enough protein for keratin, hair grows more slowly, and the individual strands that do grow will be weaker. Second, the iron found in meat (called *heme iron*) is more easily absorbed by the body than the iron in plant foods (non-heme iron). Vitamin C improves the body's ability to absorb non-heme iron, so vegetarians should eat iron-rich vegetables and foods rich in vitamin C *at the same meal.* Before menopause, women may want to consider taking a multivitamin that contains iron. (See the section on supplements below for more information.)

> **BEST FOODS FOR IRON-RICH PROTEIN:** *Clams, oysters, lean beef, turkey (dark meat), duck, lamb, turkey (light meat), chicken (dark and light meat), pork, shrimp, egg yolks*

> **BEST IRON-RICH PROTEIN (vegetarian sources):** *Fortified whole grain cereals, tofu, soybeans, lentils, beans (kidney, garbanzo, lima, navy, black, pinto), black-eyed peas*

> **BEST IRON-RICH VEGETABLES (low in protein, but offer ample iron):** *Spinach, seaweed, Swiss chard, asparagus, Brussels sprouts, mustard greens, kale, broccoli*

VITAMIN C

Vitamin C is necessary for hair health for many reasons. Vitamin C helps the body use non-heme iron—the type found in vegetables—to assure that there is enough iron in red blood cells to carry oxygen to hair follicles. Vitamin C is also used to form collagen, a structural fiber that helps our bodies—quite literally—hold everything together. Hair follicles, blood vessels, and skin all require collagen to stay healthy for optimal growth. For example, one of the first signs of severe vitamin C deficiency is tiny bumps and red spots around the base of body hair on the arms, back, buttocks, and legs, caused when tiny blood vessels leak around the follicles. Hair growth is also affected. On the body, the small hairs on arms and legs can become misshapen, curling in on themselves. On the head, even minor vitamin C deficiencies can lead to dry, splitting hair that breaks easily.

BEST FOODS FOR VITAMIN C: *Guava, bell peppers (yellow, red, green), orange juice, hot chile peppers, oranges, grapefruit juice, strawberries, pineapple, kohlrabi, papaya, lemons, broccoli, kale, Brussels sprouts, kidney beans, kiwi, cantaloupe, cauliflower, red cabbage, mangos, grapefruit (pink, red), white potatoes (with skin), mustard greens, cherry tomatoes, sugar snap peas, snow peas, clementines, rutabagas, turnip greens, tomatoes, raspberries, Chinese cabbage, blackberries, green tomatoes, cabbage, watermelon, tangerines, lemon juice, okra, lychees, summer squash (all varieties), persimmons*

FAQS

My husband was bald when I met him in our 20s. He tried Rogaine, but it didn't work for him. He's doing this weird comb-over thing with his remaining hair, and it looks hideous. Are you sure there's nothing that can help him?

Nutritional cures can't fix male pattern baldness. I always recommend that men who are uncomfortable with their baldness talk with their doctors. Rogaine is not the only medication available anymore. But I must say that there has never been a better time to be bald! Instead of a comb-over, many men opt to shave their heads entirely for a sleek, modern look. And I wish more men would understand that many women think that confident bald men are sexy. I love my husband's bald head. The measure of a man is not his hair, but his loving nature and the strength of his character.

BETA CAROTENE

Beta carotene in foods is converted to vitamin A in the body, and vitamin A is necessary for all cell growth, including hair. A deficiency can lead to dry, dull, lifeless hair, and dry skin, which can flake off into dandruff. Note that you can have too much of a good thing when it comes to vitamin A—too much can cause hair loss. My advice is to add more beta carotene–rich foods to your meals rather than take vitamin A supplements. If you should choose to take a multivitamin, check the label to make sure that your brand supplies no more than 50% DV of vitamin A in the form of retinol. Retinol is listed on supplement labels as palmitate or acetate, and should never exceed 2,000 IU. The other 50% or more should come in the form of beta carotene, which is converted to vitamin A as we need it.

BEST FOODS FOR BETA CAROTENE: *Sweet potatoes, carrots, kale, butternut squash, turnip greens, pumpkin, mustard greens, cantaloupe, red peppers, apricots, Chinese cabbage, spinach, lettuce (romaine, green leaf, red leaf, butterhead), collard greens, Swiss chard, watercress, grapefruit, watermelon, cherries, mangos, red ripe tomatoes, guava, asparagus, red cabbage*

NAILS

Like hair, nails are made mainly of the hardened protein keratin, which means that the foods that create beautiful hair also help nails stay strong. For example, protein is necessary for nail growth and strength, zinc keeps nails from weakening, and iron keeps nails from distorting into spoon shapes. Just as high doses of selenium can cause hair loss, too much selenium can also lead to nail loss (yikes!).

Although many people believe that calcium supplements help build strong nails, research doesn't support the notion. Researchers from New Zealand tested the effects of calcium on nail health. Nearly 700 postmenopausal women took 1,000 milligrams of calcium every day for a year, and demonstrated that taking calcium supplements made no difference in reported nail strength. So although I heartily recommend calcium for so many different health issues, nail health isn't among them.

ZINC

The mineral zinc is involved in tissue growth and repair, including hair growth. It also helps keep the oil glands around the hair follicles working properly. Low levels of zinc can cause hair loss, slow growth, and dandruff. The amount you get from eating foods rich in zinc is plenty to keep your tresses gorgeous. Aside from a multivitamin which provides up to 100% DV, I don't recommend taking extra zinc supplements because excess zinc can inhibit the body's ability to absorb copper, a minor but necessary mineral.

BEST FOODS FOR ZINC: *Oysters, lean beef, crab, ostrich, pork tenderloin, peanut butter, wheat germ, turkey, veal, pumpkin seeds, chicken, chickpeas (garbanzo beans), fat-free yogurt, fortified whole grain cereals, pine nuts, cashews, sunflower seeds, lima beans, lentils, pecans, cheese (fat-free, reduced-fat), fat-free milk, almonds, walnuts, peanuts, black-eyed peas, green peas*

BONUS POINTS

- **Drink enough water.** Water helps the body transport vitamins, minerals, and other nutrients throughout the body, including to the scalp and hair follicles. Plus, dehydrated cells don't work as well as they should, which means that the cells in follicles can't build healthy hair. I recommend staying well hydrated throughout each day—no need to count glasses or ounces, just drink whenever you feel thirsty.
- **See a doctor about unusual hair loss,** such as seeing more than the typical number of hairs collecting on your shower floor, or if you notice more scalp than you're used to seeing, or any other worrisome signs. Maybe it's nothing . . . but maybe it's an early indicator of a treatable disorder. Better to be safe than sorry.
- **Don't abuse your hair.** Pulling hair tight in braids or ponytails, over-treating hair with perms or bleach, or manually tugging or twisting on hair can cause loss or breakage. Unfortunately, nutrition can't help repair that kind of trauma. Be kind to your hair.

SUPPLEMENTS

I don't recommend taking any individual supplements for gorgeous hair. Food is still your best bet. If you feel the need to take a supplement, the only one I would recommend is a multivitamin that contains 100% DV for zinc, copper, vitamin C, the B vitamins (specifically B_6, B_{12}, and folic acid), and vitamin A (optimally 50 to 100% should come from beta carotene and/or mixed carotenoids, and certainly no more than 2,000 IU from retinol, typically listed as palmitate or acetate). If you are a woman of childbearing age, look for a multivitamin that contains up to 100% DV iron. All men and non-menstruating women should look for a multi that contains no iron. Unless you've been diagnosed with anemia, you won't need it or want it because too much iron can be toxic. Hint: Look for vitamins labeled "For Men" or "Senior Formula"—those are typically iron-free.

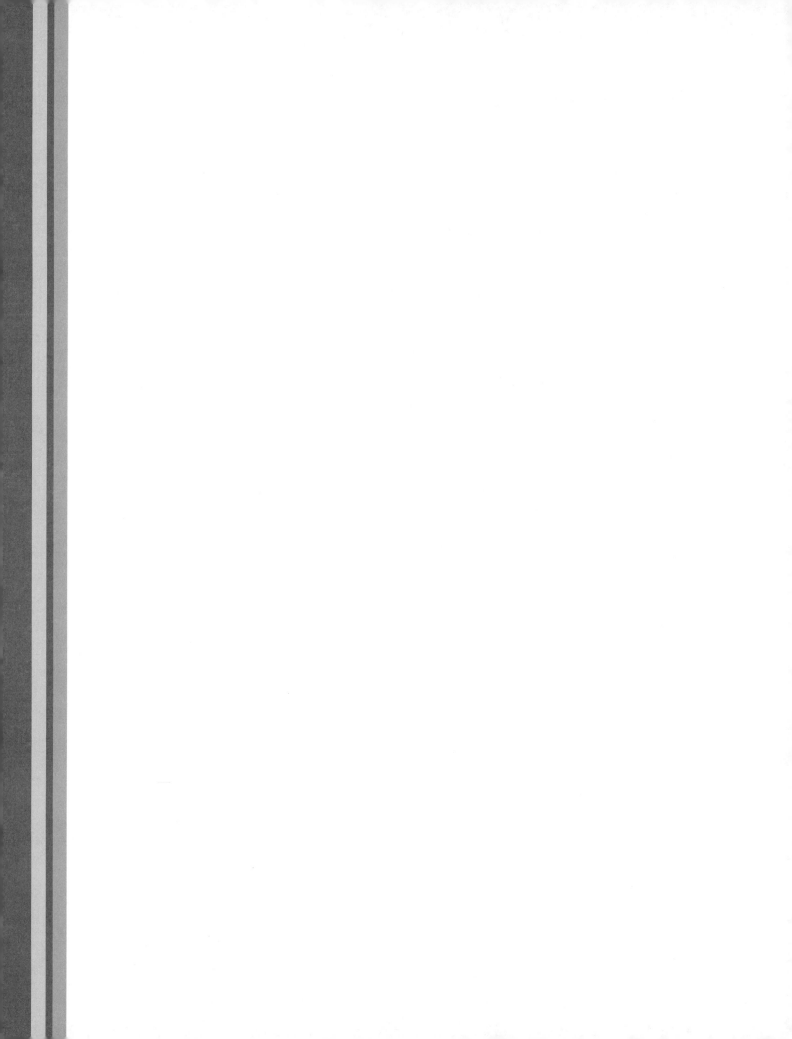

JOY'S 4-STEP PROGRAM
FOR HEALTHY HAIR

Follow this program if you have experienced unusual hair loss, or if you want healthier, more beautiful hair.

STEP 1 ... START WITH THE BASICS

These are the first things you should do to assure healthy hair:

- See your doctor if you've been losing more hair than usual to rule out a medical cause.

- Stay well hydrated—drink water whenever you feel thirsty. On the average, men require 13 8-ounce cups of fluid per day, and women require 9 8-ounce cups per day.

STEP 2 ... YOUR ULTIMATE GROCERY LIST

This list contains foods with high levels of nutrients that help make hair strong and lustrous, plus some foods used as ingredients in the meal plans and recipes. You don't have to purchase every item . . . but these foods should make up the bulk of what you eat for the week.

FRUIT

Apricots	Cantaloupe	Lemons (and juice)	Persimmons
Bananas	Cherries	Limes (and juice)	Pineapple
Berries (boysenberries,	Clementines	Lychees	Tangerines
blackberries,	Grapefruit (and juice)	Mangos	Watermelon
raspberries,	Guava	Oranges (and juice)	
strawberries)	Kiwi	Papaya	

VEGETABLES

Artichokes	Chickpeas (garbanzo	Parsnips	Squash, summer
Asparagus	beans)	Peas (green,	Squash, winter
Avocado	Collard greens	sugar snap)	(especially acorn
Beans (black, pinto,	Corn	Peas, black-eyed	and butternut)
kidney, lima,	Green beans	Peppers (hot; yellow/	Swiss chard
garbanzo, navy)	Kale	red/green)	Tomatoes (including
Beets	Kohlrabi	Potatoes, sweet	green tomatoes,
Broccoli	Lentils	Potatoes, white	red ripe tomatoes,
Broccoli raab	Lettuce (romaine,	Pumpkin	cherry tomatoes,
Brussels sprouts	green leaf, red leaf,	Rutabagas	tomato paste)
Cabbage (including red,	butterhead)	Scallions	Turnip greens
Chinese)	Mustard greens	Seaweed	Watercress
Carrots	Okra	Snow peas	
Cauliflower	Onions (including red,	Soybeans (edamame)	
Celery	Vidalia)	Spinach	

SEAFOOD

Salmon, wild (fresh,	Shellfish (shrimp,	Trout(rainbow, wild)
canned)	clams, oysters, crab)	Tuna (canned light)

LEAN MEATS/EGGS/SOY FOODS

Beef, lean	Ham, lean	Pork (including	Turkey burgers
Chicken	Lamb	tenderloin)	Veal
Duck	Liver	Tofu, extra firm	Veggie burgers
Eggs	Ostrich	Turkey	

NUTS AND SEEDS (PREFERABLY UNSALTED)

Almonds	Peanuts	Pistachio nuts	Walnuts
Cashews	Pecans	Pumpkin seeds	
Peanut butter	Pine nuts	Sunflower seeds	

WHOLE GRAINS

Barley	Cereal, fortified whole	Oatmeal	Rice (brown, wild)
Bread, whole grain	grain	Pasta, preferably whole	Wheat bran
Bread crumbs,	English muffin, whole	wheat	Wheat germ
whole wheat	wheat	Pita, whole wheat	

DAIRY

Cheese (fat-free,	cheese (preferably	Milk (fat-free,	
reduced-fat)	reduced-fat)	1% reduced-fat)	
Cheese (for meal	Cottage cheese	Soy milk, enriched/	
plan): reduced-fat,	(fat-free, 1% reduced-	fortified	
Cheddar; goat	fat)	Yogurt (fat-free, low-fat)	

MISCELLANEOUS

Broth, beef and chicken	Ginger, fresh	Oil, canola	Satay dipping sauce
(fat-free, reduced-	Guacamole	Oil, olive	Soup, lentil or black
sodium)	Ketchup	Oil, sesame	bean
California roll,	Margarine spread, soft	Orange juice concentrate	Soy sauce,
six-piece	tub, reduced fat,	Parsley, flat-leaf	reduced-sodium
Chili powder, sweet	trans fat–free	Pepper, black	String cheese, reduced-
Cinnamon, ground	Mayonnaise, reduced-	Pepper, cayenne	fat
Cornstarch	fat	Salad dressing, reduced-	Vinegar, balsamic or
Cumin	Mustard	calorie	red wine
Garlic	Nonstick cooking spray	Salt, sea	

STEP 3 ...GOING ABOVE AND BEYOND

If you want to do everything you can for hair health, here are some additional things you might try:

- If you like, feel free to take a multivitamin. Men and nonmenstruating women should choose a vitamin without iron.

- Be gentle with your hair—limit the pulling, processing, coloring, and even brushing.

IS A CUT IN YOUR FUTURE?

The next time you go to a hair stylist, ask for an honest assessment of the state of your tresses. If your hair is dry, split, or poorly nourished, it will never recover. And if your hair is fine, too much length can put stress on fragile strands, causing breakage and a flat, lifeless appearance. In both cases, you may need to cut several inches off to make your hair look as healthy and vibrant as possible. Don't think of it as losing length—instead, consider it a beauty investment. Cut your losses (so to speak), and be patient while your new, glossy, healthy hair grows in.

STEP4 ...MEAL PLANS

These sample menus include foods that are full of nutrients that contribute to healthy, strong, shiny hair, including high-quality protein, iron, zinc, beta carotene, B vitamins and vitamin C.

Every day, choose *one* option for each of the three meals—breakfast, lunch, and dinner. Then, one or two times per day, choose from a variety of my suggested snacks. Approximate calories have been provided to help adjust for your personal weight management goals. If you find yourself hungry (and if weight is not an issue), feel free to increase the portion sizes for meals and snacks. Beverage calories are *not* included.

BREAKFAST OPTIONS

(Approximately 300 to 400 calories)

Cantaloupe with Vanilla Yogurt and Sunflower Seeds

½ cantaloupe filled with 6 to 8 ounces fat-free vanilla yogurt and topped with 2 tablespoons sunflower seeds (or slivered almonds or chopped walnuts) and 1 tablespoon wheat germ.

Broccoli-Cheddar Omelet with Toast

Sauté 1 cup chopped broccoli in nonstick cooking spray (or 1 teaspoon canola or olive oil) until soft. Beat 1 whole egg and 2 egg whites and add to broccoli; cook until edges brown. Add 1 ounce reduced-fat Cheddar and fold omelet in half. Continue cooking until the underside is golden brown. Serve with 1 slice whole wheat bread, toasted (with optional 1 teaspoon soft tub, trans fat–free margarine spread).

Banana-Walnut Oatmeal

½ cup dry instant oatmeal prepared with 1 cup water (and/or optional fat-free milk), topped with 2 tablespoons chopped walnuts and ½ sliced medium banana.

Tropical Cottage Cheese with Almonds

Mix 1 cup fat-free or 1% reduced-fat cottage cheese with ½ cup each chopped papaya, pineapple, and mango. Top with 1 tablespoon chopped almonds (or walnuts, pecans, or sunflower seeds).

Whole Grain Cereal with Milk and Fruit

1 cup whole grain cereal (120 calories or less) with 1 cup fat-free milk and 1 tablespoon wheat germ. Enjoy with 1 whole grapefruit (or 1 cup blackberries, raspberries, or sliced strawberries).

LUNCH OPTIONS

(Approximately 400 to 500 calories)

Turkey Sandwich with Avocado and Baby Carrots

4 ounces turkey breast (or ham), romaine lettuce leaves, tomato, and 2 thin slices avocado on 2 slices whole grain bread (or in 1 whole wheat pita or wrap) with optional 1 tablespoon reduced-fat mayo or mustard. Enjoy with 1 cup baby carrots and/or bell pepper sticks.

Japanese Spread: Edamame with California Roll

1 cup boiled edamame (soybeans in the pod) with 1 six-piece California roll and unlimited steamed vegetables sprinkled with reduced-sodium soy sauce.

Turkey Burger with Salad

1 cooked 5-ounce turkey burger or veggie burger (if store-bought, any brand, 250 calories or less) topped with tomato, onion, and 2 tablespoons ketchup in a whole grain bun (or toasted whole grain English muffin or pita). Enjoy with a green salad (spinach, dark lettuce, turnip greens, mustard greens) tossed with 1 teaspoon olive oil and 2 tablespoons balsamic vinegar or fresh lemon juice (or 2 tablespoons reduced-calorie dressing).

Spinach Salad with Beets, Goat Cheese, and Walnuts

Large bed of spinach leaves topped with ½ cup sliced beets, ½ cup sugar snap peas, 2 ounces goat cheese (preferably reduced-fat), and 2 tablespoons chopped walnuts; toss with 2 teaspoons olive oil and unlimited vinegar or fresh lemon juice (or 2 to 4 tablespoons reduced-calorie dressing).

Lentil Soup with Tomato Cheese Melt

2 cups lentil or black bean soup (if store-bought, any brand, 300 calories or less). Serve with 1 toasted slice whole grain bread topped with sliced tomato and 1 ounce reduced-fat cheese, heated in a 350°F oven until cheese melts.

DINNER OPTIONS

(Approximately 500 to 600 calories)

Turkey Chili with Black Beans

1 serving (2 cups) Turkey Chili (page 367) or prepared turkey or vegetarian chili (if store-bought, any brand, less than 400 calories) topped with 1 ounce shredded fat-free Cheddar. Serve with tossed salad (leafy greens and other preferred vegetables) tossed with 1 teaspoon olive oil and unlimited balsamic vinegar or fresh lemon juice (or 2 to 3 tablespoons reduced-calorie dressing).

Chicken with Satay Sauce and Brown Rice

5 ounces chicken breast, grilled with 2 teaspoons canola or sesame oil and served with Satay dipping sauce (1 level tablespoon creamy peanut butter mixed with 1 tablespoon reduced-sodium soy sauce and 1 teaspoon minced garlic). Enjoy with 1 cup steamed Chinese cabbage (or green beans, Swiss chard, broccoli, spinach, asparagus, Brussels sprouts, or cauliflower) and ½ cup cooked brown rice.

Spiced Pork Tenderloin with Black-Eyed Peas, Caramelized Onions, and Cauliflower

Spiced Pork Tenderloin with Black-Eyed Peas, Caramelized Onions, and Cauliflower (page 102).

Sautéed Tofu with Peanuts, Peppers, Sugar Snap Peas, and Scallions

6 ounces cubed extra-firm tofu, ½ cup sliced bell peppers, ½ cup sugar snap peas, and 2 chopped scallions (plus 1 tablespoon peanuts) sautéed in 2 teaspoons canola or sesame oil and 1 tablespoon reduced-sodium soy sauce. Enjoy with ½ cup cooked whole wheat pasta (or ½ baked sweet or white potato) and 1 cup steamed broccoli (or Swiss chard or asparagus).

Orange Pepper Beef Stir-Fry with Fresh Fruit

1 serving Orange Pepper Beef Stir-Fry (page 101) with 1 cup fresh berries (or ½ mango, ½ grapefruit, or ¼ cantaloupe).

SNACK OPTIONS

100 calories or less

- *Best vegetables:* 1 cup raw or cooked bell peppers (red, green, yellow), broccoli, broccoli raab, kale, Brussels sprouts, cabbage, sugar snap peas, tomatoes, okra, zucchini squash, carrots, lettuce and leafy greens, spinach, collards, Swiss chard, watercress, asparagus, kohlrabi, okra, artichokes, beets, cauliflower, or seaweed
- *Best fruits:* 1 orange, tangerine, kiwi, or guava; 2 clementines; ½ papaya, mango, grapefruit, or cantaloupe; 1 cup boysenberries, blackberries, raspberries, cherries, sliced strawberries, watermelon, or pineapple; ½ cup lychees; 4 apricots; 20 strawberries
- 1 hard-boiled egg (or 3 egg whites)
- ½ cup fat-free or 1% reduced-fat cottage cheese with celery sticks
- 1 reduced-fat string cheese

100 to 200 Calories

- 1 cup boiled edamame (soybeans in the pod)
- 1 slice whole grain bread, toasted and topped with 1 level tablespoon peanut butter

- ¼ cup guacamole with pepper sticks

- 1 banana with 2 level teaspoons peanut butter

- 1 ounce (about ¼ cup) almonds, walnuts, pecans, peanuts

- ¼ cup sunflower seeds or pistachio nuts in the shell

- ½ baked sweet potato

- 1 cup fat-free, flavored yogurt topped with ½ cup berries

- ½ cup fat-free or 1% reduced-fat cottage cheese mixed with ½ cup berries (blackberries, sliced strawberries, or raspberries) and topped with optional 1 tablespoon wheat germ

ORANGE PEPPER BEEF STIR-FRY

What could be fresher and brighter than orange juice, lime juice, and a rainbow of peppers? Add broccoli, beef, and a few Asian tastes, and you've got a quick and easy dinner that everyone enjoys.

Makes 2 servings

½	pound stew beef or top round
½	cup fat-free, reduced-sodium beef broth
¼	cup reduced-sodium soy sauce
¼	cup orange juice concentrate
2	tablespoons lime juice
1	tablespoon sesame oil
1	tablespoon minced garlic
1	tablespoon minced fresh ginger
1	tablespoon cornstarch
1	tablespoon canola oil
1	small red pepper, thinly sliced
1	small green bell pepper, thinly sliced
1	small yellow bell pepper, thinly sliced
1	small Vidalia or red onion
1	cup broccoli florets
	Salt
3	scallions, thinly sliced

1. Place the beef in the freezer for 15 to 20 minutes, until firm but not totally frozen, for easy slicing. Cut into paper-thin slices against the grain.

2. In a large bowl, whisk the broth, soy sauce, orange juice concentrate, lime juice, sesame oil, garlic, and ginger. Stir in the cornstarch until no lumps remain. Set aside.

3. Spray a wok or large skillet with cooking spray. Add the oil and warm over medium heat. Add the peppers, onion, and broccoli and cook, stirring, 4 to 5 minutes, until the vegetables begin to soften but are still crisp. Increase the heat to high and add the beef. Cook, stirring, 3 to 4 minutes, until the beef begins to take on color.

4. Reduce the heat to low and add the broth mixture. Cook 2 to 3 minutes longer, until the sauce thickens and the beef is no longer pink inside. Season with salt if needed and garnish with scallions. Serve immediately.

PER SERVING
485 calories, 43 g protein, 32 g carbohydrate, 21 g fat (4 g saturated), 74 mg cholesterol, 1,284 mg sodium, 5 g fiber; plus 5 mg iron (30% DV), 392 mg vitamin C (653% DV), 3,628 IU vitamin A (73% DV), 7 mg zinc (45% DV), 117 mcg folic acid (30% DV), 1 mg vitamin B_6 (58% DV), 2 mcg vitamin B_{12} (34% DV)

SPICED PORK TENDERLOIN WITH BLACK-EYED PEAS, CARAMELIZED ONIONS, AND CAULIFLOWER

Don't let the long list of ingredients put you off—the prep is simple, the taste is sublime. And how many do recipes you know that deliver almost the entire alphabet of vitamins and minerals, from vitamin A to zinc?

Makes 4 servings

¼	teaspoon sweet chili powder
¼	teaspoon ground cinnamon
¼	teaspoon cumin
¼	teaspoon sea salt, plus more to taste
¼	teaspoon ground black pepper, plus more to taste
⅛	teaspoon cayenne pepper
1	pork tenderloin (about 3½ pounds), cut into four 1"-thick steaks
	Nonstick cooking spray
2	tablespoons olive oil
1	large red onion, thinly sliced
¼	to ½ cup fat-free, reduced-sodium chicken broth
1	can (16 ounces) black-eyed peas, drained and rinsed
1	small head cauliflower, cut into florets
1	tablespoon whole wheat bread crumbs
2	tablespoons minced fresh flat-leaf parsley
	Zest of 1 lemon
1	tablespoon lemon juice

1. In a small bowl, combine the sweet chili powder, cinnamon, cumin, salt, black pepper, and cayenne pepper. Spray the pork with cooking spray. Rub the spice mixture over the surface of the meat. Wrap in plastic wrap and refrigerate for at least 3 hours, or overnight.

2. Coat a large skillet with cooking spray. Add 1 tablespoon olive oil and heat over high heat. Add the onion and cook, stirring, until it begins to brown, 3 to 4 minutes. Add ¼ cup broth and reduce the heat to medium. Cook, stirring occasionally and adding more broth as needed to keep the onion from burning, 15 to 20 minutes, until the onion is a deep caramel color. Stir in the black-eyed peas and set aside.

3. In a steamer or saucepan with a lid, steam the cauliflower over 1 inch of water until tender, 4 to 5 minutes. In a bowl, mix the bread crumbs, parsley, lemon zest, and juice. Season with salt and pepper. Sprinkle over the cauliflower.

4. Coat a large skillet with cooking spray. Heat the remaining 1 tablespoon olive oil over high heat. Add the tenderloin steaks and reduce the heat to medium-high. Cook, turning once, until the steaks are browned and the centers are no longer translucent pink, 7 to 8 minutes. Serve immediately with the onion mixture and cauliflower.

PER SERVING
555 calories, 66 g protein, 32 g carbohydrate, 17 g fat 4(g saturated), 184 mg cholesterol, 363 mg sodium, 0 g fiber; plus 14 mg iron (77% DV), 54 mg vitamin C (89% DV), 1,052 IU vitamin A (>20% DV), 7 mg zinc (49% DV), 57 mcg folic acid (14% DV), 6 mg vitamin B_6 (295% DV), 9 mcg vitamin B_{12} (153% DV)

CHAPTER 6

FEEDING A BEAUTIFUL SMILE

S mile.

Go ahead, try it. Smile . . . right now, wherever you are.

Psychologists have discovered that when people smile, they can activate brain centers that signal happiness, even if they didn't feel particularly happy to begin with. Imagine all the feel-good moments you'll miss out on if you're too self-conscious about your teeth to smile.

Many of us are more concerned with how our smiles look than how healthy our teeth are. Don't believe me? Take a look at these numbers: About 80 percent of adults have some form of periodontal disease, which often goes untreated. Most people don't even floss every day let alone visit the dentist regularly. On the other hand, tooth whitening is a huge and growing business, a market estimated to be about $1 billion in the United States alone.

But there's more to dental health than white teeth. It takes understanding some unpleasant truths about the dynamics of food, plaque, decay, tartar, and gum disease. None of it is pretty. Except your teeth, which will be beautiful with just a few changes to your diet and dental routine.

WHAT AFFECTS TOOTH HEALTH?

A tooth has a structure similar to a Tootsie Pop. As just about anyone knows, a Tootsie Pop has a hard lollipop outer shell, a soft Tootsie Roll center, and a supporting stick that extends out from the middle of the pop. A tooth has a hard enamel outer shell, a softer dentin center, and a root canal that extends from the middle of the tooth into the jaw. This root canal contains nerves and blood vessels that feed the tooth and keep it alive.

Enamel surrounds the exposed part of the tooth, stopping just inside the gum line. Made primarily of calcium, it is the hardest substance in the body—harder, even, than bone. But unlike bone, enamel cannot regenerate. If the outer shell is breached, the inner part of the tooth becomes vulnerable, and can erode down to the root. That's why any cracks or areas of decay need to be filled by a dentist.

Just under the enamel is the dentin, which contains millions of fluid-filled tubules, tiny canals that lead to the nerve—the extremely sensitive nerve. When the protective enamel wears away then you've got trouble. Cavities, cracks, gum recession, tooth-grinding, brushing too hard, or even eating too many acidic foods can all provide access to the tubules and consequently a tooth's nerve center. Hot foods, cold drinks, sugary foods, or even sudden puffs of air can ride the tubules into the core of your tooth. Anyone with tooth sensitivity knows this is no minor problem . . . it is both uncomfortable and embarrassing—there's nothing sexy about that pained grimace after a sip of ice water.

So the first key to good tooth health is keeping your enamel shell strong. That can be a challenge all by itself. Consider this: Every minute of every day, our teeth are collecting a film of plaque—a combination of naturally occurring mouth bacteria, food sugars, and other substances. Food sugars come not just from the obvious sources—the sugar in candy, soft drinks, and other sweets—but also from the natural sugars created during the breakdown of fruits, whole grain foods, and other carbohydrates. All these sugars feed the bacteria, which, in turn, produce acid that leeches calcium salts from enamel thereby weakening it. The process is called *demineralization*. As long as the bacteria and sugars remain in your mouth, the acid level will remain high—which is why sticky foods like raisins, jam, or gummy bears can wreak havoc on enamel long after you finish eating. Once you stop eating a meal and clear food remnants out of your mouth (by, say, brushing), acid levels remain high for about 30 minutes or so before your saliva slowly returns everything back to normal. If you sip sugary drinks or snack continuously, your teeth may remain bathed in acid all day long . . . and if you have dry mouth from low saliva flow, the acid remains higher longer.

Plaque remains on the teeth unless you brush or floss it away. After about 24 hours, the soft plaque begins to harden into *tartar,* which cannot be removed by simple brushing. If tartar forms at or under the gum line, it can cause the gums (also called *gingiva*) to become inflamed, causing redness, puffiness, and bad breath. This inflammation (or *gingivitis*) might not sound like a big deal—until you take the long view.

Gingivitis is just the first stage of gum disease. Teeth are embedded in the jaw, held in place by connective tissue and surrounded by your gums. If tartar is not removed, toxins destroy the connective tissue, and bacteria can invade the bone around the teeth, creating infection and causing bone loss (a condition known as periodontal disease). If periodontal disease is left untreated, the tooth becomes unanchored, loosens, and eventually falls out.

For healthy teeth, then, start with some basic dental hygiene:

- Limit the number of sugary foods (and low-quality carbohydrates) you eat during the day. Dried fruits, crackers, pretzels, cookies, and other foods that get stuck on or between teeth can be particularly devastating to enamel over time. Lollipops and hard candies are also detrimental since they bathe your back teeth in sugars for prolonged periods of time.
- Limit the number of "eating episodes" during the day. If you eat once every 30 minutes, your mouth will always contain acid, and your enamel will be under constant attack. Of course, eating every few hours is normal and perfectly fine.
- Avoid sugary drinks altogether . . . but when it comes to your teeth, the key is to specifically avoid sodas, fruit juices, sweetened coffee or tea, and sweetened sports drinks *between meals*. In fact, many dentists recommend avoiding all carbonated beverages, even sugar-free varieties, because they often contain other ingredients that can be acidic. If you must drink them, use a straw to bypass your teeth.
- Brush your teeth as soon as possible after every meal. If you cannot brush, at least rinse your mouth with water to remove some food debris. Chewing sugarless gum can also help.
- Floss at least once a day to remove food particles and plaque from above the gum line.
- Visit the dentist regularly for a professional cleaning—at least once a year, or more frequently if your dentist recommends it. Many dentists recommend twice yearly visits to keep on top of tartar, but some people who are more susceptible to tooth decay and/or tartar build-up may need to go even more often.

FAQS

I'm bleaching my teeth to make them whiter. Is there anything I should eat or not eat to get the best results?

During the active phase of bleaching—especially after in-office bleaching—the enamel is much more susceptible to stains and demineralization. Be especially careful to avoid eating sugary foods, dried fruits, or other sticky carbohydrates that can also cause demineralization. In addition, avoid foods that can easily stain your teeth, such coffee, tea, red wine, tomato sauce, and grape juice—basically, if it can stain your clothes, it might stain your newly whitened teeth. Dentists recommend staying away from staining foods for three days after each bleaching procedure. And because all whitening products are *not* created equal, always ask your dentist about the safest way to whiten your teeth.

HOW FOOD AFFECTS TOOTH HEALTH

Although it seems like tooth health is all about what not to eat, there are some foods that contribute to good tooth health.

CALCIUM AND VITAMIN D

Most people understand that calcium and vitamin D are important for strong bones, but many of us fail to make the connection between our bones and our teeth. Teeth are embedded in the jaw bone, so if bone density falls, your teeth won't have a firm footing. If periodontal disease sets in and begins to erode bone, strong bones will be your first defense against tooth loss. Plus, a calcium-poor diet seems to increase the overall risk of developing periodontal disease. Research has shown that women who get less than 500 milligrams of calcium per day from their diet have a 54 percent greater risk of periodontal disease compared with those who get more than 800 milligrams of calcium per day. But calcium cannot be absorbed and used by bone without vitamin D, so both are important. I highly recommend eating foods rich in calcium and vitamin D. In addition, women of all ages (especially those who don't get enough through diet) should consider taking a supplement that contains calcium plus D$_3$ (cholecalciferol, the most potent form of vitamin D). See the Supplements section (page 111) for more information.

BEST FOODS FOR CALCIUM: *Yogurt (fat-free, low-fat), milk (fat-free, 1% reduced-fat), enriched/fortified soy milk, calcium-fortified fruit juice, cheese (fat-free, reduced-fat), tofu with calcium, sardines (with bones), wild salmon (fresh, canned with bones), soybeans, frozen yogurt (fat-free, low-fat), low-fat ice cream, calcium-fortified whole grain waffles, bok choy, kale, white beans, broccoli, almonds*

BEST FOODS FOR VITAMIN D: *Wild salmon (with bones), mackerel (not king), sardines (with bones), herring, fortified milk (fat-free, 1% reduced-fat), enriched/fortified soy milk, egg yolks, mushrooms (especially shiitakes), vitamin-D–fortified margarine (soft tub, trans fat–free), fortified whole grain cereals*

VITAMIN C

Vitamin C is critical for keeping gums healthy because it strengthens blood vessels and connective tissue—including the connective tissue that holds your teeth in your jaw. The

INFLAMMATION AND DISEASE

Many dentists are finding themselves in a position to save lives, thanks to research that has linked periodontal disease with an increased risk of heart disease. What do the two have in common? In a word, inflammation.

You know that if a skunk sprays its scent in your neighbor's yard, the stink will soon be in your yard, too. The same type of thing happens with inflammation. When there is an infection or disease in the gums, the body responds with an immune response that increases levels of inflammatory chemicals designed to fight the problem. But these chemicals don't stay just in the mouth, they circulate throughout the body. One of the side effects of inflammatory chemicals is that they can do collateral damage—and the delicate lining of blood vessels is often in the line of fire. Over time, this can lead to atherosclerosis, blood clots, and heart disease.

Although no one knows exactly which comes first, the mouth inflammation or the heart disease, the link is clear. A 2006 study of middle-aged men in Northern Ireland showed that those with periodontal disease had a risk of heart disease *three times higher* than that of men with healthy gums. If your dentist tells you that your gums are in trouble, see your primary care physician for a full work-up, including a test for a chemical called *C-reactive protein* (CRP), which is a marker of inflammation levels in the body. It just might save your life.

antioxidant properties of vitamin C also help reduce inflammation, so this vitamin may help prevent or slow the progression of gingivitis. In a study published in 2000, researchers found that people who did not get enough vitamin C in their diets had about 20 percent increased risk of developing periodontal disease than people who ate plenty of vitamin C–rich foods.

BEST FOODS FOR VITAMIN C: *Guava, bell peppers (yellow, red, green), calcium-fortified orange juice, hot chile peppers, oranges, calcium-fortified grapefruit juice, strawberries, pineapple, kohlrabi, papaya, lemons, broccoli, kale, Brussels sprouts, kidney beans, kiwi, cantaloupe, cauliflower, red cabbage, mangos, grapefruit (pink, red), white potatoes (with skin), mustard greens, cherry tomatoes, sugar snap peas, snow peas, clementines, rutabagas, turnip greens, tomatoes, raspberries, Chinese cabbage, blackberries, green tomatoes, cabbage, watermelon, tangerines, lemon juice, okra, lychees, summer squash, persimmons*

WATER AND TEA

Water not only helps wash away food debris that can get trapped in teeth, it also helps keep saliva levels high. This is important because saliva is the body's best defense against tooth decay. The proteins and minerals in saliva counteract enamel-eating acids, keeping your teeth strong. That's why people with dry mouth, no matter what the cause, need to see the dentist more frequently than others. If you have dry mouth, hard candies can be disastrous! Chew sugarless gum instead. Saliva is more than 95 percent water, so if you become dehydrated, saliva flow will be reduced. The best way to stay hydrated is to drink plenty of water throughout the day.

Another good drink option is unsweetened green tea. Tea is thought to help prevent tooth decay due to its ability to kill certain types of mouth bacteria, and possibly through its fluoride content. Black tea is good, too, but it can stain the teeth.

BONUS POINTS

■ **Talk with your dentist about the importance of fluoride.** Fluoride is one of the most effective measures available for preventing tooth decay. Its effects are so powerful that many public water supplies provide safe levels of fluoridation. Studies have consistently found that children who receive fluoride from their water or dental treatments have less than half the number of dental caries (more commonly known as cavities) as children who don't get fluoride. This mineral occurs naturally in some foods, such as tea and seafood, and in foods cooked in fluoridated water. With the popularity of bottled water and water filtration systems, many people are not getting as much fluoride as they might think. (To find out whether your drinking water contains fluoride, call your county water department, and the public information phone number published on the bottle of your favorite brand of bottled water or on your filter packaging.) Dentists recommend that everyone brush with a fluoride toothpaste, and suggest that many people can benefit from using a fluoride rinse. Don't take fluoride supplements without a doctor's recommendation, and don't swallow toothpaste—too much fluoride can be toxic and cause tooth discoloration.

- **If you have heartburn from reflux disease, or if you are bulimic, talk with your dentist.** Stomach acids that make their way into the mouth, either from reflux or vomiting, can eat away tooth enamel. While you are working on solving your medical problem, make sure your dentist knows about it so you can work together to keep your teeth as healthy as possible.

- **Stop using tobacco products.** People who smoke or use other tobacco products are more likely to have tartar, periodontal disease, and tooth loss compared with people who don't use tobacco. One Swedish study of smokers and nonsmokers found that smokers were more than twice as likely to have periodontal disease—and more severe disease—than nonsmokers. It also stains your teeth, which is never attractive.

- **Go for crunchy.** Raw vegetables and crunchy fruits (like apples) are not only jam-packed with vitamins and minerals, they help clean your teeth of plaque and bacteria. Think of them as nature's tasty toothbrushes!

- **Chew sugarless gum if you can't brush after a meal or snack.** Chewing sugarless gum protects teeth because it stimulates saliva to wash away food particles, acts as a natural tooth brush, and buffers acids to protect enamel. In addition, the artificial sweetener xylitol can inhibit tooth decay by actually remineralizing teeth. Many dentists recommend that their patient chew a piece of xylitol-containing gum after every meal. Read labels, but brands that contain xylitol include most flavors of Trident (except Trident White), Orbit sugar-free gum, Arm & Hammer Dental Care Sugar Free Baking Soda. (Because formulations can change, always check the ingredient list for xylitol before buying sugarless gum.)

- **Drink soft drinks wisely.** I do not recommend drinking sodas or sugared soft drinks at all (big surprise!). However, I recognize that some of you may have an ingrained soda habit. While you are weaning yourself off them, here are some tips for safer (but not safe) teeth:

    Use a straw. Sipping through a straw will keep the soda further in the back of the mouth, instead of hitting every tooth.

    Choose root beer. People tend to think that cola drinks are the worst for teeth. Not true. Non-cola sodas and canned ice tea contain tartaric acid, malic acid, and other additives that erode teeth. Of all the drinks out there, root beer has the fewest additives, and therefore harms teeth the least.

    Drink with meals. If you drink sodas between meals, that sugar and acid combination prolongs the amount of time your enamel can be demineralized.

SUPPLEMENTS

If you want to do everything possible to improve tooth health, you may want to consider these supplements *in addition to* the food fixes:

1. **Multivitamin.** Tooth health depends on the health of the body. To be assured that you get the vitamins and minerals you need to keep your beautiful smile, consider taking a multivitamin that contains 100% DV for vitamins C and D.

2. **Calcium plus vitamin D₃.** Most people don't get enough calcium in their diets. Vitamin D can be scarce, too. If you're not getting your daily dose through food (that's at least 1,000 milligrams calcium and 400 IU vitamin D), I recommend that women take a supplement that contains 500 to 600 milligrams of calcium *with* 100 to 400 IU of vitamin D₃ (cholecalciferol, the most potent form) twice a day. This should be taken in addition to a multivitamin (which already provides 100% DV for vitamin D—that's 400 IU), if you choose to take one. Men should never take a calcium supplement without first checking with their physician.

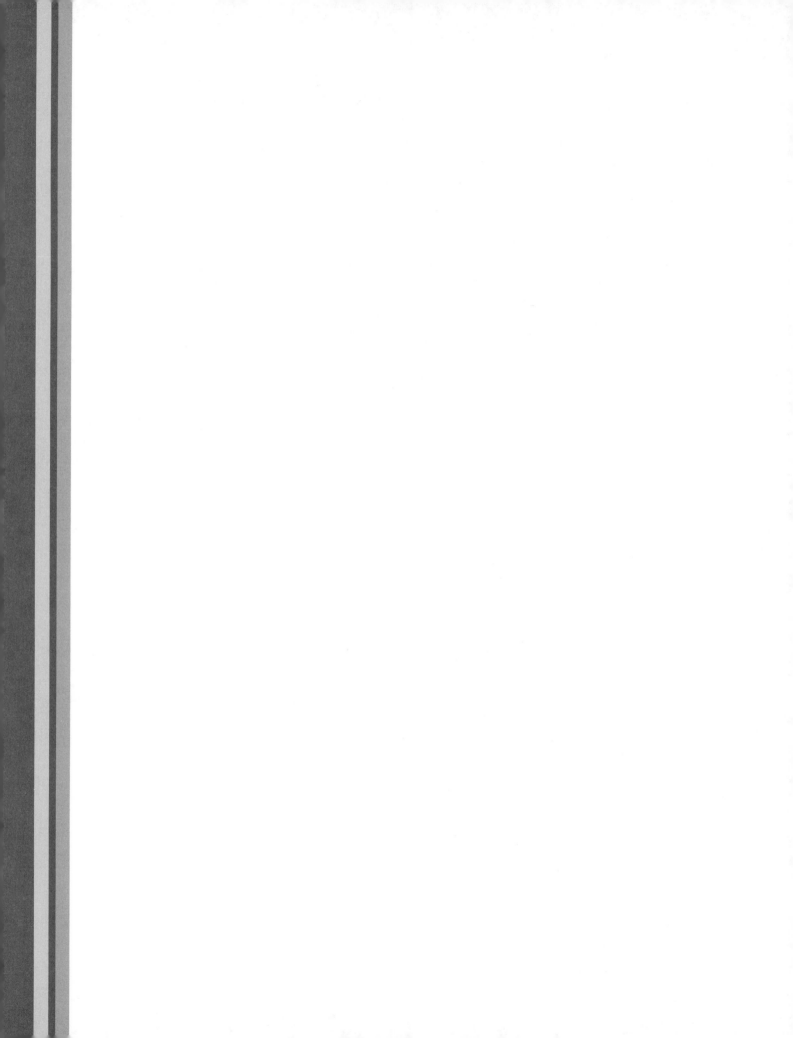

JOY'S 4-STEP PROGRAM
FOR FEEDING A BEAUTIFUL SMILE

Follow this program if you want to maintain a gorgeous smile.

STEP1 ...START WITH THE BASICS

These are the first things you should do to keep your teeth healthy:

- See your dentist. If you haven't been in more than a year, see your dentist immediately for a checkup and cleaning, and to prevent gum disease. Some people with extensive disease can have no symptoms at all, so let a professional check out your mouth.

- If you smoke or use other tobacco products, quit.

- Chew sugarless gum if you can't brush after meals.

- Limit the number of sugary foods and unnecessary, nutrient-less carbohydrates in your diet.

STEP2 ...YOUR ULTIMATE GROCERY LIST

This list contains food with high levels of nutrients that contribute to tooth health (specifically foods rich in calcium and vitamins D and C), plus some foods used as ingredients in the meal plans and recipes. Although fruit and whole grain products are incredibly healthy, they are also carbohydrates and can increase the level of acid in the mouth. Therefore, make sure to brush after eating or at least drink plenty of water and/or unsweetened green tea. Also, consider chewing sugarless gum following meals and snacks.

FRUIT

Berries (blackberries, strawberries, raspberries)	Guava	Oranges	Pineapple
	Juice, calcium-fortified	Oranges, mandarin (canned in light syrup)	Tangerines
	Kiwi		Watermelon
Cantaloupe	Lemons (and juice)		
Clementines	Lychees	Papaya	
Grapefruit (pink, red)	Mangos	Persimmons	

VEGETABLES

Beans, kidney	Kohlrabi	yellow/red/green)	Tomatoes (including
Bok choy	Mushrooms (especially shiitake)	Potatoes, white	green tomatoes, cherry tomatoes)
Broccoli		Rutabagas	
Brussels sprouts	Mustard greens	Shallots	Turnip greens
Cabbage (including Chinese, red)	Okra	Snow peas	
	Onions	Soybeans (edamame)	
Cauliflower	Peas, sugar snap	Squash, summer (all varieties)	
Kale	Peppers (hot;		

SEAFOOD

Herring	Salmon (wild with bones)	Sardines (canned with bones)
Mackerel (not king)		

LEAN MEATS/EGGS/SOY FOODS

Eggs
Tofu with calcium

NUTS AND SEEDS (PREFERABLY UNSALTED)

Almonds

WHOLE GRAINS

Cereal, fortified whole grain	English muffins, whole grain	Pita bread, whole grain	Waffles, calcium-fortified whole grain
		Pizza crust, whole grain	

DAIRY

Cheese (fat-free, reduced-fat)	Parmesan, ricotta, Swiss	soft tub, trans fat-free	Soy milk, enriched/fortified
Cheese (for meal plan): fat-free or reduced-fat Mozzarella,	Ice cream (low-fat)	Milk, fortified (fat-free, 1% reduced-fat)	Yogurt (fat-free, low-fat)
	Margarine spread, vitamin D–fortified,		Yogurt, frozen (fat-free, low-fat)

MISCELLANEOUS

Flour	Marinara sauce	Nutmeg	Salt
Ginger, fresh	Mayonnaise, reduced-fat	Oil, sesame	Sugar, granulated, or sugar substitute
Hot cocoa, diet (100 calories or less)	Mint, fresh	Paprika	Sugarless gum
Maple syrup, reduced-calorie	Mustard, Dijon	Pepper, black	Tea (green, black)
	Nonstick cooking spray	Salad dressing, reduced-calorie	

STEP 3 ...GOING ABOVE AND BEYOND

If you want to do everything you can for tooth health, here are some additional things you might try:

- Consider taking a multivitamin for general nutrition, and women should consider taking a supplement of calcium plus vitamin D_3 for strong bones and teeth. Men should consider taking a vitamin D_3 supplement.

- If you have heartburn from reflux disease, or if you're bulimic (and self-induce vomiting), see your primary care physician to get treatment.

- Add crunchy fruits and vegetables into your daily diet.

HALITOSIS HELP

Worried about bad breath? Your first step should be to visit your dentist to make sure you don't have gum disease. If your mouth is healthy, you might need to alter your diet. Nearly everyone knows that garlic can cause odor problems—it's not called the "stinking rose" for nothing. But other common foods can also foul your breath. The worst offenders are coffee, cheese, and onions. If you brush your teeth or chew some sugarless gum, you'll take care of most of the problem. But keep in mind that onions and garlic contain smelly compounds that are absorbed into the bloodstream and exhaled from your lungs for hours after you eat them. And note that extremely low-carb diets can cause "ketone breath" from the metabolism of large quantities of fat. I consider this another good reason to add some healthy high-quality carbs to your diet, so feel free to enjoy your share of vegetables, fresh fruit, and whole grains.

STEP4 ...MEAL PLANS

These sample menus include foods that have been shown to contribute to good tooth health.

Every day, choose *one* option for each of the three meals—breakfast, lunch, and dinner. Then, one or two times per day, choose from a variety of my suggested snacks. Approximate calories have been provided to help adjust for your personal weight management goals. If you find yourself hungry (and if weight is not an issue), feel free to increase the portion sizes for meals and snacks. Beverage calories are *not* included.

BREAKFAST OPTIONS

(Approximately 300 to 400 calories)

Broccoli-Cheese Soufflé

1 serving Broccoli-Cheese Soufflé (page 121).

Strawberry-Kiwi Smoothie with Cottage Cheese

1 serving (2 cups) Strawberry-Kiwi Smoothie (page 122) with 1 cup fat-free or 1% reduced-fat cottage cheese.

Waffles with Maple Yogurt and Fresh Fruit

2 calcium-fortified, whole grain frozen waffles, toasted and topped with maple yogurt (2 tablespoons reduced-calorie maple syrup mixed with ½ cup plain, fat-free or low-fat yogurt). Enjoy with 1 orange or ½ grapefruit.

English Muffin with Eggs, Tomato, and Cheese

Toasted whole grain English muffin, each half topped with 1 thin slice tomato, 1 egg (scrambled or sunny side up), and 1 (¾-ounce) slice fat-free cheese.

Hard Boiled Egg with Cereal, Milk, and Berries

¾ to 1 cup fortified, whole grain cereal (120 calories or less) mixed with 1 cup fat-free milk and topped with ½ cup sliced strawberries (or raspberries or blackberries). Enjoy with one hard-boiled egg.

LUNCH OPTIONS

(Approximately 400 to 500 calories)

Edamame with Wild Salmon Dijonnaise

1 cup boiled edamame (soybeans in the pod), lightly salted. Enjoy with 5 ounces canned wild salmon with bones, drained, mashed, and mixed with 1 tablespoon reduced-fat mayonnaise, 1 to 2 teaspoons Dijon mustard, minced onion, and black pepper. Serve the salmon on a large bed of lettuce drizzled with lemon juice and your choice of seasonings (or 1 to 2 tablespoons reduced-calorie dressing).

Broccoli-Cheese Soufflé with Cottage Cheese and Almonds

1 serving Broccoli-Cheese Soufflé (page 121). Serve with ½ cup fat-free or 1% reduced-fat cottage cheese topped with 1 tablespoon slivered almonds.

Tomato-Cheese Omelet with Tropical Mango-Citrus Smoothie

Beat 1 whole egg with 2 to 3 egg whites. Cook in small skillet coated with nonstick cooking spray. When bottom is cooked, gently flip and add 3 tablespoons chopped tomato and 1 ounce reduced-fat or fat-free cheese. Fold omelet in half and continue cooking until egg mixture firms and cheese melts. Enjoy with 1 serving (2 cups) Tropical Mango-Citrus Smoothie (page 123).

Mixed Vegetable Salad with Sardines

4 ounces (about 8) sardines with bones (canned in oil or tomato sauce) tossed with unlimited leafy greens, chopped tomatoes, carrots, sweet pepper, onion, and ½ cup white or navy beans. Drizzle with 2 to 4 tablespoons reduced-calorie salad dressing (or 1 teaspoon olive oil and 1 to 2 tablespoons vinegar or fresh lemon juice). Season with a pinch of optional salt and ground black pepper to taste.

Tofu Salad with Snow Peas, Almonds, and Mandarin Oranges

4 ounces extra-firm tofu, cubed and chilled, tossed with 2 cups leafy greens or lettuce, 1 cup steamed and chilled snow peas, ½ chopped tomato, and ½ cup mandarin oranges (canned in light syrup). Drizzle with 1 to 2 teaspoons sesame oil and 1 tablespoon reduced-sodium soy sauce and top with 1 to 2 tablespoon slivered almonds.

DINNER OPTIONS

(Approximately 500 to 600 calories)

Wild Salmon Salad with Parmesan Baked Potato

1 serving Wild Salmon Salad (page 322) with unlimited leafy greens. Enjoy with ½ plain baked potato topped with 2 tablespoons grated Parmesan cheese.

Breakfast for Dinner: Almond-Berry Oatmeal

¾ cup dry instant oatmeal prepared with 1½ cups fat-free milk, topped with 2 tablespoons slivered almonds and 1 cup mixed berries (sliced strawberries, raspberries, and blackberries). Sweeten with optional 1 teaspoon sugar, honey, or artificial sweetener.

Whole Wheat Pita Pizza with the Works

Toast 1 split whole wheat pita bread (or use 200 calories of whole wheat pizza crust). Top each pita half with 2 to 3 heaping tablespoons marinara sauce and ¼ cup reduced-fat ricotta cheese, plus ½ cup sweet pepper sticks and unlimited chopped broccoli florets pre-sautéed in nonstick cooking spray. Top each half with 2 tablespoons shredded reduced-fat mozzarella cheese. Heat in 350°F oven until cheese melts and bubbles. Season with crushed red pepper and oregano.

Healthy Chicken Parmesan and Broccoli

1 serving Healthy Chicken Parmesan and Broccoli (page 252).

Sweet and Sour Tofu-Veggie Stir-Fry

1 serving Sweet and Sour Tofu-Veggie Stir-Fry (page 251). Serve with 1 cup cooked brown rice.

SNACK OPTIONS

100 calories or less

- *Best Vegetables:* 1 cup raw or cooked turnip greens, mustard greens, broccoli, kale, bell peppers, kohlrabi, Brussels sprouts, cauliflower, cabbage, tomatoes, sugar snap peas, snow peas, rutabaga, summer squash, or okra
- *Best Fruits:* 1 guava, orange, kiwi, or tangerine; 2 clementines; ½ mango, grapefruit, papaya, or cantaloupe; 20 strawberries; 1 cup watermelon, raspberries, sliced strawberries, blackberries, or pineapple
- 1 hard-boiled egg
- 1 cup fat-free milk
- 1 cup diet hot cocoa (100 calories or less)
- ½ cup fat-free or 1% reduced-fat cottage cheese
- 10 almonds

100 to 200 calories

- ½ cup frozen yogurt or ice cream (fat-free or low-fat)
- 1 cup (6- to 8-ounce container) fat-free, flavored yogurt
- 1 serving (2 cups) Tropical Mango-Citrus Smoothie (page 123)
- 1 serving (2 cups) Strawberry-Kiwi Smoothie (page 122)
- ¾ cup whole grain cereal with 1 cup fat-free milk
- 1 cup fat-free milk with 1 cup berries (sliced strawberries, raspberries, or blackberries)
- 20 almonds

BROCCOLI-CHEESE SOUFFLÉ

This guilt-free soufflé provides twice the amount of vitamin C you need every day, and more than 40 percent of your daily requirement for calcium. The delicious flavor (and healthy ingredients!) will have you smiling.

Makes 2 servings

2	teaspoons grated Parmesan cheese
6	egg whites plus 3 yolks, at room temperature
¼	teaspoon salt, plus more to taste
2	tablespoons reduced-fat, soft tub, trans fat–free margarine spread
2	tablespoons all-purpose flour
1	cup fat-free milk, heated just to a simmer on stovetop or in microwave
½	teaspoon paprika
¼	teaspoon nutmeg
	Ground black pepper to taste
1	bunch broccoli, cut into florets (about 3 cups)
¼	cup reduced-sodium chicken broth (or water)
1	shallot or 1 small onion, minced
¼	cup plus 1 tablespoon finely grated reduced-fat Swiss cheese

1. Preheat the oven to 375°F. Coat a 6- or 8-cup ceramic gratin dish with nonstick cooking spray and sprinkle the inside with the Parmesan cheese.
2. In a large metal bowl, beat the egg whites and salt on high speed until the egg whites become stiff but not lumpy, 4 to 6 minutes. Set aside.
3. In a medium saucepan over medium-high heat, melt the margarine until it begins to foam. Add the flour and mix vigorously until the flour turns to a paste without browning, 2 to 3 minutes. Off the heat, pour in the hot milk, and whisk quickly until the mixture is smooth. Add the paprika, nutmeg, and salt and pepper to taste. Bring the mixture to a slow boil over medium-high heat. Cook, stirring constantly, for 2 to 3 minutes, until the sauce becomes heavy and thick. Remove from the heat. Add the egg yolks, one at a time, mixing well after each addition.
4. In a blender, puree the broccoli and broth or water. Stir the broccoli mixture, shallot or onion, and ¼ cup Swiss cheese into the milk mixture. With a spatula, gently fold in one-third of the egg whites, lifting the milk mixture from the bottom of the pan. Transfer the milk mixture to the bowl with the remaining egg whites and continue to fold until just combined, without deflating the egg whites.
5. Pour into the prepared gratin dish and sprinkle with the remaining 1 tablespoon Swiss cheese. Bake, uncovered, 25 to 30 minutes, until the soufflé puffs and is golden on the top. Serve immediately.

PER SERVING
343 calories, 29 g protein, 24 g carbohydrate, 14 g fat (5 g saturated), 317 mg cholesterol, 788 mg sodium, 4 g fiber; plus 77 IU vitamin D (20% DV), 470 mg calcium (48% DV), 120 mg vitamin C (200% DV)

STRAWBERRY-KIWI SMOOTHIE

Refreshing and easy to make, one serving provides almost twice the amount of vitamin C you need for an entire day! This smoothie also provides tooth-strengthening calcium and vitamin D from the milk . . . and all for only 155 calories.

Makes 2 servings, 2 cups each

1 ½	cups fat-free milk
1	cup strawberries, hulled and quartered
2	kiwis, peeled and quartered (about ½ cup)
2	tablespoon fresh mint, chopped, plus two sprigs for garnish
1	tablespoon granulated sugar or sugar substitute
1	cup crushed ice

In a blender or food processor, combine the milk, strawberries, kiwis, chopped mint, sugar or sugar substitute, and ice and blend until smooth. Garnish with fresh mint sprigs.

PER SERVING
155 calories, 8 g protein, 32 g carbohydrate, 0 g fat, 0 mg cholesterol, 81 mg sodium, 4 g fiber; plus 75 IU vitamin D (19% DV), 270 mg calcium (27% DV), 113 mg vitamin C (188% DV)

TROPICAL MANGO-CITRUS SMOOTHIE

Here's another fabulous smoothie recipe you can enjoy anytime, for health or just for pleasure.

Makes 2 servings, 2 cups each

1½	cups fat-free milk
1	medium mango, peeled and chopped (about 1 cup)
1	medium orange, zest, peeled and chopped (about ½ cup), plus 1 sliced orange for garnish
1	lime, zest and juiced
1	teaspoon minced fresh ginger
1	cup crushed ice

1. Zest the orange (can use vegetable peeler), and set aside the zest. Peel the orange, and chop.
2. Zest the lime, and set aside the zest. Juice the lime.
3. In a blender or food processor, combine the milk, mango, chopped orange, lime juice, lime and orange zest, ginger, and ice and blend until smooth.

PER SERVING
171 calories, 8 g protein, 30 g carbohydrate, 0 g fat, 0 mg cholesterol, 80 mg sodium, 4 g fiber; plus 75 IU vitamin D (19% DV), 277 mg calcium (28% DV), 73 mg vitamin C (122% DV)

PART FOUR

LIVING LONG
AND STRONG

CHAPTER 7

CARDIOVASCULAR DISEASE

One spring day, Wendy noticed the world's longest conga line of ants traveling across her driveway, heading into her garage. From there, the ants disappeared into an almost imperceptible crack near an interior wall. She called an exterminator, expecting to get a bill for a hundred dollars or so for spraying around the garage. Instead, she ended up with an estimate of $12,000. As with heart disease, what looked to be a small isolated problem from the outside turned out to be a sign of a much bigger problem developing out of sight.

You see, seven years earlier, Wendy and her husband decided to do a little home remodeling, including an upstairs bathroom. It turns out that there was a tiny hole in the floor of their newly installed shower—a hole that dripped water onto the beams holding up the second floor. At first, that small amount of water had no noticeable effect but over the years it added up to a couple *billion* drops. The subflooring and wood studs had rotted—ambrosia to carpenter ants, which knew a good thing when they found it and made a nest. So, in addition to the cost of fumigating the whole house, the shower stall had to be removed, tile pried up, subfloor and studs ripped out and replaced, new tile installed, et cetera, et cetera. Many thousands of dollars worth of "et cetera."

Cardiovascular disease is a lot like Wendy's house. Many people ignore their doctors' warnings about high cholesterol or blood pressure numbers because they feel perfectly healthy. But those numbers are just the ants on your body's metaphoric driveway, the thing that clues you in to what's going on *inside*. By the time you get diagnosed with high cholesterol or high blood pressure or high triglycerides, you may already have significant structural damage.

I often tell my clients to take nutritional changes at a pace that feels comfortable to them. That's not good enough when it comes to cardiovascular disease. The consequences of doing too little are severe—heart attack, stroke, pain, debility, death. Sadly, not everyone gets a second chance. So don't wait until after your next vacation, or your daughter's wedding, or that anniversary dinner to start. My advice is to start immediately and go for broke! Change your diet, change your habits, change your lifestyle. I'll show you the how in this chapter. No matter what your risk factors, there are things you can start doing now.

WHAT AFFECTS CARDIOVASCULAR DISEASE?

Oxygen enters the blood stream through the lungs. The blood goes through the heart, which pumps it throughout the body to carry oxygen and nutrients to every cell, from the hair follicles on your head to your toes. Because blood has to travel to such remote areas, blood vessels have to come in various sizes, from the thick arteries and veins that branch off from the heart, to the tiny capillaries that feed the tiniest, most distant parts of your body. Cardiovascular disease, also commonly called *heart disease,* can affect any part of this vast network, from the heart (*cardio-*) through all the blood vessels (*-vascular*).

Healthy blood vessels are flexible and strong, capable of containing the pulsing pressure of rushing blood, heartbeat after heartbeat, year after year, for a lifetime. We'd like to think that they are durable, too, but the reality is that vessels are relatively fragile. Think about Monarch butterflies. They migrate hundreds of miles in a single season—some more than 1,500 miles—on wings that are so fragile that they can be destroyed with a single touch. That's what blood vessels are like: tough but delicate, sturdy but vulnerable. If anything goes wrong and blood can't get to all parts of the body, cells won't receive the nutrition and oxygen they—and you—need to survive. If blood can't get to the heart, the result is a heart attack. If blood can't get to all to portions of the brain, the result is a stroke. In other words, the blood must keep flowing.

HIGH BLOOD PRESSURE (HYPERTENSION)

As the heart contracts to pump blood through the arteries, the force of that rushing blood against the vessel walls is called *systolic blood pressure.* As the heart relaxes between beats, the blood presses less forcefully against the vessel walls, as reflected by *diastolic blood pressure.* When you go to the doctor, your blood pressure is given in two numbers: systolic pressure over diastolic pressure, measured in millimeters of mercury (mmHg).

Physicians recommend that you maintain blood pressure at or below 120/80 mmHg, but high blood pressure (HBP) is medically defined as any reading higher than 140/90 mmHg. Readings of 121 to 130 systolic or 81 to 89 diastolic are considered prehypertension, a warning that blood pressure may soon rise into the danger zone. The higher your blood pressure, the greater your risk of disease, including heart attack, stroke, kidney failure, and other blood vessel disorders. Even prehypertension causes physiologic changes that can be thought of as *pre-atherosclerosis*. That's because when blood pressure is higher than normal, it pummels the delicate lining of blood vessels. Left untreated, HBP can cause structural damage and inflammation. In addition, HBP can trigger a condition called *atherosclerosis*—the formation of plaque, a fatty substance that builds up on the inside of the vessels, making them narrower and less flexible, and choking the blood supply to every part of the body. Mind you, these narrow vessels must still carry the same amount of blood as they did when they were healthy, which only adds to the pressure the vessel walls must bear. So high blood pressure is a risk factor for even higher blood pressure. That's why blood pressure problems never really go away—once you have damage from HBP, you'll have to fight to control it forever.

FAQS

I have high cholesterol, and I've heard that red yeast rice works the same as some of the statin drugs. I'll do anything to avoid taking medication. Does red yeast rice work? Is it safe?

Red yeast rice does work to lower cholesterol, but only because it contains naturally occurring chemicals that are identical to medicinal statins. They work the same, and they have the same risks and side effects—including possible liver toxicity and muscle pain or weakness. The difference is that prescription medications are standardized, regulated, and produced in a sterile environment. The amount of active ingredient in each dose of red yeast rice can vary from package to package, or even from capsule to capsule in the same package. Worse, red yeast rice may contain contaminants, some of which may cause serious illness. This is one of those cases when *natural* doesn't mean better. If you want the benefits of red yeast rice, talk with your doctor about whether you should start taking a statin medication.

If you've been diagnosed with HBP, your doctor has probably already told you the basics. You can control blood pressure by getting to and maintaining a healthy weight, reducing your bad cholesterol (LDL) if it's high, limiting the salt in your diet, exercising, and adding calcium, vitamin D, magnesium, and potassium to your diet (discussed below).

HIGH LDL CHOLESTEROL, LOW HDL CHOLESTEROL

Cholesterol is a natural fat-like substance found in all animal tissue—humans included—because it is part of all cell membranes. Cholesterol is also part of the myelin sheath that surrounds and protects nerves, and it is used to make vitamin D, bile, and some hormones. Our bodies make all the cholesterol we need for health, but we also get cholesterol from eating meat, poultry, and fish. (Incidentally, cholesterol is *never* found in plant-based foods, so "cholesterol-free!" labels on products like peanut butter are really just stating the obvious.)

Cholesterol comes in two main varieties: low-density lipoprotein (LDL) cholesterol (commonly called *bad cholesterol*—remember L for *lousy*), and high-density lipoprotein (HDL) cholesterol (*good cholesterol*—remember H for *hero*). LDL cholesterol is one of the components of vessel-clogging plaque. Over time, plaque can incorporate calcium and other substances that make the plaque hard and brittle. If the plaque deposits grow large enough, they can block a blood vessel. In addition, the brittle plaque can break off, travel through the blood stream, and form a clot anywhere in the body.

The higher your LDL cholesterol, the greater your risk of developing life-threatening plaque. So, you want your *low*-density *low*. According to the National Institutes of Health (NIH), the optimal level of LDL cholesterol is below 100 mg/dL. High LDL cholesterol is defined as 160 mg/dL and higher—but certainly anything above 130 is worth treating.

HDL cholesterol, on the other hand, is like nature's plaque vacuum cleaner—it picks up the vessel-clogging cholesterol and carries it away to the liver, where it is disposed of in the form of bile. The higher your HDL levels, the cleaner your blood vessels will be. So, you want your *high*-density *high*. According to the NIH, people with HDL of 60 mg/dL or higher have a lower risk of heart disease, whereas HDL below 40 mg/dL is considered too low.

Because HDL is so important to the health of blood vessels, some physicians prefer to talk about the cholesterol ratio—your total cholesterol divided by your HDL cholesterol. For example, if your total cholesterol number is 250 and your HDL is 50, your ratio is 250/50 or 5. A ratio of 3.5 is considered optimal, and people are urged to aim for a ratio of 5 or less.

Interestingly, men and women may need to pay attention to different numbers. With women, LDL cholesterol and the cholesterol ratio are equally valuable for predicting risk of atherosclerosis. With men, the ratio may be more important—having near optimal levels of LDL may still be dangerous if HDL is too low and the cholesterol ratio is too high. If any of your numbers are high (or if your HDL is low), it's important to make cholesterol control a priority.

High cholesterol can be caused by several factors, some you can change, and some you can't. Heredity can play a big part. Some people can have a perfect heart-healthy lifestyle, and still have skyrocketing cholesterol because their bodies naturally make too much of it—our bodies' production of cholesterol is independent from what we eat. Also, LDL cholesterol increases naturally with age, so even if you put up all-star numbers when you were younger, each passing year has made you that much more likely to have problems. Men naturally have higher cholesterol than women, but the female advantage fades when the hormonal changes of menopause lead to a steep rise in women's LDL cholesterol.

And as if high LDL cholesterol wasn't dangerous enough on its own, results of a study published in a 2006 issue of the journal *Hypertension* showed that people who had high LDL cholesterol or a high cholesterol ratio had an increased risk of developing high blood pressure. People with a level of bad cholesterol (non-HDL cholesterol, which includes LDL and other dangerous cholesterol forms, such as very low-density lipoprotein and intermediate-density lipoprotein) higher than 190 had about a 30 percent greater risk of developing HBP compared with people with bad cholesterol levels of less than 160. Even worse, people with a cholesterol ratio of 6 or higher had a 47 percent increased risk of HBP compared with people who had ratios of 4 or less. On the other hand, people with HDL (our hero) of 53 or higher, had a 32 percent *decreased* risk of developing hypertension. Really, these results make sense. High LDL cholesterol leads to atherosclerosis . . . which causes narrowing of the blood vessels . . . which means your heart has to pump that much harder to squeeze blood through them . . . which means increased blood pressure. You can improve your cholesterol profile by reducing body weight (if you are overweight), increasing physical activity, and following my cholesterol-busting nutrition program.

HIGH TRIGLYCERIDES

Triglyceride is just a fancy word for *fat*—the fat in our bodies is stored in the form of triglycerides. Triglycerides are found in foods and manufactured in our bodies. As with cholesterol, eating too much of the wrong kinds of fats (more about that in the sections on saturated and trans fats below) will raise your blood triglycerides, but some people also have a genetic predisposition that causes them to manufacture way too much triglycerides on their own, no matter how carefully they eat. Triglyceride levels can shoot up after eating foods that are high in saturated fats or carbohydrates, or after drinking alcohol. That's why triglyceride tests require an overnight fast. Triglycerides can become elevated because of genetics, or in reaction to having diabetes, hypothyroidism, or kidney disease. As with most other heart-related factors, being overweight and inactive also contribute to abnormal triglycerides.

There are so many reports about cholesterol-lowering supplements, especially policosanol. How can I tell what is valuable and what isn't?

You're right—it seems that every time you open a magazine there's a story about another miracle supplement. Policosanol is a sugar cane extract that has been touted as a way to reduce cholesterol. But a rigorous 2006 study showed that even 80 milligrams of high-quality policosanol per day didn't have any effect on cholesterol. As I write, there is preliminary information that says that cinnamon and cloves (in supplement form only, not from food) may help lower cholesterol. This is potentially good news, but it is too early to recommend seeking out cinnamon supplements. You don't want to be a guinea pig, one of the first to test out some new treatment—there may be undiscovered side effects or you may waste money on a worthless treatment. On the other hand, you also don't want to miss out on a treatment that the medical community has embraced. My advice is to read everything, and if you see something interesting, make a copy and take it to your doctor. It can't hurt to ask a professional, and most doctors are happy when their patients are proactive about improving their health.

High triglyceride levels make blood thicker and stickier, which means that it is more likely to form clots. Normal triglyceride levels are defined as less than 150 mg/dL; 150 to 199 is considered borderline high; 200 to 499 is high; and 500 or higher is officially called very high. To me, anything over 150 is a red flag indicating my client needs to take immediate steps to get the situation under control.

Studies have shown that triglyceride levels are associated with increased risks of cardiovascular disease and stroke—in both men and women—alone or in combination with other risk factors (high triglycerides combined with high LDL cholesterol can be a particularly deadly combination). For example, in one ground-breaking study, triglycerides alone increased the risk of cardiovascular disease by 14 percent in men, and by 37 percent in women. But when the test subjects also had low HDL cholesterol and other risk factors, high triglycerides increased the risk of disease by 32 percent in men and 76 percent in women. Fortunately, triglycerides are relatively easily controlled with the diet and lifestyle changes outlined in this chapter. To lower triglycerides, lose weight if you're overweight, reduce saturated fat and trans fat, avoid foods that are concentrated in sugar (even dried fruit and fruit juice), cut way back on alcohol (when triglycerides are high, sugar and alcohol will keep them high), and incorporate omega-3 fats.

HIGH HOMOCYSTEINE

Homocysteine is an amino acid naturally produced when the body breaks down proteins that contain another amino acid, methionine. No one knows exactly what role homocysteine plays in heart disease. It could be that homocysteine directly damages blood vessels. In the laboratory, homocysteine causes inflammation, damages blood vessel linings, and encourages blood clots. Or, it could be that homocysteine is just a marker—a sign that other things are going wrong in the body to create heart disease. Many scientists agree on one point, however: People with blood levels of homocysteine higher than 10 micromol/L may have an increased risk of heart attack and stroke.

The research picture gets cloudy when it comes to the benefits of lowering homocysteine. Early studies suggested that lowering abnormally high levels of homocysteine reduced the risk of heart disease and heart attack, especially when there were other risk factors at work, such as smoking or hypertension. More recent studies found that when people with normal homocysteine levels lowered them even more, there was no heart-related benefit. So, what's a person to do? If homocysteine treatment required a prescription medication, making a decision could be difficult. But the best treatment isn't new, risky, or expensive; it's making sure you're getting enough of the ultimate *B trio* of folic acid, vitamin B_6, and vitamin B_{12} in the food you eat. So although research results may be murky, my advice is simple: Eat more of these healthful foods, as described in the next section.

C-REACTIVE PROTEIN

When the body is exposed to infection, allergens, or even physical damage, it reacts by releasing chemicals designed to fight off the invasion or fix the damage. While working to protect us, these substances create inflammation. One of the body's markers for inflammation is C-reactive protein (CRP).

Inflammation feeds atherosclerosis. Your immune system's response to atherosclerosis is to rush white blood cells to the site of the damage. But the plaque gobbles up the white cells and grows bigger. Once plaque matures, it becomes fragile, and inflammation can cause this brittle plaque to rupture. These shattered pieces of plaque get carried along the blood stream, and can form clots that cause heart attacks or strokes.

The value of CRP is that it tells us when inflammation is present, possibly causing cardiovascular disease. If we know that, we can take steps to reduce the inflammation and prevent blood vessel damage. The nutrition and lifestyle changes in this chapter can help reduce inflammation.

THE METABOLIC SYNDROME

As you might imagine, having one risk factor for heart disease is bad enough, but having more than one amplifies the threat. The metabolic syndrome describes a cluster of risk factors that, when taken together, create a toxic environment in blood vessels. The metabolic syndrome is characterized by having at least three of the following symptoms: high blood pressure, high triglycerides, low HDL cholesterol, large waist circumference (greater than 35" for women, 40" for men), or fasting blood sugar greater than 110 mg/dL. People with the metabolic syndrome have an increased risk of heart disease, stroke, and diabetes. Fortunately, the 4-step plan in this chapter can help improve each of the risk factors, so you can solve all *five* problems with one approach.

HOW FOOD AFFECTS CARDIOVASCULAR DISEASE

Eating well for heart health means knowing which foods to limit, and which to embrace.

FOODS TO LIMIT OR AVOID

The top dietary recommendation for cardiovascular health is to eliminate or at least drastically limit the foods you eat that contain saturated fats, trans fats, cholesterol, refined carbohydrates, and salt.

SATURATED FATS

Saturated fats are found in animal-based foods, including meats, butter, whole milk dairy products (including yogurt, cheese, and ice cream), and poultry skin. They are also found in some high-fat plant foods, such as palm oil. The Nurses' Health Study, which included more than 80,000 participants, showed that saturated fats increase the risk of coronary artery disease. It was estimated that if you replace just 100 calories of saturated fat in your diet every day with unsaturated fats (found in as olive oil or nuts), you can reduce your risk of heart disease by about 40 percent. Just 100 calories! That's about the total number of calories in one homemade chocolate chip cookie, so swap that cookie for 5 macadamia nuts or 12 almonds and you're on your way to a healthier heart. By making a few simple changes, you can improve your risk profile:

- Avoid butter, cream cheese, lard, sour cream, doughnuts, cakes, cookies, chocolate bars, chocolate chips, ice cream, fried foods, pizza, cream- or cheese-based salad dressings, cheese sauce, cream sauces, animal shortenings, high-fat meats (including hamburgers, bologna, pepperoni, sausage, bacon, salami, pastrami, spareribs, and hot dogs), high-fat cuts of beef and pork, whole-milk dairy products.
- Choose lean meats only (including skinless chicken and turkey, lean beef, lean pork), fish, reduced-fat or fat-free dairy products. Try soy foods as a substitute for meat at least some of the time. Although soy itself may not reduce risk of heart disease, it replaces hazardous animal fats with healthier proteins. Choose high-quality soy foods, such as tofu, tempeh, enriched/fortified soy milk, and edamame.
- Always remove skin from poultry.

■ Prepare foods by baking, roasting, broiling, boiling, poaching, steaming, grilling, or stir-frying. No deep-fat frying.

TRANS FATS

Trans fats were developed in a laboratory to improve the shelf life of processed foods—and they do. But calorie for calorie, trans fats are more dangerous than the saturated fats I just advised you to avoid. Most stick margarines contain trans fats, and trans fats are found in many packaged baked goods, potato chips, snack foods, fried foods, and fast food that use or create *hydrogenated oils*. (All food labels must now list the amount of trans fats, right after the amount of saturated fats—good news for consumers.) By substituting olive oil or vegetable oil for trans fats in just 2 percent of your daily calories, you can reduce your risk of heart disease by 53 percent. In a 2,000-calorie-a-day diet, that's about *40 calories*. Think of it this way—an average serving of French fries contains about 5 grams of trans fats, or about 45 calories worth of evil trans fats, and a daily serving would be enough to *double* your risk of heart disease. There is no safe amount of trans fats, so try to keep them as far from your plate as possible.

CHOLESTEROL-RICH FOODS

Years ago, doctors used to recommend that people with heart disease avoid all high-cholesterol foods. But dietary cholesterol does not harm health as much as saturated fats and trans fats do. Research into the effects of dietary cholesterol have been mixed, which is not surprising—different people have different susceptibilities. Still, if you want to take a firm hand to reduce your risk factors, you may want to consider cutting down on all high-cholesterol foods, including egg yolks, shellfish, liver, and other organ meats like sweetbreads and foie gras. You'll notice whole eggs and shellfish on a couple of my best food lists—that's because they're high in other heart healthy nutrients—as well as cholesterol. That said, if your LDL cholesterol is high, limit your intake of egg yolks to no more than three per week (whites are unlimited), and limit shellfish to no more than one portion twice weekly. You may also want to speak with your cardiologist about personal limitations.

REFINED CARBOHYDRATES

Refined carbohydrates include sugary foods, sugared soft drinks, fruit juice, sweet baked goods, anything baked with white flour (including white bread, rolls, cereal, buns), and white rice. These low-quality carbs cause a sudden rise in insulin, which may lead to a spike in triglycerides. Whenever possible, aim for high-quality instead of low-quality carbs. That means limiting sweets, and choosing whole grain foods, such as oatmeal, healthy cereals, brown and wild rice, whole wheat pasta, and bread products that include the word *whole* or *oats* in the first ingredient.

SALT

For decades, the science has been pretty clear: Salt increases blood pressure in people who are salt sensitive, and the more salt you eat, the greater the potential rise in blood pressure.

Sodium in small doses is necessary for the body to function properly, but too much will draw excess fluid into the blood, effectively raising blood pressure. Salt is a hard habit to break—it actually dulls your sense of taste, which means that, over time, you'll be reaching for that shaker more often to get the same taste. The best thing to do is go cold turkey. Well, almost. First, take the salt shaker off the kitchen table, and try not to add salt to foods you prepare at home. If you miss the flavor, experiment with some of the salt substitutes on the market (such as Mrs. Dash and Morton salt-substitute seasonings). Second, when reading food labels, choose brands that have less sodium. Third, limit hidden sources of sodium, such as ketchup, soy sauce, teriyaki sauce, salad dressings, prepared marinades, pickles, sauerkraut, deli meats, canned vegetables, canned soups, and broth. Go out of your way to buy brands that offer lower-sodium varieties, especially when it comes to canned goods. If you buy canned beans, choose low-sodium brands whenever possible, and always rinse thoroughly before using—the liquid they are packed in can be very high in sodium.

GOOD FOODS TO CHOOSE

FRUITS AND VEGETABLES

I know you're probably sick of hearing advice about eating plenty of fruits and vegetables, but it really is important, especially for people fighting cardiovascular disease. The scientific data all support the same claim: People who eat five or more servings of fruits and vegetables daily have a reduced risk of heart attack and stroke compared with people who eat less than three servings daily. Specifically, heart attack risk is about 15 percent lower, and stroke risk is about 30 percent lower! On average, the risk of coronary artery disease is reduced by about 5 percent for each additional serving of fruits and vegetables you eat every day.

What's the magic in fruits and vegetables? No one really knows. Sure, they're full of vitamins, minerals, fiber, and antioxidants, but we don't know which ones are most helpful because whenever scientists try to mimic the effects of foods with supplements, their formulations simply don't produce the same protective effects as the real thing. That means that you have to eat the foods, the whole foods (and nothing but the foods) in order to reap the benefits of fruits and vegetables. *Two large caveats:* If you're taking any cardiac medication, avoid eating grapefruit and drinking grapefruit juice (a compound in grapefruit interferes with the breakdown of many medications). Also, if you're taking a blood thinner like Coumadin, have your doctor monitor your blood and medication dosage as you increase your intake of dark leafy green vegetables. These vegetables are rich in vitamin K which plays a key role in blood clotting (see full list of Vitamin K–rich foods in the Osteoporosis chapter on page 234).

SOLUBLE FIBER

Soluble fiber, especially the viscous type, may help reduce cholesterol by grabbing onto cholesterol and escorting it through your digestive system and out of your body. It also may reduce the intestinal absorption of cholesterol, and it can lower blood pressure. Research has shown that eating an additional 5 to 10 grams of soluble fiber a day can reduce LDL cholesterol by 3 to 5 percent. If you eat a few foods rich in soluble fiber every day, you'll get *at least* 5 grams. It is a small improvement, but every percentage point counts!

BEST FOODS FOR SOLUBLE FIBER: *Psyllium seeds (ground), oat and rice bran, oatmeal, barley, lentils, Brussels sprouts, peas, beans (kidney, lima, black, navy, pinto), apples, blackberries, pears, raisins, oranges, grapefruit, dates, figs, prunes, apricots, cantaloupe, strawberries, bananas, peaches, broccoli, carrots, cauliflower, cabbage, spinach, sweet potatoes, yams, white potatoes, tomatoes, avocado, raspberries, corn, almonds, flaxseed (ground), sunflower seeds*

HEALTHY FATS

There was a time when heart researchers slapped the same label—*bad*—on every kind of fat. Now, we know that trans fats and saturated fats are amazingly dangerous for cardiovascular health, but omega-3 fats and monounsaturated fats are actually good for your heart.

Heart-healthy fish oils are especially rich in omega-3 fatty acids. In multiple studies over the past 15 years, people who ate diets high in omega-3s had 30 to 40 percent reductions in heart disease, and fewer cases of sudden death from arrhythmia. Although we don't yet know why fish oil works so well, there are several possibilities. Omega-3s seem to reduce inflammation, reduce high blood pressure, decrease triglycerides, raise HDL cholesterol, and make blood thinner and less sticky so it is less likely to clot. So omega-3s affect nearly every risk factor for heart disease. It's as close to a food prescription for heart health as it gets. I recommend eating at least three servings of one of the omega-3–rich fish every week. If you cannot manage to eat that much fish, try taking fish oil capsules, which have the same effect. (See the Supplements section, page 000, for more information.)

BEST FOODS FOR OMEGA-3 FATTY ACIDS: *Wild salmon (fresh, canned), herring, mackerel (not king), sardines, anchovies, rainbow trout, Pacific oysters, omega-3–fortified eggs, flaxseed (ground and oil), walnuts, butternuts (white walnuts), seaweed, walnut oil, canola oil, soybeans*

Monounsaturated fats, found mainly in olive oil, are thought to protect people against heart disease by reducing blood pressure. Scientists discovered the benefits of olive oil by observing Mediterranean populations. They use olive oil more than any other form of fat and typically have low rates of coronary artery disease. Research shows it doesn't help to just *add* monounsaturated fats to your diet—you need to replace some of the unhealthy fats that are already in your diet (all those saturated and trans fats mentioned earlier) with better choices. There is some evidence that substituting olive oil for some carbohydrates in your diet (particularly those unhealthy low-quality refined carbohydrates!) can increase HDL.

BEST FOODS FOR MONOUNSATURATED FATS:
Olive oil, canola oil, avocado, macadamia nuts, hazel-nuts, pecans, almonds, peanuts, cashews, Brazil nuts, pistachio nuts, pine nuts, peanut butter, olives

B VITAMINS: FOLATE, B_6, B_{12}

If this book had been written just a year earlier, this section on B vitamins would have read much differently. Folate, vitamin B_6, and vitamin B_{12} are known to reduce levels of homocysteine, and high homocysteine often means a higher risk of coronary artery disease. So to reduce homocysteine, it is important to eat plenty of vitamin B–rich foods.

But then came three studies involving more than 9,000 participants who had a very high risk of a coronary artery event; they had either documented heart disease or a history of heart attack or stroke. This research showed that taking these vitamins in the form of supplements lowered homocysteine, but didn't actually reduce the risk of heart attacks or strokes. Those who took the vitamins had the same number of heart attacks and strokes as those who did not. While some scientists believe that this casts doubt on the value of B vitamins for heart health, other experts still consider them essential. It could be that food will work where supplements don't. Or perhaps the vitamins work best before cardiovascular disease is so advanced that it can't be reversed. I believe that it is too early to cast the B vitamins aside. There's more research underway, but in the meantime, I recommend getting your folate, vitamin B_6, and vitamin B_{12} from food sources, which are delicious and generally good for health. If they also help keep your heart pumping, that's even better.

FAQS

I did everything right—I saw a nutritionist, I started exercising, and stopped smoking—but my LDL cholesterol is still high. My doctor put me on a statin medication. Is there anything I should do differently with my diet?

First, keep following all of your doctor's advice. Second, follow all the diet recommendations in this chapter. If your cholesterol returns to normal levels, don't stop—the change means the program is working, and it's a lifestyle change not a temporary one-time fix. Statins are valuable medications, but they are just one tool for keeping cholesterol under control. The nutrition and lifestyle changes in this chapter can help turn your risk factors around, which will mean better health in the long run. However, some people have a genetic predisposition to make cholesterol and may still require medications in addition to lifestyle changes. Finally, many health experts (including me) recommend that their clients who take one of the cholesterol-lowering statin medications also take a supplement called *Coenzyme Q_{10}*. CoQ_{10} is an antioxidant necessary for energy production in cells. Without CoQ_{10}, cells can't function properly. Our bodies usually make sufficient CoQ_{10} to keep us healthy. Statins work by inhibiting the mechanism that allows the liver to make cholesterol, but they also slow the body's production of CoQ_{10}, leading to deficiency. To counteract these effects, I recommend taking 100 milligrams of CoQ_{10} once a day in a soft gel formulation. Although most people can take CoQ_{10} safely and without side effects, it is always a good idea to talk with your doctor before taking any supplement.

BEST FOODS FOR FOLATE: *Fortified whole grain cereals, lentils, black-eyed peas, soybeans, oatmeal, turnip greens, spinach, mustard greens, green peas, artichokes, okra, beets, parsnips, broccoli, broccoli raab, sunflower seeds, wheat germ, oranges and juice, Brussels sprouts, papaya, seaweed, berries (boysenberries, blackberries, strawberries), beans (black, pinto, kidney, garbanzo, navy), cauliflower, Chinese cabbage, corn, whole grain bread, pasta (preferably whole wheat)*

FAQS

I had blood tests done recently. My LDL cholesterol is normal, my triglycerides are normal, but my HDL cholesterol is abnormally low. Is there anything I can do to improve my HDLs?

Some people have a genetic tendency to low HDL, even when all their other cardiovascular risk factors are normal. Although this might seem harmless, it can throw off your cholesterol ratio, and may indicate a future risk of heart problems. I recommend you incorporate a daily exercise regimen (exercise has been shown to boost HDL levels) and follow the diet and lifestyle recommendations in this chapter—these steps will help assure that your blood vessels stay as healthy as possible.

In addition, I recommend taking low dosages of omega-3 fatty acids (see Supplements section, page 144, for more information), and extended release formulations of niacin (such as Niaspan, which is only available by prescription). Extended-release niacin has been shown to raise HDL cholesterol by about 14 percent in men, and by about 20 percent in women. In addition, niacin can help lower triglycerides and LDL cholesterol.

It is important to talk with your doctor before beginning niacin treatment. Although niacin is a powerful treatment for boosting HDL cholesterol, it can be dangerous for people with diabetes, gallbladder disease, gout, glaucoma, peptic ulcer, or impaired liver function, or who are pregnant or have had a recent heart attack. In addition, niacin can interact with other medications, and it may cause some uncomfortable side effects, including flu-like symptoms, rash, and flushing so intense that it can temporarily leave you looking sunburned and feeling like you're having a hot flash.

Ask your doctor for a specific recommendation for the type of niacin to choose—it comes in extended-release, controlled-release, sustained-release, or regular formulations, so it isn't as easy as picking just any supplement off the shelf.

BEST FOODS FOR VITAMIN B₆: *Fortified whole grain cereals, chickpeas (garbanzo beans), wild salmon (fresh, canned), lean beef, pork tenderloin, chicken breast, white potatoes (with skin), oatmeal, bananas, pistachio nuts, lentils, tomato paste, barley, rice (brown, wild), peppers, sweet potatoes, winter squash (acorn), broccoli, broccoli raab, carrots, Brussels sprouts, peanut butter, eggs, shrimp, tofu, apricots, watermelon, avocado, strawberries, whole grain bread*

BEST FOODS FOR VITAMIN B₁₂: *Shellfish (clams, oysters, crab), wild salmon (fresh, canned), fortified whole grain cereal, enriched/fortified soy milk, trout (rainbow, wild), tuna (canned light), lean beef, veggie burgers, cottage cheese (fat-free, 1% reduced-fat), yogurt (fat-free, low-fat), milk (fat-free, 1% reduced-fat), eggs, cheese (fat-free, reduced-fat)*

CALCIUM AND VITAMIN D

Calcium and vitamin D work as a team—vitamin D helps the body absorb and use calcium. These two nutrients have been shown to help reduce blood pressure by 3 to 10 percent. Although this doesn't sound like much, it could add up to about 15 percent reduction in risk for cardiovascular disease. Some research suggests that milk proteins may act similarly to antihypertensive (blood pressure–lowering) medications called *ACE inhibitors.*

BEST FOODS FOR CALCIUM: *Yogurt (fat-free, low-fat), milk (fat-free, 1% reduced-fat), enriched/fortified soy milk, calcium-fortified fruit juice, cheese (fat-free, reduced-fat), tofu with calcium, sardines (with bones), wild salmon (with bones), soybeans, frozen yogurt, low-fat ice cream, calcium-fortified whole grain waffles, bok choy, kale, white beans, broccoli, almonds*

BEST FOODS FOR VITAMIN D: *Wild salmon (with bones), mackerel (not king), sardines (with bones), herring, fortified milk (fat-free, 1% reduced-fat), enriched/fortified soy milk, egg yolks, mushrooms (especially shiitake), vitamin D–fortified margarine (soft tub, trans fat–free), fortified whole grain cereal*

MAGNESIUM

Although more research is needed, magnesium may turn out to be a potent ally for reducing the risk of cardiovascular disease. In lab animals, magnesium reduces inflammation and alters the way fats are metabolized. Human studies suggest that eating lots of magnesium-rich foods may reduce triglycerides, lower blood pressure, and increase HDL cholesterol. In a long-term, 15-year study, eating plenty of magnesium-rich foods reduced the risk of developing the metabolic syndrome by about 30 percent.

> **BEST FOODS FOR MAGNESIUM:** *Pumpkin seeds, spinach, Swiss chard, amaranth, sunflower seeds, cashews, almonds, quinoa, tempeh, sweet potatoes, white potatoes, soybeans, millet, beans (black, white, navy, lima, pinto, kidney), artichoke hearts, peanuts, peanut butter, chickpeas (garbanzo beans), brown rice, whole grain bread, sesame seeds, wheat germ, flaxseed*

POTASSIUM

Your blood levels of potassium and sodium are inextricably linked. When potassium is low, the body retains sodium (and, as discussed above, too much sodium raises blood pressure). When potassium is high, the body gets rid of sodium. Eating potassium-rich foods is important for maintaining a healthy balance of both minerals, and, by extension, for keeping blood pressure low. *Important note:* Do *not* take potassium supplements unless specifically prescribed by your doctor. Too much potassium will upset the balance, and could have serious, even life-threatening consequences.

> **BEST FOODS FOR POTASSIUM:** *White potatoes, yams, fat-free and low-fat yogurt, soybeans, Swiss chard, snapper, sweet potatoes, avocado, cantaloupe, artichokes, bananas, spinach, lettuce (especially romaine), radicchio, arugula, endive, black cod (sablefish), honeydew melon, pumpkin, milk (fat-free, 1% reduced-fat), carrots, beans (white, black, navy, kidney, pinto), lentils, lima beans, apricots, papaya, split peas, pistachio nuts, winter squash (acorn, butternut), enriched/fortified soy milk, watermelon, beets, tomatoes (including sauce, juice), kale, mushrooms, raisins, peanuts, plums, almonds, sunflower seeds, prunes (and juice), chickpeas (garbanzo beans), oranges (and juice), broccoli*

GARLIC

The naturally occurring compound called *allicin* is the active part of garlic that seems to help lower cholesterol. It acts as a powerful antioxidant, and may also affect the way LDL cholesterol is used in the body and reduce triglycerides. There is some evidence that garlic may also lower homocysteine and reduce blood pressure. Although most studies of garlic use garlic supplements, some have shown similar good results for raw garlic. Unfortunately a great many of my clients don't like or can't tolerate raw garlic. Either they don't like the taste or it upsets their stomachs. Still, I recommend adding garlic to your cooking—as much as you like, as often as your family and friends can stand. Gently sauté the garlic separately from other foods to avoid burning it, or bake it and enjoy it as a rich, nutty-flavored paste. Garlic can act as a blood thinner, so if you are already taking aspirin or warfarin, please make your doctor aware that you've added garlic to your diet. (See the Supplements section, page 144, for more information about garlic supplements.)

PLANT STEROLS OR STANOLS

Sterols and stanols are natural substances found in small amounts in the cell membrane of plants, including fruits, vegetables, legumes, nuts, and seeds. Sterols are found in relatively high amounts in pistachio nuts, sunflower seeds, sesame seeds, and wheat germ. In terms of their effects on the human body, plant sterols and stanols are virtually the same.

Sterols and stanols have a structure similar to cholesterol, and they compete with cholesterol for access to receptors in the small intestines. (Imagine 15 people all hoping to get a ride in their friend's Volkswagen Beetle—not everyone is going to be riding in the car.) Sterols/stanols compete with cholesterol, effectively blocking its access. Research has shown that sterols and stanols have been shown to cut the amount of cholesterol absorbed by the small intestines by about 50 percent, and to reduce LDL cholesterol levels by between 5 and 14 percent.

You can reap these cardiovascular benefits with just 2 grams of sterol/stanol per day, though you can't get that much eating fruits and vegetables alone. Sterols and stanols have been added to certain heart-healthy spreads that taste and cook just like margarine, including Take Control and Benecol spreads. These spreads have been found to be safe, with very few side effects (although some people complained of upset stomach). That said, they're only for those with cholesterol problems, who should consume no more than the amounts recommended: 2 to 3 tablespoons per day (each tablespoon provides 1 gram of sterol/stanol). You can use it on whole grain bread, melt it on heart-healthy vegetables, or use it in cooking. I recommend trying the *light* versions of these spreads to save yourself 30 calories per tablespoon. If you're not a bread eater, please don't start just to have a vehicle for these spreads! Instead, consider the plant stanol/sterol supplements. (See the Supplements section, page 144, for more information about nonfood sources of plant sterol/stanols.)

ALCOHOL

The benefits of alcohol depend, in part, on exactly what your cardiovascular risk factors are. If your problem is high triglycerides, alcohol should be considered a rare treat, if you indulge at all. Even small amounts of alcohol can increase triglyceride levels dramatically.

For other risk factors, research suggests that one or two servings of alcohol per day may be good for your heart—that's no more than one serving per day for women, and no more than two servings per day for men. Studies have shown that drinking moderate amounts of alcohol reduces the risk of coronary artery disease by about 25 percent, and reduces the risk of death from heart disease by about 12 percent. Alcohol seems to increase the good HDL cholesterol and prevent clots.

There are right ways and wrong ways to use alcohol for heart health. The right ways are to drink moderately, and with a meal. The optimal amount of alcohol is one or two drinks per day (one serving is 12 ounces of beer; 5 ounces of wine; or one shot of hard alcohol). Although all alcohol has heart-healthy benefits, red wine also contains antioxidants called *flavonoids* and *resveratrol*—an extra boost of nutrition. Studies show that people who drink these moderate amounts of alcohol have a lower risk of disease than abstainers . . . although I can't recommend starting to drink if you're a teetotaler.

The wrong way to use alcohol is to drink heavily. People who regularly drink five or more servings of alcohol per day have a higher risk of disease than people who drink moderately or who abstain completely. Even three or more drinks per day raises blood pressure and increases triglycerides. The worst risks are for binge drinkers—people who occasionally consume large amounts of alcohol. Women who have five or more drinks and men who have nine or more drinks in a single drinking episode put themselves at risk of what scientists call *major coronary events*—heart attacks, strokes, and death. No one wants to see a big celebration—a Super Bowl or bachelorette party—end that way. If your team makes it to the Super Bowl and loses, it's a bummer, but it doesn't have to be fatal.

If you are currently taking medication for lowering blood pressure or cholesterol, or if you have diabetes, *always* talk with your doctor about whether drinking alcohol makes sense for you. There are some questions about whether alcohol might interact with medications, or complicate potential liver problems.

FAQS

I can't tell you how happy I was when I read that chocolate may help improve blood pressure . . . is it true?

Yes, but with limitations. Scientists have discovered that the antioxidant flavonoids in chocolate can lower blood pressure, reduce inflammation, improve the elasticity of blood vessels, increase HDL, and limit the negative effects of LDL cholesterol. Dark chocolate contains more than double the amount of flavonoids as milk chocolate, and—another strike against it—the milk may stop the intestines from absorbing the flavonoids. So if you're going to eat chocolate, choose a variety that is at least 60 percent dark chocolate. Of course, chocolate is also rich with calories and fat that will lead to weight gain if you overdo it, so make sure that you eat chocolate only in 1-ounce snack-sized portions . . . and remember to account for the extra 150 calories in your daily calorie allotment.

MULTIPLE CHANGES, MEGA BENEFITS

I saved my client story for this point in the chapter because I'm guessing you're probably feeling a little overwhelmed right now. Take heart . . . as Sean did.

Sean was 36 years old, and about 35 pounds overweight. He had high blood pressure, LDL cholesterol of 170, HDL cholesterol of 48, and triglycerides of about 300. His internist was also a cardiologist, and wanted to put Sean on medication before he developed serious heart disease. Sean couldn't stand the thought of going on medication, so he made a deal with his doctor—if he didn't get his numbers down within two months, he would fill his prescription.

When Sean came to see me, his diet was a mess. He ate and partied like he was still in college. Weekends were orgies of buffalo wings, beer, pizza, and ice cream, all things he was loathe to give up . . . but he did. We made a game of his deal with the doctor—Beat

FAQS

I'm confused about coffee. Is it OK for me to have a cup in the morning, or will it increase my risk of cardiovascular disease?

I understand the confusion. It seems as though there is always something new being written about the benefits or risks of coffee. I can show you research that says that coffee might be dangerous, and I can show you research that says the exact opposite. Most important is to follow whatever your doctor tells you. If your doctor says no coffee, then that's your final answer. There might be something special about your medical history that requires limiting caffeine. No doubt the debate will continue as study results come in. In 2006, for example, researchers released the results of a large-scale study conducted at Harvard that followed more than 44,000 men and 84,000 women for nearly 20 years. They discovered that coffee didn't make any difference in the risk for heart attack or heart disease, regardless of whether the participants drank less than one cup of coffee per month or more than five cups per day. The one cautionary note: Drink only filtered coffee—unfiltered preparations such as percolated or French press coffee (including espresso and cappuccino) may cause an increase in homocysteine and LDL cholesterol.

the Medication. Sean did everything in this program. He stopped smoking. He started walking every evening with his wife and baby. He took fish oil capsules and plant stanol supplements. And he started eating only heart-healthy foods, including those with plenty of calcium and magnesium. He cut out salt and fruit juice and even stopped drinking beer. That was the hardest part, and it was a real struggle for Sean, but he was playing for keeps.

After two months, Sean had lost 17 pounds. His LDL cholesterol dropped 30 points to 140, his HDLs stayed the same, and his triglycerides—slashed by more than half—were down to 120. His doctor was thrilled and gave him another two months to get his LDLs closer to 100.

For the next two months, Sean continued the program and dropped another 16 pounds. At the end of four months, he got all his risk factors under control. His blood pressure was normal, his HDL was the same, his LDL was down to 124, and his triglycerides fell to 105. He did it! He beat the medication. Even better, he felt fabulous, energetic, and empowered. Ultimately, his doctor and I would love to see his LDL cholesterol come down even more, and I am optimistic it will happen.

Want to be like Sean? It is never too late to make these healthy changes. Study after study has shown that the more heart-healthy living you do, the greater the benefits. With cardiovascular disease, you don't want to wait. don't forget we're talking about stroke, heart attack, and the possibility of sudden death. Be like Sean. Do it all. You may be able to heal yourself. But even if you need to take medications, that doesn't diminish the good that you're doing for yourself. Some people need medication, even if they do everything right, and that group includes two of my own relatives! Even then, this program is important.

BONUS POINTS

- **Know all your numbers.** Don't rely on your doctor to keep track of your blood pressure, triglycerides, and cholesterol levels—they don't do much good sitting in a medical file drawer. Every time you have your blood tested, write down your numbers, and track your progress. Most doctors recommend follow-up blood work every year or every six months, depending on your individual health concerns. There's nothing more motivating than results—in this case seeing your numbers drop steadily lower and lower. Work with your doctor to set goals for each of the following tests: Blood pressure, LDL cholesterol, HDL cholesterol, cholesterol ratio (total cholesterol divided by HDL cholesterol), triglycerides, homocysteine, and C-reactive protein.

■ **Ask about iron and thyroid.** Heart disease risk can be affected by elevated ferritin (a measure of iron), and high cholesterol can be a side effect of low levels of thyroid hormones. Talk with your doctor about whether you need to have these additional tests.

■ **If you smoke, quit.** Smoking causes inflammation, not just in your lungs, but throughout your body. Inflammation can contribute to atherosclerosis, blood clots, and risk of heart attack. Smoking makes all heart health indicators worse. If you have high cholesterol, high triglycerides, or high blood pressure, smoking magnifies the danger.

■ **If you are overweight, focus on losing weight.** Body fat produces and secretes hormones and other types of biochemicals, including inflammatory chemicals. People who are overweight have higher levels of C-reactive protein, a marker for inflammation. And as already discussed, inflammation contributes to atherosclerosis and heart attacks. In addition, being overweight increases blood pressure and decreases HDL cholesterol. In 2006, researchers found that the more overweight you are, the greater your risk of death . . . not just from heart disease, but from all causes. Even if you have normal blood pressure, normal cholesterol and don't smoke, being overweight increases the risk of death from heart disease by more than 40 percent. You don't have to return to your high school weight to see a benefit—every little bit helps. Research has shown that losing just 10 pounds can reduce LDL cholesterol by 5 to 8 percent. (See Weight Loss on page 19 for more information on how to lose weight while following this heart-healthy program.)

■ **Become more physically active.** Even moderate exercise can help improve cholesterol, triglycerides, and blood pressure. Aerobic exercise seems to be able to stop the sharp rise of triglycerides after eating, perhaps because of a decrease in the amount of triglyceride released by the liver, or because active muscle clears triglycerides out of the blood stream more quickly than inactive muscle. If you haven't exercised regularly (or at all) for years, I recommend starting slowly, by walking at an easy pace for 15 minutes a day, five days a week. Then, as you feel comfortable, increase the amount of time by five minutes each day. Strive to work up to 45 minutes each day. (Always get clearance from your doctor before beginning an exercise program.) If you are relatively healthy and are cleared for exercise, research shows that you might get optimal heart benefit from moderate-intensity exercise that burns about 500 calories or more. This means brisk walking for about 90 minutes, three to five times per week. I know it sounds like a lot, but your life may depend on it.

■ **If you also have diabetes, control your blood sugar.** Uncontrolled blood sugar can increase your risk of coronary artery disease, heart attack, and stroke. Part of your heart care is diabetes care. (For more information about nutritional advice for diabetes, see Type 2 Diabetes on page 191.)

■ **Manage stress.** High blood pressure has been linked to emotional stress and anxiety. It is so common that the phrase *white-coat hypertension* has been used to describe the spike in blood pressure some people experience in the stressful setting of the doctor's office. The best stress reducers are meditation (especially Transcendental Meditation), going to church or temple, biofeedback, guided relaxation, and cognitive-behavioral therapy. Taking time to play with or pet a dog or cat also seems to help. (In case you're wondering, watching TV does not work as a stress reliever—scientists actually checked.) Research has shown that reducing stress can reduce blood pressure by as much as 10 percent. It may not seem like much, but it's not bad for a few minutes of meditation or quiet relaxation every day.

- **If you have hypertension, avoid hot tubs.** Well, not just hot tubs, but also saunas, steam rooms, hot baths, and other activities that relax your body with heat. They can raise your heart rate and cause dizziness, while raising blood pressure even higher.
- **Get enough sleep.** Research shows that people who get six to eight hours of sleep per night have less risk of developing hypertension than people who got five hours or less per night. It could be that people who sleep too little have a lot of stress, and their lack of rest may make them too tired to follow through on healthy diet and exercise plans. When you make time for sleep, you may also find that it's easier to make time for everything else, too.

SUPPLEMENTS

If you are trying to get your cholesterol under control, and want to consider supplements *in addition to* the food fixes, I recommend:

1. **Multivitamin.** To assure that you're getting all the vitamins and minerals necessary for good health, consider taking a daily multivitamin. Choose a senior formula, which typically provides extra amounts of the B vitamins involved in homocysteine reduction *without* any iron. There is no need to take mega doses—100% DV of most vitamins and minerals is sufficient.

2. **Soluble fiber.** I recommend getting as much soluble fiber from the foods in your diet as possible. However, if you can't regularly eat five to eight servings of fruits and veggies a day, I recommend adding a psyllium soluble fiber supplement. Take 5 to 10 grams per day with a full glass of water. Common and respected brands include Metamucil, Fiberall, and Konsyl. Because fiber supplements can interfere with some medications, talk with your doctor before taking them. Common side effects include bloating and flatulence. Severe allergic reactions have been reported in rare circumstances.

3. **Omega-3s from fish oil.** If you can't get enough fish oil from your diet, I recommend taking fish oil capsules. I recommend a standard 1 gram (1,000 milligrams) daily for raising HDL or fighting general heart disease. These supplements also have been shown to lower triglycerides by 20 to 50 percent, but this effect requires a higher dosage of 2 to 4 grams. *Important note:* Dosages this high should only be taken under a doctor's supervision. (It is possible to get a prescription for these higher doses, so you may want to check to see if your medical prescription plan will cover it.) There are two types of omega-3s: EPA (eicosapentaenoic acid) and DHA (docosahexaenoic acid).

Check the label to ensure that each gram contains at least 220 milligrams from EPA and 240 grams from DHA. (The remainder can be from either.) Store in the fridge to prevent rancidity. To prevent fishy burps, buy enteric-coated varieties, take with food, and split doses throughout day. Because fish oil acts as a blood thinner, it should *not* be taken by people who have hemophilia, or who are already taking blood thinning medications or are on aspirin therapy (unless approved by their doctor). People with diabetes should talk with their doctors before trying fish oil supplements because they may affect blood sugar.

4. **Garlic.** Some studies show that taking garlic supplements for at least 4 to 25 weeks may reduce LDL cholesterol by 4 to 12 percent—not a mind-blowing reduction, but you may want to consider garlic if you want to try absolutely everything. Look for products standardized to provide 1.3% allicin, or aged-garlic extracts. I recommend taking 200 to 400 milligrams three times per day (for a total of 600 to 1,200 milligrams/day). *Important note:* Garlic can affect the way other medications work and some individuals may have adverse reactions, so always talk with your doctor before starting to take garlic supplements. Because garlic acts as a blood thinner, do *not* take garlic supplements if you are currently on aspirin therapy or blood thinning medications or supplements (unless approved by your doctor).

5. **Sterols/stanols.** If you don't use spreads and want to get the benefits of plant sterols and stanols without extra calories, you might consider taking supplements. My favorite is Cholest-Off by Nature Made. You have to take two tablets in the morning and two tablets at night (a total of four tablets a day), 15 to 30 minutes before a meal. If you are taking a prescription cholesterol-lowering medication, talk with your doctor before taking sterol/stanol supplements.

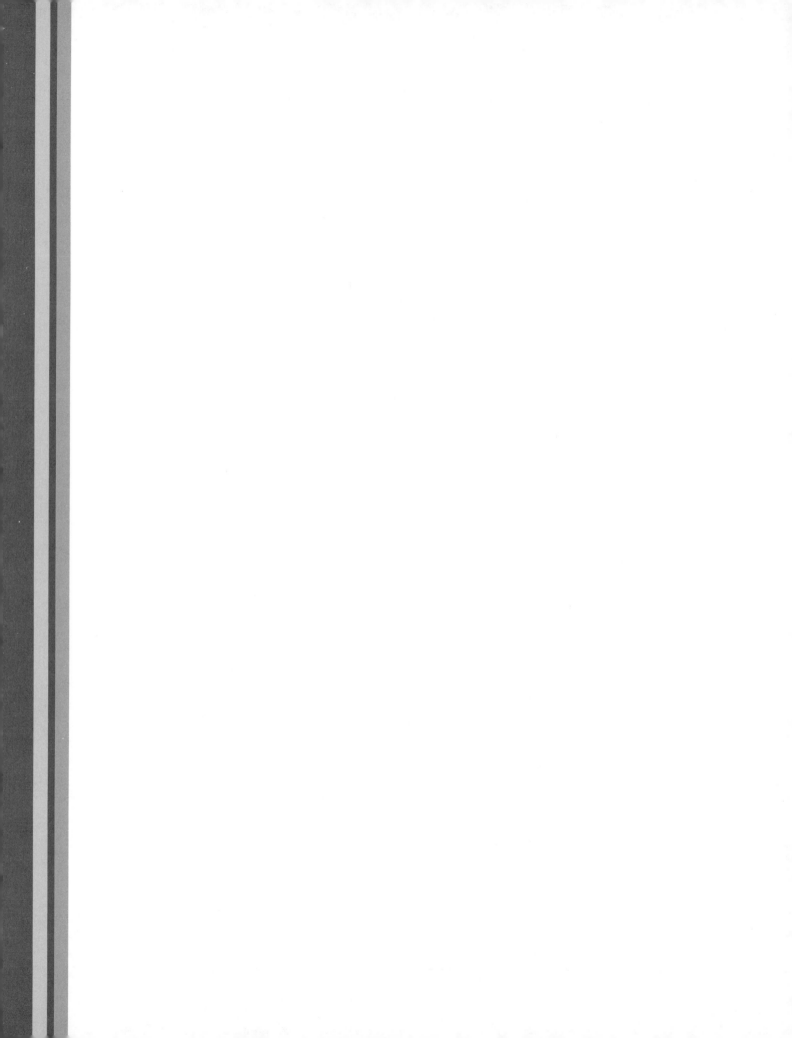

JOY'S 4-STEP PROGRAM
FOR CARDIOVASCULAR DISEASE

Follow this program if you high cholesterol, high blood pressure, if you have been told you have cardiovascular disease, or if you have had a heart attack or stroke. If you have a family history of cardiovascular disease, you may want to follow this program to help prevent future problems.

STEP1 ...START WITH THE BASICS

These are the first things you should do to get control over your cardiovascular risk factors:

- If it has been more than a year since your last doctor visit, consider going in for a heart disease check up. Blood levels of cholesterol, triglycerides, and other risk factors can change dramatically in one year. Get your most recent numbers. Ask about whether you also should be checked for blood ferritin, thyroid, and blood sugar levels.

- If you smoke, quit.

- If you are overweight, lose weight.

- Begin a program of regular exercise. Always talk with your doctor before starting, and consult your doctor immediately if you experience unusual chest pain, left arm pain or tingling, or general weakness during or after exercise.

STEP 2 ... YOUR ULTIMATE GROCERY LIST

The foods you choose are critical for good cardiovascular health. This list contains foods with high levels of nutrients that can help you get your risk factors under control, including magnesium, calcium, vitamin D, potassium, B vitamins, soluble fiber, and omega-3 fatty acids—plus some foods used as ingredients in the meal plans and recipes. You don't have to purchase every item . . . but these foods should make up the bulk of what you eat for the week. If you find yourself getting bored, try some unfamiliar foods from these groups—they may become favorites. Skip dried fruit, fruit juice, and alcohol if you have high triglycerides. Skip grapefruit and grapefruit juice if you're on any cardiac medication. Look for low-salt alternatives for canned and packaged favorites.

FRUIT

ALL fruits, but especially:	blackberries, raspberries, strawberries)	if you're taking medication)	Pears
Apples	Cantaloupe	Juice, calcium-fortified	Plums
Apricots	Dates	Melon, honeydew	Prunes (and juice)
Bananas	Figs	Oranges (and juice)	Raisins
Berries (boysenberries,	Grapefruit (skip	Papaya	Watermelon
		Peaches	

VEGETABLES

ALL vegetables, but especially:	Cabbage (including Chinese)	Mustard greens	Soybeans (edamame)
Artichokes (including hearts)	Carrots	Okra	Spinach
Arugula	Cauliflower	Olives	Squash, winter (acorn, butternut)
Asparagus	Chickpeas (garbanzo beans)	Onions, especially red	Swiss chard
Avocado	Collard greens	Parsley	Tomatoes (including tomato sauce, juice, paste)
Beans (black, kidney, lima, navy, pinto, white, garbanzo)	Corn	Parsnips	Turnip greens
Beets	Endive	Peas (black-eyed, split)	Watercress
Bok choy	Escarole	Peas	Yams
Broccoli	Kale	Peppers	
Broccoli raab	Lentils	Potatoes, sweet	
Brussels sprouts	Lettuce (all varieties, especially romaine)	Potatoes, white	
	Mushrooms (especially shiitake)	Pumpkin, fresh and canned 100% pure pumpkin puree	
		Radicchio	
		Seaweed	

SEAFOOD

Anchovies	Mackerel (not king)	Sardines (with bones)	Snapper
Black cod (sablefish)	Salmon, wild (with	Shellfish (shrimp, clams,	Trout (rainbow, wild)
Herring	bones)	Pacific oysters, crab)	Tuna (canned light)

LEAN MEATS/EGGS/SOY FOODS

Beef, lean	Pork tenderloin	Turkey breast, ground	Veggie burgers
Chicken breast	Tempeh	lean	
Eggs (especially omega-	Tofu (with calcium)	Turkey breast, sliced	
3–fortified)	Turkey bacon, lean	Turkey burgers	

NUTS AND SEEDS (PREFERABLY UNSALTED)

MOST nuts, but	Cashews	Pecans	Sunflower seeds
especially:	Flaxseed, ground	Pine nuts	Walnuts
Almonds	Hazelnuts	Pistachio nuts	
Brazil nuts	Macadamia nuts	Psyllium seeds, ground	
Butternuts (white	Peanut butter	Pumpkin seeds	
walnuts)	Peanuts	Sesame seeds	

WHOLE GRAINS

Amaranth	Millet	Pita bread, whole	Tortillas, whole grain
Barley	Oat bran	wheat	or spinach
Bread, whole grain	Oatmeal	Quinoa	Waffles, calcium-
Cereals, fortified whole	Pasta (preferably whole	Rice (brown, wild)	fortified whole grain
grain	wheat)	Rice bran	Wheat germ

DAIRY

Cheese (fat-free,	Cottage cheese (fat-free,	(fat-free, 1% reduced-	Yogurt (fat-free,
reduced-fat)	1% reduced-fat)	fat)	low-fat)
Cheese, fat-free Cheddar	Ice cream, low-fat	Soy milk, enriched/	Yogurt, frozen (fat-free,
(for meal plan)	Milk	fortified	low-fat)

MISCELLANEOUS

Artificial sweetener	Mayonnaise, reduced-	Paprika	Salt substitute
Basil, fresh and dried	fat	Parsley, fresh	Stanol/sterol spread,
Garlic	Mustard, Dijon	Pepper, black	soft tub (regular or
Hot sauce	Nonstick cooking spray	Pepper flakes, hot red	light)
Hummus	Oil, canola	Rosemary, fresh	Thyme, fresh and dried
Margarine spread,	Oil, flaxseed	Sage, fresh	Vinegar, balsamic or
reduced-fat vitamin	Oil, olive	Salad dressing,	red wine
D–fortified, soft tub,	Oil, walnut	reduced-calorie	
trans fat–free	Oregano, dried	Salsa	

STEP3...GOING ABOVE AND BEYOND

If you want to do everything you can to reduce your risk factors, here are some additional things you might try:

- Consider taking a senior formula multivitamin.

- Avoid eating foods high in saturated fats, trans fats, cholesterol, salt, and refined carbohydrates.

- Talk with your doctor about whether omega-3, sterol/stanol, garlic, or soluble fiber supplements might be right for you.

- Try to get enough sleep.

SALT SUBSTITUTES

If you need to be on a sodium-controlled diet, salt substitutes (such as Mrs. Dash and Morton) are a way to enjoy food without having to endure blandness. Some salt substitutes use potassium chloride (instead of sodium chloride found in regular salt); the taste is similar, but it is not for everyone. People with kidney problems or who are taking certain medications should not use potassium chloride, so ask your doctor if you can use it. But everyone can enjoy the many other seasonings out there. Instead of salt, experiment with cayenne (hot) pepper, lemon or lime juice, garlic powder (not garlic salt), herb blends (without salt), flavored vinegars, wine, dill, nutmeg, cilantro, celery seed (not celery salt), curry powder, and wasabi powder (very hot!).

STEP4 ...MEAL PLANS

These sample menus include foods that have been shown to be protective against cardio-vascular disease, and none of the dangerous foods.

Every day, choose *one* option for each of the three meals—breakfast, lunch, and dinner. Then, one or two times per day, choose from a variety of my suggested snacks. Approximate calories have been provided to help adjust for your personal weight management goals. If you find yourself hungry (and if weight is not an issue), feel free to increase the portion sizes for meals and snacks. Beverage calories are *not* included.

BREAKFAST OPTIONS

(Approximately 300 to 400 calories)

Oatmeal with Milk and Fresh Berries

½ cup dry instant oatmeal prepared with 1 cup water or milk (fat-free, 1% reduced-fat, or enriched/fortified soy); top with 2 tablespoons ground flaxseed (or wheat germ) and ½ cup berries (sliced strawberries, raspberries, blackberries). Sweeten with optional 1 teaspoon sugar, honey, or artificial sweetener.

Hearty Eggs with Vegetables and Toast

Beat 1 whole omega-3–fortified egg plus 2 egg whites. Cook in a hot skillet coated with nonstick cooking spray, adding 2 tablespoons chopped tomato and unlimited spinach, mushrooms, peppers, and onion. Serve with toasted whole grain English muffin (or 2 slices whole wheat toast), dry or with 2 teaspoons soft tub stanol/sterol spread. Instead of ½ of the English muffin or 1 slice toast, you may substitute 1 serving fruit (1 orange, 1 plum, 1 apple, 1 small banana, ½ grapefruit, or ¼ cantaloupe).

Apple Slices with Peanut Butter

2½ level tablespoons peanut butter spread on 1 sliced apple (or banana).

Cereal with Milk, Nuts, and Wheat Germ

1 cup whole grain fortified cereal mixed with 1 cup milk (fat-free, 1% reduced-fat, or enriched/fortified soy), topped with 1 tablespoon chopped walnuts and 1 tablespoon wheat germ (or ground flaxseed). Enjoy with 1 orange (or ½ banana or ½ grapefruit).

Breakfast Burrito

Beat 1 whole omega-3–fortified egg with 2 egg whites. Cook on griddle coated with nonstick cooking spray. Mix cooked eggs with ¼ cup black beans and 2 tablespoons shredded fat-free or reduced-fat cheese. Wrap in a whole grain or spinach tortilla (150 calories or less). Serve with optional onions, peppers, salsa, and/or hot sauce.

Strawberry-Banana Cottage Cheese with Almonds

1 cup 1% reduced-fat or fat-free cottage cheese (or 8 ounces fat-free plain or flavored yogurt) mixed with ½ sliced banana, ½ cup chopped strawberries, and 1 tablespoon slivered almonds.

Broccoli-Cheese Egg White Omelet with Turkey Bacon

Sauté 1 cup broccoli florets in skillet coated with nonstick cooking spray until soft. Beat 1 whole egg with 3 egg whites and add to broccoli. When bottom is cooked, gently flip and cook other side. Top with 2 tablespoons shredded fat-free cheese. Fold omelet over and cook until cheese melts; season with salt substitute and ground black pepper. Enjoy with 2 strips lean turkey bacon and ½ grapefruit (or ¼ cantaloupe or 1 orange).

LUNCH OPTIONS

(Approximately 400 to 500 calories)

Turkey-Avocado Sandwich

4 ounces sliced turkey breast (or lean ham or grilled chicken breast), 2 to 3 thin slices avocado, romaine lettuce or spinach leaves, tomato, and onion on 2 slices whole grain bread or pita. Spread with optional mustard, 2 teaspoons reduced-fat mayonnaise, or hummus. Enjoy with large handful baby carrots or pepper sticks (red, yellow, green).

Hearty Grilled Chicken Salad

4 ounces grilled skinless chicken breast on a large bed of mixed leafy greens (romaine, spinach, mustard greens, collard greens, endive), topped with ½ cup cherry tomatoes, 1 chopped bell pepper, mushrooms, artichoke hearts, 2 tablespoons chickpeas (garbanzo beans), 2 tablespoons beans (kidney, black, navy, or soybeans), and ¼ chopped avocado. Toss with 2 teaspoons olive oil and unlimited vinegar or fresh lemon juice (or 2 to 4 tablespoons reduced-calorie dressing).

Edamame with Wild Salmon Dijonnaise

1 cup boiled edamame (soybeans in the pod), lightly sprinkled with salt substitute. Enjoy with 5 ounces canned wild salmon with bones, drained, mashed, and mixed with 1 tablespoon reduced-fat mayonnaise, 1 to 2 teaspoons Dijon mustard, minced onion, and black pepper. Serve on large bed of leafy greens (spinach, romaine, etc.) tossed with fresh lemon juice or 2 tablespoons reduced-calorie dressing.

Vegetable-Cheese Omelet with Baked Potato

Beat 1 whole egg with 2 to 3 egg whites. Cook in skillet coated with nonstick cooking spray. Add 3 tablespoons chopped tomato, ½ cup sliced mushrooms, and optional dried basil. When bottom is cooked, gently flip and cook some more. Top with 1 ounce shredded reduced-fat or fat-free cheese. Fold omelet and continue cooking until egg mixture firms and cheese melts. Enjoy with 1 plain medium baked white or sweet potato.

Heart-Smart Turkey Burger with Veggies

1 (5-ounce) lean turkey burger (or any store-bought turkey or veggie burger 200 calories or less) with optional 2 tablespoons guacamole, tomato, onion, and salsa. Enjoy on ½ whole grain bun (or in 70-calorie pita pocket). Serve with 1 cup raw or cooked vegetables (broccoli, cauliflower, carrots, kale, Brussels sprouts, green beans, mushrooms, Swiss chard, beets, artichokes, spinach, collard greens, or asparagus).

Mixed Vegetable Salad with Sardines

4 ounces (about 8) sardines with bones (canned in oil or tomato sauce), tossed with unlimited leafy greens, tomatoes, carrots, mushrooms, peppers, onions, and ½ cup beans (choose from white, navy, kidney, chickpeas, or soybeans). Drizzle with 2 to 4 tablespoons reduced-calorie salad dressing (or 1 teaspoon olive oil and unlimited vinegar or fresh lemon juice); season with salt substitute and fresh ground pepper.

Hearty Yogurt Fruit Fiesta

1 cup fat-free vanilla yogurt (or 1% reduced-fat or fat-free cottage cheese) mixed with ½ chopped apple (or pear), ½ sliced banana, and ½ cup berries (or substitute favorite fruits). Top with 2 tablespoons ground flaxseed, 1 tablespoon sunflower seeds, and 1 tablespoon chopped walnuts.

DINNER OPTIONS

(Approximately 500 to 600 calories)

Heart-Smart Surf and Turf

1 serving Tuscan Bean Dip (page 159) with unlimited carrots, celery, and pepper sticks. Serve with 5 ounces grilled or baked tilapia (or wild salmon, trout, or red snapper) seasoned with 1 teaspoon olive oil, preferred herbs, pepper, optional salt substitute, and fresh lemon juice.

Pork Tenderloin with Roasted Balsamic Carrots and Potato

5 ounces grilled, baked, or broiled pork tenderloin. Enjoy with 2 servings Roasted Balsamic Carrots (page 158) and ½ plain medium baked potato (or ½ cup brown or wild rice).

Whole Wheat Penne with Sea Bass and Green Peas

1 serving Whole Wheat Penne with Sea Bass and Pea Sauce (page 324; feel free to substitute fish of choice). Serve with side salad of leafy greens, mushrooms, carrots, and 1 tablespoon chopped walnuts tossed with 2 teaspoons olive oil and vinegar or fresh lemon juice (or 2 to 4 tablespoons reduced-calorie dressing).

Hearty Turkey Meat Loaf with Salad

1 serving Hearty Turkey Meat Loaf (page 156). Enjoy with large tossed salad of leafy greens, sliced peppers, mushrooms, carrots, tomatoes, optional beets, and artichokes, tossed with ½ cup beans (choose from black, navy, chickpeas, pinto, kidney) and 2 teaspoons olive oil and unlimited vinegar or fresh lemon juice (or 2 to 4 tablespoons reduced-calorie salad dressing).

Pesto Salmon with Roasted Artichoke Hearts

1 serving Pesto Salmon with Roasted Artichoke Hearts (page 157). Serve with ½ plain medium baked white or sweet potato topped with optional 1 tablespoon reduced-fat plant stanol spread (such as Benecol Light or Take Control Light).

Chopped Chicken Salad with Apples and Walnuts

1 serving Chopped Chicken Salad with Apples and Walnuts (page 325; use Red Delicious apple in salad).

Turkey Chili with Black Beans, Corn, and Brown Rice

1 serving (2 cups) Turkey Chili (page 367), topped with 1 ounce shredded fat-free Cheddar cheese. Serve with mixed salad of leafy greens (optional peppers, carrots, beets, and artichokes) tossed with 1 teaspoon olive oil and unlimited balsamic vinegar or fresh lemon juice (or 2 tablespoons reduced-calorie dressing); and ½ cup cooked brown rice (or ½ plain medium baked white or sweet potato).

SNACK OPTIONS

100 calories or less

- *Best Vegetables:* 1 cup raw or cooked bell peppers (red, green, yellow), broccoli, broccoli raab, chili peppers, kale, Brussels sprouts, Chinese cabbage, red cabbage, tomatoes, mushrooms, green beans, okra, carrots, lettuce and leafy greens (mustard greens, turnip greens, endive, escarole), spinach, collards, Swiss chard, watercress, asparagus, okra, artichokes, beets, cauliflower, or seaweed

- *Best Fruits:* 1 apple (especially Red Delicious with skin), small banana, orange, pear, or peach; 2 plums; ½ papaya, grapefruit, or cantaloupe; 1 cup boysenberries, blackberries, raspberries, sliced strawberries, watermelon, or honeydew; 4 apricots or prunes; 2 dates or figs; 20 strawberries; 2 tablespoons raisins

- 1 level tablespoon peanut butter with celery sticks

- 6 ounces fat-free, flavored or plain yogurt

- 10 almonds, unsalted

- 1 cup Vegetable Oatmeal Bisque (page 323)

- 1 cup fat-free milk

100 to 200 calories

- 10 almonds plus 1 serving fruit

- Edamame: 1 cup boiled soybeans in the pod, seasoned with salt substitute

- Unsalted whole nuts: 1 ounce (about ¼ cup) of your choice of almonds, cashews, toasted pecans, walnuts, or peanuts

- ¼ cup pistachio nuts or sunflower seeds in the shell

- 8 macadamia nuts

- ½ cup fat-free or 1% reduced-fat cottage cheese mixed with 2 tablespoons ground flaxseed (or wheat germ)

- 1 slice whole grain toast (or 70-calorie pita bread) with 1 level tablespoon peanut butter

- 1 cup fat-free, plain yogurt mixed with ½ cup berries and 1 tablespoon ground flaxseed or wheat germ

- 1 cup baby carrots or pepper sticks with ¼ cup hummus or guacamole

- 1 sliced apple with 1 level tablespoon peanut butter

- Frozen banana: peel banana, slice into several ½ inch wheels, place in a small plastic bag, and freeze. Enjoy with optional 1 cup fat-free milk.

- Strawberry-Banana Fruit Smoothie: in blender, mix 1 cup fat-free milk, 1 cup frozen strawberries, ½ frozen banana

- 1 serving Warm Dark Chocolate Sauce with Fresh Fruit (page 81)

- Vanilla Pumpkin Yogurt Pudding: 1 cup vanilla fat-free flavored yogurt mixed with ½ cup canned 100% pure pumpkin puree

HEARTY TURKEY MEAT LOAF

You won't miss the high-fat beef in my heart-smart version of meat loaf. It's got great flavor and health-boosting ingredients—even oatmeal (instead of white bread crumbs), which adds soluble fiber and creates the perfect consistency.

Makes 4 servings

1	pound lean ground turkey breast
1	small summer zucchini, grated
1	cup instant oatmeal
½	cup shiitake mushrooms, chopped
¼	cup fat-free milk
¼	cup fresh basil, thinly sliced
3	tablespoons reduced-sodium soy sauce
2	egg whites
4	cloves garlic, minced
½	teaspoon dried thyme
½	teaspoon dried oregano
	Salt substitute
	Ground black pepper to taste

1. Preheat the oven to 350°F. Coat a 1-quart loaf pan with cooking spray or line with aluminum foil.
2. In a large bowl, mix the turkey, zucchini, oatmeal, mushrooms, milk, basil, soy sauce, egg whites, garlic, thyme, and oregano and season with salt substitute and pepper.
3. Press the turkey mixture into the loaf pan and cover with aluminum foil. Bake 40 minutes. Remove foil and bake 5 to 10 minutes longer, until the top begins to brown and the center is no longer pink. Serve immediately.

PER SERVING
239 calories, 33 g protein, 20 g carbohydrate, 3 g fat (0 g saturated), 45 mg cholesterol, 569 mg sodium, 3 g fiber; plus 61 IU vitamin D (15% DV), 46 mg magnesium (12% DV)

PESTO SALMON WITH ROASTED ARTICHOKE HEARTS

Swimming with omega-3 fats, salmon is one of the world's most heart-healthy foods. You'll up the ante with my pesto variation, which incorporates walnuts, garlic, olive oil, and artichokes—ingredients that will satisfy your ticker as well as your taste buds.

Makes 2 servings

- 2   cups fresh basil leaves
- 1   tablespoon walnuts, chopped
- 3   cloves garlic, minced
-      Salt substitute
- 1   can (16 ounces) artichoke hearts, rinsed and drained, or 1 package (9 ounces) frozen artichoke hearts, rinsed and thawed
- 1   large tomato, diced
- 1   teaspoon fresh thyme leaves, chopped
-      Ground black pepper
- 2   fillets (6 ounces each) wild salmon, skin removed
- 1   tablespoon olive oil

1. Preheat the oven to 350°F. Line an 8" × 11" baking pan with parchment paper or aluminum foil.
2. In a blender or food processor, combine the basil, walnuts, one-half of the garlic, and salt substitute to taste. Blend until the mixture resembles a coarse meal.
3. Arrange the artichoke hearts in 2 separate mounds in the prepared pan. Top with the tomato and sprinkle with the thyme and salt substitute and pepper to taste. Place one salmon fillet on top of each artichoke mound and season with salt substitute and pepper. Spread the basil mixture on the fillets. Drizzle each fillet with ½ tablespoon olive oil.
4. Bake 20 to 25 minutes, until the fillets are no longer translucent in the center and the fish flakes when pressed with a fork. Serve immediately.

PER SERVING
430 calories, 41 g protein, 22 g carbohydrate, 20 g fat (2.7 g saturated), 93 mg cholesterol, 500 mg sodium, 5 g fiber

ROASTED BALSAMIC CARROTS

When it comes to heart health, carrots alone provide soluble fiber, potassium, and vitamin B$_6$. In this recipe, the addition of olive oil and garlic makes it that much more potent. Just another way to enjoy one of our all-time favorite vegetables!

Makes 4 servings

1	pound carrots, peeled and cut into wedges
1/4	cup balsamic vinegar
2	tablespoons minced fresh rosemary
2	cloves garlic, minced
1/4	teaspoon paprika
	Salt substitute
	Ground black pepper
1	tablespoons olive oil

1. Preheat the oven to 400°F.
2. Tear a large piece of aluminum foil, about 24" long. Spread the carrots out evenly over one half. Sprinkle with the vinegar, rosemary, garlic, and paprika. Season with salt substitute and pepper. Drizzle with the olive oil and fold the opposite end over, folding around the edges to make a neat package with no openings. Place the package on a baking sheet and bake 20 to 25 minutes, until the carrots are tender when pierced with a knife. Serve immediately.

PER SERVING
90 calories, 1 g protein, 15 g carbohydrate, 4 g fat (0 g saturated), 0 mg cholesterol, 79 mg sodium, 4 g fiber; plus 540 mg potassium (15% DV)

TUSCAN BEAN DIP

Vegetables go down easy when you have something delicious to dip them in. A friend once watched in shock as her vegetable-hating daughter cleared a plate of crudités with this dish. Give it a try—it's loaded with taste and, thanks to the beans, provides lots of protein and fiber.

Makes 3 servings, ½ cup each

1	can (16 ounces) cannellini or navy beans, rinsed and drained
2	tablespoons balsamic vinegar
2	teaspoons olive oil
2	tablespoons thinly sliced basil leaves
½	teaspoon chopped fresh sage or rosemary
2	cloves garlic, minced
⅛	teaspoon hot red pepper flakes
	Ground black pepper
	Salt substitute

In a large bowl, mash the beans with the back of a fork or a hand-held potato masher. Stir in the vinegar, olive oil, basil, sage or rosemary, garlic, and pepper flakes. Season to taste with salt substitute and pepper. Serve immediately with vegetable sticks.

PER SERVING
210 calories, 12 g protein, 33 g carbohydrate, 3.5 g fat (0 g saturated), 0 mg cholesterol, 30 mg sodium, 8 g fiber; plus 75 mg magnesium (20% DV), 462 mg potassium (13% DV), 96 mcg folic acid (25% DV)

CHAPTER 8

ARTHRITIS

As anyone with arthritis can tell you, arthritis sufferers truly suffer. Osteoarthritis can wear down the knees. Rheumatoid arthritis can twist and deform the fingers. And gout can make walking an exercise in masochism.

Arthritis is not a single disease, but a category that includes about a hundred joint-related disorders. According to the National Institutes of Health, arthritis affects about one in every five people in the United States—most of whom don't realize how much nutrition can improve the way they feel. In some cases, such as with gout, a change in diet can often dramatically reduce symptoms. Because arthritis can have such debilitating effects, stumbling on even a single piece of helpful information can feel like unearthing a buried treasure. I remember the first time I talked about arthritis on the *Today* show, I got an overwhelming number of phone calls—hundreds of them!—asking for more details. That's what this chapter is all about . . . helpful details that could bring your pain level down a few critical notches.

WHAT AFFECTS ARTHRITIS?

In medical lingo, the suffix *–itis* means *inflammation*. Arthritis, then, means any disease that involves inflammation of the joints. But let's start at the very beginning and talk about what joints are made of.

Joints are places where bones come together. Some, such as the joints that connect the bones of the skull, are stable and immovable. Others have minimal mobility, such as the joints connecting the vertebrae of the spine. But most joints of the body are *synovial joints,* which allow for varying degrees of movement, depending on their structure. For example, shoulders and hips are able to move freely in every direction because of their ball-and-socket design, while elbows and knees bend in a single direction, like a hinge.

All synovial joints share certain features:

1. The ends of the bones are coated with a soft, smooth substance called *cartilage,* which helps to cushion the bone and reduce friction.
2. The joint is encased by a ligament that holds the bones together. This ligament forms a capsule around the entire joint.
3. The inside of the capsule is covered by a special lining called the *synovial membrane.*
4. The synovial membrane secretes a lubricating fluid called, you guessed it, *synovial fluid.*

Of all the different types of arthritis, the two most common are *osteoarthritis* and *rheumatoid arthritis.*

OSTEOARTHRITIS

Osteoarthritis (OA) occurs when the cartilage covering the end of the bone deteriorates, causing pain and swelling when the bones rub against each other. Over time, the bones can become misshapen from wear, and small bone spurs can grow at the bone ends, causing even more pain. If pieces of bone or cartilage break off, they can remain in the joint, causing still greater pain. In some people, the damage can be so extensive that the joint may have to be replaced.

Although we tend to think of OA as the logical outcome of wear and tear on the joints, scientists aren't so sure. Yes, wear and tear can affect some people's joints, but not everyone's. OA is due to a combination of factors, including genetics, past injury, joint use and overuse, and the aging process in general. We can't help our genetics, past injuries, or the aging process. And I'm certainly not going to recommend that you stop walking or participating in your favorite sport just to preserve your joints. In fact, exercise can help keep joints mobile. (More about that later!) However, there is something you can do to protect your joints from overuse. The word *overuse* implies that it's a problem for serious athletes—and it is—but it also happens when there is too much stress placed on the joint . . . the kind of stress caused by excess body weight.

Being overweight can compress joints. Imagine that you are balancing a book on your head, and someone comes along and places another book on top . . . and then another, and then another. With each book, the vertebrae in your neck will become jammed closer and closer together. When you carry too much weight, that same kind of compression affects your knees and hips. Weight loss can help . . . in a big way. Every 1 pound of weight you lose equates to 4 pounds less stress and pressure on your knees.

The benefits of weight loss go beyond knees. For example, one study followed 48 men and women who had gastric bypass surgery for extreme weight loss. Before surgery, all 48 had musculoskeletal pain, including joint pain, usually in more than one part of their bodies. After surgery, only 11 of them (23 percent) reported musculoskeletal pain, and there was improvement in pain in the spine, neck, arms, hands, legs, and feet. Osteoarthritis stiffness and joint function improved significantly, and the participants reported better quality of life. Surgery for weight loss is a drastic step, and it isn't necessary for most people. The vast majority of overweight people can lose enough weight to reduce their osteoarthritis symptoms through dietary changes alone. (See Weight Loss on page 19 for more information about the best ways to lose weight.)

RHEUMATOID ARTHRITIS

Rheumatoid arthritis (RA) is a disease that causes inflammation of the lining of the joint capsule—the *synovial membrane*. Early in the disease process, affected joints can feel swollen, painful, hot, and tender to the touch. As the disease progresses, the synovial membrane thickens and begins to release enzymes that can dissolve bone and cartilage inside the joint. If these enzymes eat away at enough tissue, the joint can become deformed—and the pain can be excruciating. Although some people have constant active disease, others have periods of rest or remission when symptoms may ease up or disappear.

RA is an autoimmune disease, which means that the immune system, which typically defends the body against foreign invaders (such as bacteria or viruses), suddenly turns on itself. In this case, the immune system attacks synovial membranes. Scientists don't know what triggers the process, why it goes into remission, or why it flares up periodically. Genetics play at least some role. Hormones may also play a part, as RA affects women more often than it affects men, and because flares often occur after a pregnancy. Some researchers believe that a bacterial or viral infection may set the wheels in motion, but that has not been proven. What we do know is that although RA cannot be cured, it can be managed with medication and lifestyle changes.

HOW FOOD AFFECTS ARTHRITIS

Because arthritis is a disease of inflammation, the most effective—and logical—treatment is anything that fights inflammation. Medical management of arthritis usually starts with ibuprofen and other anti-inflammatory medications, and nutritional care starts with anti-inflammatory foods.

Inflammation is a complex physiological reaction that begins whenever there is some assault to the body, such as injury, viral or bacterial infection, or exposure to allergens or chemicals. Whenever the body senses danger, it goes on high alert and bursts into action—it begins manufacturing and pumping out interleukins, cytokines, and other substances that rush to the site of the problem. The purpose of those substances is to protect tissue from the assault of foreign invaders.

Most of the time, this defensive system works marvelously well, but not always. Imagine that your house has an infestation of houseflies. If you wanted to be certain to eliminate

FAQS

I keep hearing about different herbal remedies for my arthritis. How do I know which ones are worth trying?

Herbs have been used as medical treatments for thousands of years by many cultures around the world. Research, however, is limited and the results are inconsistent. Depending on which herbs you choose, they can help *or hurt* your health, sometimes in ways we can't predict. That's why I recommend that you talk with your doctor if you have specific questions or health concerns. Among the dozens of potential herbal treatments for arthritis, the most promising are boswellia, devil's claw, and cat's claw.

Boswellia comes from the boswellia serrata tree, which grows in some parts of India. Its anti-inflammatory properties may help relieve some of the pain and stiffness of both osteoarthritis and rheumatoid arthritis. If you want to try boswellia, look for extracts standardized to 60 percent boswellic acids. The typical dosage is 300 to 400 milligrams of boswellic acids, three times daily.

Devil's claw is an African plant used to treat arthritis pain. Typical dosage is 750 milligrams, three times per day. Look for an extract standardized to contain 50 to 100 milligrams of the active ingredient harpagoside. Long-term safety hasn't been tested, and short-term side effects can include diarrhea, headache, and loss of taste. Because devil's claw can lower blood sugar, it may not be safe if you have diabetes or hypoglycemia.

Cat's claw is a vine that grows in rainforests in South America and Asia. Limited studies have shown that it may be helpful for relieving the pain of osteoarthritis and rheumatoid arthritis. It's available in capsules, tablets, liquid, and tea bags—dosage varies. The public is advised to only buy products that contain *uncaria tomentosa*. Another plant (*acacia greggi*), also called cat's claw, is highly toxic. For osteoarthritis, 100 milligrams daily of a specific freeze-dried aqueous cat's claw extract has been used. For rheumatoid arthritis, 60 milligrams daily in three divided doses of a specific cat's claw extract (free of tetracyclic oxindole alkaloids) has been used. Cat's claw can cause allergic reactions and gastrointestinal upset. There has been at least one report of kidney failure possibly triggered by cat's claw. For all these reasons, I recommend talking with your doctor before trying cat's claw.

the problem, you could buy a flyswatter, *and* set glue traps, *and* fumigate with a powerful insecticide, *and* bring in a thousand spiders to spin webs to trap the flies. But that response would be overkill. Once the flies were gone, you would have a new set of problems—namely a house full of airborne toxins and way, way too many spiders. The immune system often opts for overkill, and we're left with hot, red, swollen, painful joints. The inflammation comes and stays, and there's no way to just turn it off. That's why the best way to fight the pain of nearly any kind of arthritis is to fight inflammation with medication and/or with nutrition.

An anti-inflammatory diet excludes foods that fan the flames of inflammation . . . and embraces plenty of foods that reduce it. To get the most out of nutritional changes, you should adopt both sets of recommendations.

FOODS TO AVOID

I already mentioned that being overweight puts extra stress on the joints, which increases the risk of wear and tear. But there is another reason being overweight is a problem. Body fat is not an inert substance, it is metabolically active, capable of producing hormones and chemicals that *actually increase levels of inflammation.* By losing weight—and avoiding excess calories that can cause weight gain—you'll automatically reduce the level of inflammation in your body.

Specific food groups that increase inflammation include:

SATURATED FATS

This category includes fats in and from animal products, such as fatty beef or pork, poultry skin, ice cream, butter, whole or 2% reduced-fat milk, regular cheese, bacon, bologna, salami, pepperoni, beef sausage, and other fatty foods. Saturated fats are also found in palm oil and palm kernel oil. My guess is that you won't find bottles of any of those oils in your pantry, but chances are you will find them in the ingredient list of any number of items on your shelves, including crackers, cookies, nondairy creamers, and other packaged baked goods—try to dramatically limit your intake. In addition to carefully reading labels, choose reduced-fat or fat-free dairy products, lean cuts of beef and pork, and skinless chicken and turkey.

TRANS FATS

Trans fats are man-made. In an effort to give baked goods a longer shelf life, scientists took common vegetable oil and added hydrogen molecules in the right places. The result was that the liquid oil turned solid . . . and dangerous. Trans fats are thought to be at least as damaging as saturated fats in terms of inflammation and other health problems. Maybe worse. You won't have to go to great lengths to determine whether a food contains trans fats or not. Food producers are well aware of the dangers of these ingredients and growing public awareness of them, so companies that don't use trans fats are proclaiming it all over their product packaging. Plus, manufacturers are now required to list the amount of trans fats, right after the listing for saturated fats on the nutrition label.

OMEGA-6 POLYUNSATURATED FATS

Polyunsaturated fats come in two main varieties—omega-3s and omega-6s. Omega-3s are the healthy fish oils (discussed below), but omega-6s are another story. While they are not as overtly dangerous for health as saturated fats or trans fats, omega-6 fats are still considered inflammatory, which means that, in high doses, they could make arthritis pain worse. Omega-6 fats are found in mayonnaise, corn oil, cotton seed oil, safflower oil, soybean oil, and sunflower oil. Whenever possible, choose healthy monounsaturated olive oil instead of these omega-6 oils.

SIMPLE AND REFINED CARBOHYDRATES

Sugary foods, white flour baked goods, white rice, bread, crackers, and other refined carbohydrates set up a state of inflammation in the body, causing increases in cytokines and other pro-inflammatory compounds. Limit these foods if you want the best chance of reducing arthritis pain and progression.

FOODS TO ADD

These foods all help to reduce some aspect of inflammation:

OMEGA-3 FATTY ACIDS

The healthiest of fats for people with arthritis or other inflammatory disorders are omega-3 fatty acids, one of the polyunsaturated fats. While other foods increase levels of inflammation in the body, omega-3s actually work to decrease inflammation by suppressing the production of cytokines and enzymes that erode cartilage.

More than a dozen studies have demonstrated that omega-3 fish oils can reduce symptoms of RA. Study participants reported greater strength, less fatigue, reduced joint swelling and tenderness, less joint stiffness, and less pain.

Although the evidence is less clear about how fish oil affects osteoarthritis, the anti-inflammatory effects of omega-3s are so potent that I recommend an omega-3–rich diet and fish oil supplements to all my clients with arthritis. I've seen some amazing results.

Take Colleen—she was in her mid-40s, only about 10 pounds overweight, but she had a problem with high cholesterol. I put her on a cholesterol-lowering program, which included fish oil capsules. After a month, she returned for a follow-up appointment and I was pleased to see she had lost a couple of pounds, and her cholesterol had begun to return to healthy levels. But Colleen was ecstatic! She explained that her joint pain—which she'd never mentioned—had almost entirely disappeared. The fish oil supplements had made Colleen feel like a new person.

Emma was in her early 70s, and had diagnosed osteoarthritis. She needed to lose about 45 pounds, which contributed to her problem, but the extraordinary level of pain she felt in her knees and hands couldn't be explained by weight alone. I put her on a healthy, calorie-controlled food plan and recommended that she take fish oil capsules . . . she also began taking glucosamine plus chondroitin supplements, and she began seeing an acupuncturist. Today, Emma swims and walks on a treadmill without pain, and she is more active than she has been in years. She still has pain flare-ups, but she feels much, much better. We don't know which of the treatments was most effective, and Emma doesn't really care. She feels healthy, and she is unwilling to stop taking any of her supplements, which she sees as her lifeline. (For more information about fish oil and other supplements, see the Supplements section, page 172.)

BEST FOODS FOR OMEGA-3 FATTY ACIDS: *Wild salmon (fresh, canned), herring, mackerel (not king), sardines, anchovies, rainbow trout, Pacific oysters, omega-3–fortified eggs, flaxseed (ground and oil), walnuts, butternuts (white walnuts), seaweed, walnut oil, canola oil, soybeans*

ANTIOXIDANTS: VITAMIN C, SELENIUM, CAROTENES, BIOFLAVONOIDS

Inflammation produces free radicals, those cell-damaging molecules that are formed in response to toxins or natural body processes. The synovium is just as prone to this kind damage as the skin, eyes, or any other body tissue. Antioxidants protect the body from the effects of free radicals, and are a critical part of an anti-inflammation diet. Research has demonstrated that certain antioxidants may help prevent arthritis, slow its progression, and relieve pain. The most powerful antioxidants are vitamin C, selenium, carotenes, and bioflavonoids.

Vitamin C is one of the nutrients most responsible for the health of collagen, a major component of cartilage. In addition, research suggests that people who eat a diet low in vitamin C may have a greater risk of developing some kinds of arthritis. For those reasons, it is important to make vitamin C–rich foods an important part of your daily diet. *However,* researchers at Duke University found that long-term, high-dose vitamin C supplements may make your osteoarthritis *worse.* I say *may* because the research was conducted on guinea pigs. The researchers' assumption is that it will have the same effect in people. I wouldn't want you to risk your health with supplements, so if you have osteoarthritis, I recommend you get vitamin C from food sources only—not from an individual supplement, but multivitamins are fine.

BEST FOODS FOR VITAMIN C: *Guava, bell peppers (yellow, red, green), orange juice, hot chile peppers, oranges, grapefruit juice, strawberries, pineapple, kohlrabi, papaya, lemons, broccoli, kale, Brussels sprouts, kidney beans, kiwi, cantaloupe, cauliflower, red cabbage, mangos, grapefruit (pink, red), white potatoes (with skin), mustard greens, cherry tomatoes, sugar snap peas, snow peas, clementines, rutabagas, turnip greens, tomatoes, raspberries, Chinese cabbage, blackberries, green tomatoes, cabbage, watermelon, tangerines, lemon juice, okra, lychees, summer squash (all varieties), persimmon*

Low levels of the mineral **selenium** are related to osteoarthritis severity, and possibly to rheumatoid arthritis. In a study of more than 900 people, those who had low levels of selenium were more likely to have osteoarthritis of the knee. People who ate very few selenium-rich foods were nearly twice as likely to have severe arthritis compared with those who ate a selenium-rich diet.

BEST FOODS FOR SELENIUM: *Brazil nuts, tuna (canned light), crab, oysters, tilapia, whole wheat pasta, lean beef, cod, shrimp, whole wheat breads (including crackers, buns), turkey, wheat germ, brown rice, chicken breast, cottage cheese (fat-free or 1% reduced-fat), mushrooms, eggs*

Carotenes are a group of powerful antioxidant nutrients found in many fruits and vegetables. The best known is beta carotene, but there are many others. When it comes to arthritis, the carotene called beta cryptoxanthin may reduce the risk of developing inflammation-related disorders, including rheumatoid arthritis. Researchers from the United Kingdom found that people who ate diets high in beta cryptoxanthin were half as likely to develop a form of inflammatory arthritis as those who ate very few beta cryptoxanthin foods. They found that adding just one additional serving each day of a food high in beta cryptoxanthin helped reduce arthritis risk.

BEST FOODS FOR BETA CAROTENE: *Sweet potatoes, carrots, kale, winter squash (especially butternut), turnip greens, pumpkin, mustard greens, cantaloupe, red bell peppers, apricots, Chinese cabbage, spinach, lettuce (romaine, green leaf, red leaf, butterhead), collard greens, Swiss chard, watercress, grapefruit, watermelon, cherries, mangos, red ripe tomatoes, guava, asparagus, red cabbage*

BEST FOODS FOR BETA CRYPTOXANTHIN: *Winter squash, pumpkin, persimmons, papaya, tangerines, red chile peppers, red bell peppers, corn, oranges, apricots, carrots, nectarines, watermelon, peaches*

The **bioflavonoids** quercetin and anthocyanidins are both forms of antioxidants. The anti-inflammatory effects of **quercetin** may seem to be similar to those of non-steroidal anti-inflammatory medications (such as aspirin and ibuprofen). For example, the synovial fluid in joints of people with rheumatoid arthritis contain highly inflammatory

FAQS

There are so many different kinds of foods to avoid. I think I can figure this out for meals I cook at home, but are there guidelines for what to eat in restaurants?

You're right—it can be difficult at first, but after a few weeks, making smart food choices will become second nature. I recommend:

American Fare

- Grilled fish or skinless chicken breast in olive oil and seasonings—with brown rice or a baked or sweet potato—and lots of grilled, roasted, or steamed vegetables.
- Salad entrées: variety of vegetables (request extra red peppers) with grilled chicken, shrimp, turkey breast, or lean ham. For dressing, use vinaigrette or request olive oil and vinegar on the side, or top with fresh salsa.
- Sandwiches: Turkey breast, lean ham, or grilled chicken breast on whole grain bread, or whole wheat pita, or rolled in a whole grain wrap. Optional avocado, roasted peppers, onion, tomato, and other vegetables.
- Soups: gazpacho, black bean, lentil, vegetable, and low-fat butternut squash.

Japanese Food

- Edamame, seaweed salad, California rolls (take advantage of sliced ginger!), and steamed vegetables.

Chinese Food

- Steamed whole fish with ginger—plus steamed brown rice and sautéed or steamed vegetables.
- Steamed chicken and broccoli (or any other vegetables—request "with ginger") with 1 to 2 tablespoons black bean or garlic sauce—and steamed brown rice.

Indian Food

- Tandoori salmon or chicken—with a variety of side vegetables.

chemicals called *tumor necrosis factor* (TNF). In research, quercetin was able to limit the inflammatory effects of TNF.

BEST FOODS FOR QUERCETIN: *Onions (red, yellow, white), kale, leeks, cherry tomatoes, broccoli, blueberries, black currants, elderberries, lingonberries, cocoa powder (unsweetened), apricots, apples with skin (especially Red Delicious), grapes (red, purple, black), tomatoes, tea (green, black), red wine, beans (green, white), lettuce (butterhead, Boston, iceberg, Bibb), peppers (ancho, hot chile, green, yellow wax), celery, chives, red cabbage, lemons, grapefruit, horseradish root*

Anthocyanidins and proanthocyanidins are powerful antioxidants known to reduce inflammation. They seem to inhibit production of certain inflammatory chemicals, including cytokines and prostaglandins. They contribute to the health of connective tissue, and are more powerful than vitamin C for defusing dangerous free radicals that can irritate body tissues and cause inflammation.

BEST FOODS FOR ANTHOCYANIDINS: *Blackberries, black currants, blueberries, eggplant, elderberries, raspberries, cherries, boysenberries, grapes (red, black), strawberries, plums, cranberries, rhubarb, red wine, red onions, apples, peaches, cabbage (red, purple), red beets, blood oranges (and juice)*

GREEN TEA

Green tea's health benefits are often underestimated. Compared with regular black tea, green tea looks weak and insubstantial. But this mild-mannered drink contains a natural antioxidant called epigallocatechin-3-gallate (EGCG). Studies suggest that EGCG works to stop the production of certain inflammatory chemicals in the body, including those involved in arthritis. Green tea also contains other antioxidants called *catechins*, which may prevent cartilage from breaking down, so joints may be preserved longer.

OLIVE OIL

Olive oil contains the "good" monounsaturated fat, which protects the body against inflammation because it contains antioxidants called *polyphenols*. In animal studies, rats with arthritis were fed diets high in various kinds of oils. The researchers found that both fish oil and olive oil prevented arthritis-related inflammation. I recommend using olive oil when cooking, instead of vegetable oil or butter. Don't pour it on—just substitute one for the other in equal or lesser amounts. Ideally, you'll want to choose an olive oil high in polyphenols. That may sound like a tough call, but it is really very simple—just look for the words *extra virgin* on the olive oil label and you'll get the highest antioxidant content available.

VITAMIN D

Although we mostly think of vitamin D as important for bone strength, it is also critical for a number of other body functions, including joint health. Studies have shown that getting adequate amounts of vitamin D reduces the risk of both rheumatoid arthritis and osteoarthritis. Among people who already have osteoarthritis, those who have a vitamin D deficiency are more likely to develop worsening disability over time. Getting even the basic daily requirements of vitamin D leads to greater muscle strength, improvement in physical functioning, and preservation of cartilage (that's at least 400 IU until age 70, and at least 600 IU for folks 70 and older).

> **BEST FOODS FOR VITAMIN D:** *Wild salmon (with bones), mackerel (not king), sardines (with bones), herring, fortified milk (fat-free, 1% reduced-fat), enriched/fortified soy milk, egg yolks, mushrooms (especially shiitake), fortified soft tub trans fat–free margarine, fortified breakfast cereals*

SPICES: GINGER AND TURMERIC

Most people don't realize that spices are for more than, well, spicing things up. They're an important source of essential nutrients. Like fruits and vegetables, spices come from plant sources, and they can have powerful effects on health. Certain spices seem to have anti-inflammatory effects, and therefore should be considered for arthritis treatment. Among the most promising are ginger and turmeric.

Ginger has been shown to lessen the pain of knee osteoarthritis when taken in highly purified, standardized supplement form. Ginger contains chemicals that work similarly to some anti-inflammatory medications, so its effects on arthritis pain are not surprising. However, ginger can also act as a blood thinner, so anyone taking a blood-thinning medication should limit their ginger use. Better yet, collaborate with your physician to monitor and possibly adjust your medication while adding foods and beverages seasoned with ginger.

Turmeric, sometimes called curcumin, is a mustard-yellow spice from Asia. It is the main ingredient in yellow curry powder. Scientific studies have shown that turmeric may help arthritis by suppressing inflammatory body chemicals. Because of its effects on enzymes related to inflammation, turmeric may have the same mode of action as Celebrex

GOUT

Imagine needle-sharp shards of glass inserted between the bones of your joints, grating and grinding with every move. That not-so-happy image is the pain of gout, one of the more common forms of arthritis. Of course it's not actually glass in the joints. In some people with a genetic susceptibility—men more often than women—the body converts excess uric acid into crystals which can accumulate in joints.

In most cases, the extreme pain of gout starts in the big toe. I've known clients who have had so much swelling and agony that they can't wear shoes. At the very least, the discomfort is enough to make walking difficult (and according to one of my clients "ruin an otherwise great vacation"). Gout can also settle into other joints of the feet, ankles, knees, fingers, wrists, and elbows.

Most cases of gout are controllable. Treatment involves medication, and avoiding anything that raises levels of uric acid. Because uric acid is a byproduct of the metabolism of purine, a substance naturally found in body tissues, you'll never get rid of it entirely. However, if you have gout, or have been told you're at high risk, there are several ways to keep uric acid levels as low as possible:

- **Maintain a healthy weight.** Extra body tissue means extra uric acid production from normal processes of breakdown and turnover.

- **Avoid purine-rich meats and seafood.** The more purine-rich meats and seafood you eat, the more uric acid you'll produce, and the greater your risk of gout. Studies have shown that eating lots of these high-purine foods increases the risk of gout by about 50 percent. I've seen this in my practice. Some of my clients who never before had a gout attack found themselves suffering after following a super high-protein diet because many meats can contribute to uric acid load. (High-purine vegetables don't seem to increase risk of gout, but if you're suffering with an attack, I recommend eating them only in moderation to be safe.) High-purine foods to avoid: Anchovies, herring, mackerel, scallops, sardines, sweetbreads, liver, kidney, red meat, poultry, wild game, lentils, dried beans and peas, asparagus, cauliflower, spinach, mushrooms.

- **Eat more reduced-fat dairy foods.** People who eat two or three servings daily of reduced-fat dairy foods—especially milk and yogurt—can cut their risk of gout by about half, compared with those who eat few dairy foods. Add reduced-fat or fat-free milk or yogurt to your diet.

- **Reduce alcohol intake—especially beer.** Alcoholic beverages interfere with the body's ability to clear uric acid, increasing risk of gout. In 2004, Harvard researchers reported that beer was the greatest offender—men who drank two or more beers per day had more than twice the risk of gout compared with men who didn't drink beer. Spirits also caused an increase in gout, but to a lesser degree. Wine did not seem to increase risk of gout, but I still recommend limiting your consumption.

- **Drink plenty of water.** I recommend that my clients with gout drink at least eight glasses of water daily to help flush uric acid out of the body.

- **Use aspirin sparingly.** Salicylates—the active ingredients in aspirin—can raise uric acid levels.

- **Get a check up.** About 75 percent of people diagnosed with gout also have the metabolic syndrome, a serious condition that increases the risk of heart disease. If you receive a diagnosis of gout, insist on testing for the metabolic syndrome. (More information about the metabolic syndrome is on page 132.)

and similar medications. Note: turmeric is also used as a dye, so use caution when handling it—it can discolor clothing and some surfaces. Dig in and enjoy my curry chicken recipe on page 184!

BONUS POINTS

- **See a doctor about symptoms.** Don't be complaisant about joint pain, stiffness, swelling, or weakness, and don't assume that joint pain is a normal part of growing older. Early treatment of OA, RA, or other arthritis can help slow the disease progression and provide a lot of pain relief.

- **Work to reduce cholesterol.** Although no one knows what triggers RA, an interesting European study may provide at least one clue. Researchers analyzed 10-year-old blood samples of people who later developed RA, and compared them to blood of a random sample of individuals. They discovered that people who developed RA had higher than normal levels of low-density lipoprotein (LDL) cholesterol, triglycerides, and apolipoprotein B; and lower than normal levels of high-density lipoprotein (HDL) cholesterol. The theory is that these blood results indicate the start of atherosclerosis . . . and atherosclerosis means more inflammation in the body. (See C-Reactive Protein on page 132 for more information about how heart disease is related to inflammation.) Could it be that a higher level of inflammation could turn into inflammatory joint disease? More research is needed, but it certainly gives added reason to treat your cholesterol problem as early as possible.

- **Drink plenty of water.** Cartilage is 65 to 80 percent water, so staying hydrated is important for the health and lubrication of joints. It isn't necessary to count the number of glasses of water you drink in a day—the latest research suggests that if you drink a glass of water whenever you feel thirsty, you'll probably do fine. My biggest recommendation is that you choose water, herbal tea, or green tea instead of sugary drinks or soft drinks.

- **Exercise.** Many people stop exercising at the first twinge of pain in a joint, but this can be a big mistake. Exercise can help you lose or maintain weight, which reduces the overall stress impact on joints. Strong muscles can absorb shock from daily movements, keep joints stable, and protect against additional joint injury. Stretching and yoga can improve flexibility and range of motion. Exercise of all sorts can also help you sleep better, although you should not exercise vigorously late in the day if insomnia is a problem. Talk with your doctor about the best kind of exercise for you, because the best choices will depend on your particular medical situation and pain levels. Swimming and water aerobics are usually good for everyone because they allow free movement without added stress on the joints. No matter which exercise you choose, don't overdo it when you are just starting out, and don't do anything that threatens your balance. By all means stop if the pain worsens.

- **Try acupuncture.** Among people with osteoarthritis, studies suggest that traditional Chinese acupuncture can help reduce pain and improve function. People who had about one treatment per week felt better after just four weeks, and they felt better and better, week after week. It is important to choose a qualified, skilled acupuncturist who knows how to treat osteoarthritis. I prefer that my clients go to an acupuncturist who also has a traditional medical degree to be sure that they are receiving the best combination of Western medicine and Eastern acupuncture. (Ask your rheumatologist or primary care physician for a referral. You can also find certified acupuncturists at the website for the National Certification Commission for Acupuncture and Oriental Medicine at www.NCCAOM.org.) Also, watch out for those who are more concerned with business than with health care—the most reputable will treat you only when you have pain, and will not pressure you to come in for a set number of treatments.

- **Stop smoking.** There are so many good reasons to stop smoking, but now we can add healthy joints to the list. Smoking delivers toxins throughout the body, causing inflammation and increasing the risks of rheumatoid arthritis and osteoarthritis. In one study, smokers were more than twice as likely to develop RA than people who didn't smoke. Smokers who also had a genetic susceptibility for RA were more than seven times more likely to develop the disease than the average person. The effects of smoking on osteoarthritis are less clear, but researchers from a multi-center study reported in 2005 that smokers had a greater risk of osteoarthritis of the knee, possibly because smoking interferes with the body's ability to repair its own cartilage. If you quit smoking, you'll immediately reduce your inflammation load, and you'll improve blood flow to all parts of your body, including your aching joints.

- **De-stress.** Some experts believe that autoimmune disorders, including rheumatoid arthritis, can flare up in response to stress. Plus, people who feel stressed are more sensitive to pain. Stress reduction can be as important to your health as medication, so make it a priority. Carve out time in your schedule to relax and, if necessary, downsize your to-do list by asking others to help out. Chances are friends and family will offer to help when they learn of your condition—take them up on it. Check with your local hospital to see if it offers classes in stress reduction techniques, such as guided imagery, meditation, and progressive relaxation.

- **Control your pain.** When it comes to the pain of arthritis, don't try to be hero. You have nothing to gain by toughing it out. If you hurt, see your doctor. If your doctor prescribes medication, take it. If you still hurt, make another appointment. People in constant pain may stop doing the things they love and before long their quality of life takes a real turn for the worse. Some arthritis patients become depressed; small wonder, if they're in constant pain! If you don't have the pain under control, and your current doctor seems to have exhausted the options, research pain specialists in your area through organizations such as the American Academy of Pain Management (www.AAPainManage.org).

SUPPLEMENTS

If you have arthritis and want to consider supplements *in addition to* the food fixes, I recommend:

FOR BOTH OSTEOARTHRITIS AND RHEUMATOID ARTHRITIS

1. **Multivitamin.** If you would like to consider a multivitamin to supplement your healthy (I hope!) diet, I recommend brands that provide 100% DV of vitamin D (in the form of D_3, or cholecalciferol, the most potent form of vitamin D), vitamin C, selenium, and vitamin A (with at least 50% coming from beta carotene and/or mixed carotenoids, and no more than 2,000 IU coming from retinol). Definitely *do not choose mega-dose varieties,* because some vitamins may make certain cases of arthritis worse.

2. **Omega-3 fatty acids from fish oil.** Eat foods rich in omega-3s, but for serious arthritis relief, you'll want to try fish oil supplements. Rheumatoid arthritis studies have tested the effectiveness of various dosages, from 1.2 grams to 3.2 grams. I recommend you start with a daily dose of 2 grams. If there's no relief after 4 weeks, speak with your physician about increasing to 3 grams. Store the supplements in the fridge to prevent rancidity. To prevent fishy burps, buy enteric-coated varieties, take with food, and split doses throughout day. Because fish oil acts as a blood thinner, it should not be taken by people who have hemophilia, or who are already taking blood thinning medications or aspirin (always consult your physician). People with diabetes should talk with their doctors before trying fish oil supplements because they may affect blood sugar.

FOR OSTEOARTHRITIS

1. **Glucosamine plus chondroitin.** These nutrients are naturally found in and around cartilage cells, and are thought to strengthen and stimulate growth of cartilage. They have been rumored to be helpful for osteoarthritis pain for years, but until 2006 there was no research to back up those claims. The large-scale Glucosamine Arthritis Intervention Trial (GAIT) showed that arthritis sufferers with moderate-to-severe pain had significantly reduced pain after taking a combination of glucosamine plus chondroitin compared with those who took either supplement singly or a placebo. Arthritis sufferers with mild pain did not benefit from taking the glucosamine/chondroitin combo. The amounts generally recommended are 1,500 milligrams glucosamine and 1,200 milligrams chondroitin sulfate daily. These supplements are available anywhere you buy vitamins, and are sold individually or in pre-packaged combinations. This treatment is slow-acting—you may not feel any difference for 4 weeks. In Europe, where glucosamine and chondroitin are more commonly recommended by doctors, they are used in addition to other medical treatments and medications. So if you want to try glucosamine plus chondroitin, talk with your doctor to see how it might fit in with your current treatment. *Important note*: Glucosamine is extracted from shellfish shells (chitin), so if you have an allergy to shellfish, seek your doctor's advice. If you develop a rash or other symptoms of allergy, discontinue taking it immediately. Plus, these supplements may thin the blood. If you are already taking blood thinners, or if you have a clotting disorder, consult your doctor.

2. **SAMe.** Some studies have shown that SAMe (S-adenosylmethionine) may be as effec-

tive as nonsteroidal anti-inflammatory medications. One study conducted by researchers from the University of California, Irvine, compared the effects of SAMe with the anti-inflammatory medication celecoxib (Celebrex) in 56 people with osteoarthritis. After one month, people who took celecoxib had greater pain relief, but after two months, celecoxib and SAMe reduced pain to the same degree. Joint function also improved. So although SAMe took longer, it ended up working just as well as a prescription pain reliever. Recommended dose of SAMe for arthritis is 1,200 milligrams per day. Even though SAMe is generally thought to be safe, it can have side effects, including insomnia, rash, allergy, and gastrointestinal problems. To be safe, talk with your doctor before starting treatment with SAMe.

FOR RHEUMATOID ARTHRITIS

GLA (gamma-linolenic acid). This fatty acid is found in evening primrose oil, borage oil, and black current oil. Studies show that GLA seems to reduce pain, joint tenderness, and morning stiffness of rheumatoid arthritis by suppressing certain inflammatory substances. Recommended dosage is between 1 and 3 grams per day. Because the action of this supplement may interfere with certain medications, always talk with your doctor before taking GLA.

JOY'S 4-STEP PROGRAM
FOR ARTHRITIS

Follow this program if you have osteoarthritis, rheumatoid arthritis, or other arthritis (except gout—see page 170 for more information).

STEP 1 ... START WITH THE BASICS

These are the first things you should do to take control of inflammation, which feeds your arthritis pain:

- See a doctor if you have new or uncontrolled joint pain. It is important to get early and effective treatment for arthritis.

- Ask your doctor about whether taking omega-3 fish oil supplements makes sense for you.

- If you smoke, quit.

- Begin a program of gentle, low- or no-stress exercise.

- Drink plenty of water.

- Avoid foods high in saturated fats, trans fats, and omega-6 polyunsaturated fats.

- Avoid sugary and refined carbohydrate foods.

STEP 2 ... YOUR ULTIMATE GROCERY LIST

This list contains foods with high levels of nutrients that help reduce inflammation and control arthritis pain, plus some foods used as ingredients in the meal plans and recipes. You don't have to purchase every item . . . but these foods should make up the bulk of what you eat for the week. If you find yourself getting bored with familiar items, try something new—perhaps a curry recipe like the Slow-Cooker Chicken Curry and Vegetables (page 184). If you have gout, limit your portions of foods marked with an asterisk.

FRUIT

Apples with skin (especially Red Delicious)	raspberries, strawberries)	Guava	Papaya
	Cantaloupe	Kiwi	Peaches
Apricots	Cherries	Lemons (and juice)	Persimmons
Berries (blackberries, blueberries, boysenberries, elderberries, lingonberries,	Clementines	Limes (and juice)	Pineapple
	Cranberries	Lychees	Plums
	Currants, black	Mangos	Tangerines
	Grapefruit (and juice)	Nectarines	Watermelon
	Grapes (black, red, purple)	Oranges and juice (especially blood oranges)	

VEGETABLES

Asparagus*	Chives	Onions (red, yellow, white)	Snow peas
Beans, green,	Collard greens		Soybeans (edamame)
Beans (kidney, white)	Corn	*Peas, sugar snap	*Spinach
Beets, red	Eggplant	Peppers, (hot; yellow/ red/green)	Squash, summer
Broccoli	Horseradish root	Potatoes, sweet	Squash, winter (especially butternut)
Brussels sprouts	Kale	Potatoes, white	Swiss chard
Cabbage (including Chinese, red, purple)	Kohlrabi	Pumpkin (fresh, 100% pure canned pumpkin)	Tomatoes (including red ripe tomatoes, cherry tomatoes, green tomatoes)
	Leeks		
Carrots	Lettuce		
*Cauliflower	*Mushrooms (especially shiitake)	Rhubarb	
Celery		Rutabagas	Turnip greens
Chickpeas (garbanzo beans)	Mustard greens	Seaweed	Watercress
	Okra		

SEAFOOD

*Anchovies	*Mackerel (not king)	Salmon, wild (with bones)	Tilapia
Cod			Trout, rainbow
Crab	Oysters (including Pacific)	*Sardines (with bones)	Tuna (canned light)
*Herring		Shrimp	

LEAN MEATS/EGGS/SOY FOODS

*Beef, lean
*Chicken breast
Eggs, omega-3–fortified
Turkey

NUTS AND SEEDS (PREFERABLY UNSALTED)

Brazil nuts
Butternuts (white walnuts)
Flaxseed, ground
Walnuts

WHOLE GRAINS

Breads, whole wheat
(including crackers,
buns)

Cereal, fortified whole
grain
Pasta, whole wheat

Rice, brown
Wheat germ

DAIRY

Cheese, feta, reduced-
fat
Cheese, Parmesan
Cottage cheese (fat-free,
1% reduced-fat)

Margarine spread,
vitamin D–fortified,
soft tub, trans fat–free
Milk, fortified (fat-free,
1% reduced-fat)

Soy milk, enriched/
fortified

MISCELLANEOUS

Allspice
Baking powder
Basil, fresh
Cilantro, fresh
Cinnamon, ground
Cocoa powder,
unsweetened

Flour, whole
wheat
Garlic
Ginger, fresh and
ground
Honey
Hot sauce

Mayonnaise, reduced-
fat
Oil, canola
Oil, flaxseed
Oil, olive
Oil, walnut
Pepper, black

Sugar, white and brown
Sugar substitute
Tea (black, green)
Turmeric/yellow curry
powder
Wine, red

STEP 3 ...GOING ABOVE AND BEYOND

If you want to do everything you can for arthritis pain and stiffness, here are some additional things you might try:

- If you have osteoarthritis, ask your doctor about what supplements you might try. The ones with the best track record are glucosamine with chondroitin sulfate, omega-3s, and SAMe. (See the Supplements section, page 172, for cautions and more information.)

- If you have rheumatoid arthritis, ask your doctor about what supplements you might try. The ones with the best track record are GLA and omega-3s.

- Incorporate ginger and turmeric into your recipes and meals.

- Consult a qualified acupuncturist about pain relief.

- Try to find ways to reduce stress, which can amplify pain and even trigger flares of rheumatoid arthritis.

A GINGER PRIMER

Ginger is a versatile spice that has antiinflammatory properties. It can be used in any course, from appetizers to dessert. Look for fresh ginger in the produce section of most grocery stores—it is a tan root about the size of very fat fingers. Powdered ginger, found in the spice aisle, is used most often in baking and gives a stronger taste to foods—do not automatically substitute the same amount of powdered ginger for fresh ginger. A common accompaniment to sushi, pickled ginger (also called *gari*) is made by soaking thin slices of fresh ginger in rice vinegar and sugar for a week or longer. Candied or crystallized ginger is sweet, and can be eaten as an occasional treat, or baked in cakes and muffins.

STEP4 ...MEAL PLANS

These sample menus include foods that have been shown to help ease inflammation and arthritis pain, specifically: antioxidants, omega-3 fats, vitamin D, and inflammation-reducing spices.

Every day, choose *one* option for each of the three meals—breakfast, lunch, and dinner. Then, one or two times per day, choose from a variety of my suggested snacks. Approximate calories have been provided to help adjust for your personal weight-management goals. If you find yourself hungry (and if weight is not an issue), feel free to increase the portion sizes for meals and snacks. Beverage calories are *not* included. I encourage you to drink plenty of water, and to incorporate a daily cup or two of green tea.

BREAKFAST OPTIONS

(Approximately 300 to 400 calories)

Vanilla Pumpkin Breakfast Pudding

1 cup fat-free vanilla yogurt mixed with ½ cup canned 100% pure pumpkin puree and topped with 2 tablespoons chopped walnuts and 1 tablespoon wheat germ.

Scrambled Eggs with Tomatoes, Mushrooms, and Onion

Beat 1 whole omega-3–fortified egg with 2 or 3 egg whites. Cook in hot skillet coated with nonstick cooking spray; add 2 tablespoons each chopped tomato, sliced mushrooms, and sliced onion (preferably red). Serve with toasted whole grain English muffin, dry or with 1 to 2 teaspoons soft tub, reduced-fat, trans fat–free margarine spread.

Grapefruit with Cottage Cheese

1 pink or red grapefruit (or blood orange), sectioned and mixed with 1 cup fat-free or 1% reduced-fat cottage cheese. Top with 1 to 2 tablespoons wheat germ.

Fiery Breakfast Burrito

Sauté ½ cup chopped onion, ½ cup sliced bell pepper, and 1 sliced jalapeño chile pepper (with flesh and seeds) in nonstick cooking spray until soft. Beat 1 whole omega-3–fortified egg with 2 egg whites, and scramble with the sautéed vegetables until eggs are cooked through. Wrap in a whole grain tortilla (150 calories or less) and add optional salsa and/or hot sauce.

Tropical Mango-Citrus Smoothie with Toast

1 serving (2 cups) Tropical Mango-Citrus Smoothie (page 123), with 1 slice whole wheat bread, toasted and topped with 2 heaping tablespoons fat-free or 1% reduced-fat cottage cheese and sprinkled with 1 tablespoon wheat germ.

Cereal with Milk, Nuts, and Berries

1 cup whole grain fortified cereal mixed with 1 cup fat-free milk (or enriched/fortified soy milk) and topped with 1 tablespoon chopped walnuts and ½ cup fresh berries (sliced strawberries, blueberries, raspberries, blackberries, elderberries, or lingonberries).

Pumpkin Oatmeal

½ cup dry instant oatmeal prepared with 1 cup fat-free milk (or enriched/fortified vanilla soy milk), flavored and mixed with 2 teaspoons vanilla extract, ½ cup canned 100% pure pumpkin puree, a pinch of salt, and 2 to 3 teaspoons sugar (or 1 packet artificial sweetener). Top with optional 1 tablespoon wheat germ.

LUNCH OPTIONS

(Approximately 400 to 500 calories)

The Ache-Less Salad

3 cups leafy greens topped with 4 ounces (total) of any of the following high protein options: wild salmon (with bones), sardines (with bones), mackerel (not king), crab, shrimp, Pacific oysters, tilapia, black cod, turkey breast, grilled chicken (or 2 hard-boiled eggs). Mix with ½ chopped tomato, ¼ chopped red onion, ¼ cup sliced mushrooms, 1 sliced red bell pepper, 1 sliced jalapeño chile pepper, 2 chopped beets, ½ cup chopped carrots, and ¼ cup corn. If desired, add optional red cabbage and chopped celery. Toss with 1 to 2 teaspoons olive oil and unlimited balsamic vinegar or fresh lemon juice (or 2 to 4 tablespoons reduced-calorie dressing).

Greek Chicken Pita Pocket

1 whole wheat pita, lightly toasted and filled with romaine lettuce, 3 to 4 ounces cooked chicken breast, 1 ounce crumbled reduced-fat feta cheese, and thin slices of tomato and red onion. Drizzle with plain balsamic vinegar or fresh lemon juice. Season with salt and pepper to taste. Enjoy with crunchy celery and red pepper sticks.

Turkey and Roasted Pepper Sandwich

4 ounces sliced turkey breast (or lean ham), unlimited lettuce, sliced tomato, onion, and roasted red peppers on 2 slices whole grain bread. Add optional sliced chile pepper, mustard, and 1 to 2 teaspoons reduced-fat mayonnaise. Enjoy with large handful baby carrots.

Butternut Squash Soup with Fish

2 to 3 cups Butternut Squash Soup (page 80) or any prepared low-fat soup without cream. Serve with a salad of unlimited leafy greens topped with 3 ounces canned sar-

dines, wild salmon, light tuna packed in water, or grilled chicken; drizzle with fresh lemon juice or plain vinegar and season with salt and pepper to taste.

Vegetable Omelet and Baked Potato

Beat 1 whole egg with 2 to 3 egg whites. Cook in heated skillet coated with nonstick cooking spray. When bottom is cooked, gently flip over. Top with any of the following vegetables: mushrooms, onion, peppers (bell and hot), broccoli, kale, spinach, tomato. Fold omelet over and cook until egg mixture is firm. Enjoy with 1 medium plain baked white or sweet potato (or 2 cups hearty vegetable soup).

Wild Salmon Salad

1 serving Wild Salmon Salad (page 322), or drain and mash 5 to 6 ounces canned Alaskan salmon (or lump crab meat) and mix with 2 teaspoons reduced-fat mayonnaise, minced onion, and optional mustard or horseradish. Serve over a bed of leafy greens. Enjoy with 1 (70-calorie) whole grain pita bread, split and toasted (or 100 calories of whole grain crackers).

Turkey Burger with Veggies

1 (5-ounce) lean turkey burger (or vegetarian burger) with optional sliced tomato, onion, and roasted peppers on ½ whole grain bun (or in small 70-calorie pita pocket). Enjoy with 1 cup vegetables (broccoli, cauliflower, kale, Brussels sprouts, sugar snap peas, Swiss chard, beets, spinach, or asparagus), steamed, grilled, roasted, or lightly sautéed in 1 teaspoon olive oil or nonstick cooking spray.

DINNER OPTIONS

(Approximately 500 to 600 calories)

Baked Tilapia with Vegetables and Sweet Potato

6 ounces tilapia fillet (or other fish) seasoned with 1 teaspoon olive oil, fresh ground pepper, pinch kosher salt, and fresh lemon juice. Bake, uncovered, in 400°F oven for 10 to 12 minutes. Serve with 1 cup steamed broccoli (or cauliflower, kale, Brussels sprouts, sugar snap peas, Swiss chard, beets, spinach, or asparagus) and 1 medium baked sweet potato topped with optional ground cinnamon.

Sweet and Sour Tofu-Veggie Stir-Fry with Brown Rice

1 serving Sweet and Sour Tofu-Veggie Stir-Fry (page 251). Chicken or shrimp may be substituted for the tofu. Add ½ cup sliced red onion and, if your taste buds can handle it, double up on the jalapeño peppers. Enjoy with 1 cup cooked brown rice.

Oysters Rockefeller with Grilled Salmon over Greens

1 serving Grilled Rockefeller Oysters (page 186), with 5 ounces grilled wild salmon or other fish seasoned with 1 teaspoon olive oil, pinch kosher salt, ground black pepper, and preferred seasonings. Serve salmon over a large mound of leafy greens mixed with optional sliced red onion, pepper, mushrooms, and tomato. Drizzle with 2 tablespoons reduced-calorie dressing (or plain balsamic vinegar or fresh lemon juice).

Sirloin Steak with Gingered Carrots and Baked Potato

5 ounces lean sirloin steak served with optional horseradish dip (2 teaspoons horseradish mixed with 1 tablespoon reduced-fat mayonnaise). Enjoy with ½ medium baked potato topped with 1 to 2 tablespoons warm marinara sauce, plus 1 serving Gingered Carrots (page 188).

Chicken Curry and Vegetables with Brown Rice

1 serving Slow-Cooker Chicken Curry and Vegetables (page 184) over ½ cup cooked brown basmati rice.

Angel Hair Pasta with Roasted Pumpkin, Sage, and Walnuts

1 serving Angel Hair Pasta with Roasted Pumpkin, Sage, and Walnuts (page 385) or 2 cups cooked whole wheat pasta mixed with ½ cup marinara sauce and 1 cup of any cooked Best Vegetables (below) or any vegetable from the grocery list (page 176). Serve with leafy green salad tossed with 1 teaspoon olive oil and unlimited vinegar or fresh lemon juice (or 2 tablespoons reduced-calorie dressing).

Rosemary Chicken with Sautéed Swiss Chard

5 ounces grilled Rosemary Chicken (page 347) with 2 cups Sautéed Swiss Chard (page 348). Enjoy with 1 cup baby carrots.

SNACK OPTIONS

100 calories or less

- *Best Vegetables:* 1 cup raw or cooked bell peppers (red, green, yellow), broccoli, broccoli raab, chile peppers, kale, Brussels sprouts, red cabbage, sugar snap peas, snow peas, tomatoes, mushrooms, green beans, okra, zucchini squash, carrots, lettuce and leafy greens, spinach, collard greens, Swiss chard, watercress, asparagus, kohlrabi, rhubarb, rutabagas, okra, artichokes, beets, cauliflower, or seaweed

- *Best Fruits:* 1 apple (especially Red Delicious with skin), orange, blood orange, tangerine, peach, persimmon, or guava; 2 kiwis, clementines, tangerines, or plums; ½ papaya, mango, grapefruit, or cantaloupe; 1 cup elderberries, lingonberries, black currants, cranberries, boysenberries, blackberries, blueberries, raspberries, cherries, sliced strawberries, watermelon, honeydew, red/black/purple grapes, or pineapple; ½ cup lychees; 4 apricots or 4 prunes; 20 strawberries; 2 tablespoons raisins

- 1 cup Ginger Green Tea (page 189)

- ½ cup fat-free or 1% reduced-fat cottage cheese mixed with 1 sliced jalapeño chile pepper

- ¼ cup Fiery Nectarine Chutney (page 190) with celery and red pepper sticks

100 to 200 calories

- 1 baked apple with cinnamon and 1 teaspoon sugar or honey

- 1 ounce (about ¼ cup) toasted walnuts

- Black or green tea skim latte (with fat-free milk or enriched/fortified soy milk and optional 1 teaspoon sugar or sugar substitute)

- ½ cup fat-free or 1% reduced-fat cottage cheese with 1 serving of fruit

- 1 serving (2 cups) Tropical Mango-Citrus Smoothie (page 123)

- 1 Ginger-Spiced Pumpkin Muffin (page 187)

- 1 serving Warm Dark Chocolate Sauce with Fresh Fruit (page 81)

- 1 serving Butternut Squash Soup (page 80)

- 1 cup fat-free, plain or flavored yogurt mixed with ½ cup berries and 1 tablespoon wheat germ

- 1 cup fat-free vanilla yogurt mixed with ½ cup canned 100% pure pumpkin puree

SLOW-COOKER CHICKEN CURRY AND VEGETABLES

Curry, turmeric, and ginger make this an ultimate anti-inflammatory meal. Regularly enjoyed by millions of people worldwide, this dish provides key ingredients to help fight arthritis. The traditional version incorporates whole-milk yogurt, but I use fat-free yogurt, reducing saturated fat.

Makes 4 servings (1½ cups per serving)

3	tablespoons madras curry powder
1	tablespoon olive oil
2	cloves garlic, minced
1	teaspoon turmeric
1	teaspoon minced fresh ginger
1½	pounds skinless, boneless chicken breasts, cut into 2" chunks
	Salt
1	head cauliflower (about 1½ pounds), cut into 1" florets, stem discarded
1	large onion, chopped
1	can (15 ounces) chickpeas, rinsed and drained
3	large tomatoes (about 1 pound), chopped
1	cup fat-free yogurt
2	tablespoons chopped cilantro for garnish

TO MAKE IN A SLOW COOKER

1. Combine the curry powder, oil, garlic, turmeric, and ginger in a zip-top bag. Sprinkle the chicken with salt, and place in the bag. Shake until the curry mixture evenly coats the chicken.
2. Place the cauliflower and onion in the bottom of a 4- to 5-quart slow cooker. Add the chickpeas, and arrange the chicken evenly on top. Add the tomatoes. Cover, and cook on high for 3 to 3½ hours, stirring once during cooking time, until the chicken is no longer pink in the center and the vegetables are tender.
3. Transfer the chicken curry to a large bowl and stir in the yogurt. Season with additional salt if needed, and garnish with cilantro. Serve immediately with brown basmati rice.

TO MAKE ON THE STOVETOP

1. Season the chicken with salt. In a large skillet, heat the oil over high heat. Add the chicken and cook, stirring, 3 to 4 minutes, until the chicken begins to brown. Transfer the chicken to a plate. Add the onion, and cook 3 to 4 minutes, until beginning to soften and become translucent. Add the garlic, turmeric, ginger, and curry powder and cook, stirring, 1 to 2 minutes, until the mixture becomes fragrant.

2. Add ¼ cup water, the cauliflower, chickpeas, and tomatoes. Lower the heat to a simmer, and add more water if the mixture becomes dry. Cover and cook 8 to 10 minutes, until the cauliflower is tender. Uncover and return the chicken to the pan, and cook, stirring occasionally, 10 to 15 minutes longer, until the chicken is cooked through but still tender and the liquid thickens.

3. Remove from heat. Stir in the yogurt. Season with salt if needed, and garnish with cilantro. Serve immediately with brown basmati rice.

PER SERVING
437 calories, 52 g protein, 39 g carbohydrate, 8 g fat (1 g saturated), 99 mg cholesterol, 447 mg sodium, 11 g fiber; plus 537 mcg beta carotene

GRILLED ROCKEFELLER OYSTERS

When it comes to oysters, people either love them or hate them. My own household is divided. If you're a lover, you're in luck. Pacific oysters provide omega-3 fats, which have been shown to reduce inflammation in people who suffer with swollen joints. My recipe also adds olive oil and hot sauce—two more beneficial ingredients for fighting arthritis.

Makes 4 servings, 6 oysters each

2	tablespoons olive oil
2	tablespoons all-purpose flour
1/4	cup water
	Zest and juice of 1 lemon
2	cups spinach, wilted and chopped
1/2	cup fresh basil, chopped
3	cloves garlic, minced
1/8	teaspoon hot sauce
	Salt
	Ground pepper
2	dozen large, tightly closed fresh Pacific oysters in the shell
2	tablespoons grated Parmesan cheese

1. In a small skillet, heat the oil over medium heat. Add the flour and cook 3 to 4 minutes, stirring continuously until a thick, smooth paste forms. Remove from the heat and add the water, lemon zest and juice, spinach, basil, garlic, and hot sauce. Whisk quickly until a thick sauce forms. Season with salt and pepper to taste.

2. Preheat a grill or an oven to 400°F. Shuck the oysters, reserving the shells. Arrange the oysters in the deepest reserved half-shells, one oyster per shell. Top with a spoonful of the spinach mixture and sprinkle with the Parmesan.

3. If grilling, set the half-shells on the grill, filling-side up. Cover loosely with a sheet of aluminum foil, and grill 8 to 10 minutes, until oysters are no longer translucent but still tender. If baking, place the half-shells on a baking sheet covered with aluminum foil, and bake 8 to 10 minutes, until the oysters are cooked inside and the filling begins to brown and the oysters are no longer translucent but still tender. Serve immediately.

PER SERVING
183 calories, 13 g protein, 9 g carbohydrate, 10 g fat (2 g saturated), 58 mg cholesterol, 178 mg sodium, 2 g fiber

GINGER-SPICED PUMPKIN MUFFINS

I call these Muffins with a Mission! Enjoy one as a midday snack, or couple with an egg, fat-free yogurt, or glass of fat-free milk for a balanced breakfast. Either way, it's win/win—just 131 calories and created to help ease the aches and pains of arthritis.

Makes 12

½	cup packed brown sugar
1½	cups whole wheat flour
2	teaspoons baking powder
1	teaspoon ground cinnamon
1	teaspoon ground ginger
½	teaspoon salt
1	egg
1	cup fat-free milk
½	cup canned 100% pure pumpkin
¼	cup canola oil
½	teaspoon grated orange zest

1. Preheat the oven to 375°F. Lightly spray 12 muffin cups with nonstick cooking spray.
2. In a large mixing bowl, stir together the brown sugar, flour, baking powder, cinnamon, ginger, and salt.
3. In a small bowl, beat the egg for 30 seconds, until foamy. Add the milk, pumpkin, oil, and orange zest. Beat well. Add the egg mixture to the flour mixture, and stir until the flour mixture is moistened.
4. Fill the muffin cups three-quarters full with batter. Bake for 15 minutes, until the tops spring back when you touch them with a finger. Turn out muffins onto a wire rack to cool. Once cool, you can freeze the muffins, tightly wrapped, for up to 2 months.

PER MUFFIN
131 calories, 3 g protein, 19 g carbohydrate, 5 g fat (0 g saturated), 18 mg cholesterol, 20 mg sodium, 2 g fiber

GINGERED CARROTS

I'm always looking for creative ways to prepare one of my favorite veggies—carrots. This chapter gave me a reason to experiment with ginger, and I'm thrilled with the finished product. I hope your joints, and taste buds, agree!

Makes 4 servings

1	pound carrots, peeled and cut into 1" wedges
2	tablespoons soft tub reduced-fat, trans fat–free margarine spread
¼	cup grated fresh ginger
2	teaspoons ground ginger
	Salt
	Ground black pepper

1. Preheat the oven to 400°F. Tear a large piece of aluminum foil, about 24" long. Spread the carrots evenly over one half. Rub the carrots with the margarine, fresh ginger, and ground ginger. Season with salt and pepper.

2. Fold the opposite end of the foil over, folding around the edges to make a neat package with no openings. Place the package on a baking sheet and bake 20 to 25 minutes, until the carrots are tender when pierced with a knife. Serve immediately.

PER SERVING
77 calories, 1 g protein, 12 g carbohydrate, 3 g fat (0 g saturated), 0 mg cholesterol, 129 mg sodium, 3 g fiber; plus 470 mcg beta carotene, 142 mcg beta cryptoxanthin

GINGER GREEN TEA

Swap your morning coffee or afternoon soda for a relaxing cup of pleasure. Both ginger and green tea possess potent anti-inflammatory properties. Plus, I love the sensational aroma that fills my kitchen when I make this brew. If you use the optional sugar, the calorie count will be 65.

Makes 1 serving

1	cup water
1	½-inch piece fresh ginger with skin, sliced
1	green tea bag, or 1 tablespoon loose green tea leaves in a tea ball
2	tablespoons fat-free milk
1	tablespoon sugar, honey, or sugar substitute (optional)

Bring the water to a boil. Add the ginger and boil for 30 seconds more. Remove from the heat, and add the tea bag or tea ball. Steep for 2 to 3 minutes. Add the milk. If desired, stir in sugar, honey, or sugar substitute.

PER SERVING
13 calories, 1 g protein, 2 g carbohydrate, 0 g fat, 0 mg cholesterol, 20 mg sodium, 0 g fiber

FIERY NECTARINE CHUTNEY

My sweet and spicy chutney made its debut on the *Today* show. Since then, I've discovered that it goes great with just about anything! Jalapeños and ginger possess anti-inflammatory properties, which have been shown to alleviate the aches and pains associated with arthritis. What's more, chopped onions supply quercetin . . . and the nectarines, red pepper, and orange juice provide disease-fighting antioxidants, like beta cryptoxanthin and vitamin C. Serve as a dip with crudités and baked tortilla chips, or spoon a few tablespoons on top of grilled fish, poultry, lean turkey sausages, or veggie burgers.

Makes 12 servings, ¼ cup each

2	large, ripened nectarines (about 1 pound), finely chopped with skin
1	large red bell pepper, chopped
½	cup finely chopped red onion
4	teaspoons minced jalapeño chile pepper, or more if you can take the heat (wear plastic gloves when handling)
2	tablespoons fresh lime juice
2	tablespoons orange juice
2	to 3 teaspoons sugar (optional)
¼	teaspoon ground ginger
¼	teaspoon ground allspice
¼	teaspoon salt

In medium bowl, stir together the nectarines, bell pepper, onion, jalapeño, lime juice, orange juice, sugar if you like, ginger, allspice, and salt. Refrigerate until serving time.

PER SERVING
19 calories, 0 g protein, 5 g carbohydrate, 0 g fat, 0 mg cholesterol, 49 mg sodium, 1 g fiber; plus 23 mg vitamin C (38% DV)

CHAPTER 9

TYPE 2 DIABETES

I'm not going to try to sugar-coat it—diabetes is a silent killer. Of all the disorders I treat, diabetes is among the sneakiest and nastiest.

Sneaky . . . because unless you know you're at risk and are checking for signs, symptoms might not appear until your body is damaged in some way. Nearly one-third of people who have diabetes don't know it. If you suspect there's a problem but wait until you feel sick to get help, you may be well on your to developing complications.

Nasty . . . because if it goes untreated, one or several serious complications can kill you, although the process might take years. Diabetes can lead to a heart attack or stroke, continuous pain from degenerated nerves, foot or leg amputations from gangrene, kidney failure, or blindness from retinopathy.

It's not a pretty picture, but the condition is serious, and one that deserves your serious attention if you've been diagnosed, know or even suspect you're at risk!

On a positive note, if you work with your doctor to closely monitor and control your blood sugar and commit to eating right and exercising regularly, there's great reason to believe you'll live a long, healthy life. New medications, clever blood testing devices, and breakthrough information about diabetes processes, foods, and supplements mean that near-perfect glucose control is within everyone's reach.

WHAT IS DIABETES?

Your body's primary source of energy is glucose, a simple sugar created when carbohydrates are broken down during digestion. If everything is working properly, glucose enters the blood stream . . . which triggers the pancreas to release insulin . . . which allows glucose to leave the blood and enter every cell in your body. That's how cells get their nourishment. This energy transfer at the cellular level fuels all the your bodily functions from thinking to digestion to all the fantastic physical feats the human body is capable of. Think of glucose as the electricity in a house—you have one main line which branches off into each room and branches again to supply power to the outlets within them. Skimp on the glucose, and your power goes out.

If you have diabetes, there is a problem with the way your body produces or uses insulin. If glucose can't move into the cells, it stays in the blood stream leading to the high blood sugar levels characteristic of the disease.

There are three main types of diabetes. With *type 1 diabetes,* the insulin-producing cells of the pancreas are destroyed, so there is no insulin available to let glucose enter body cells. It is as if a circuit breaker tripped, and the power is simply cut off. No insulin means no energy getting to the cells. Type 1 diabetes is an autoimmune disorder for which there is no known prevention. It requires treatment with insulin and carefully planned meals.

With *type 2 diabetes,* there are two potential insulin problems. Either 1) the pancreas can't make enough insulin; or 2) the cells have become resistant to the insulin your body produces. Either or both these conditions may be present. Going back to the electricity analogy, insulin resistance is like having a dimmer switch on your body's power supply stuck on "low"—some energy gets through to the cells, but much of the glucose is blocked from entering cells and stays in the blood stream. Treatment options vary from person to person, depending on the severity of the condition. Some people with type 2 diabetes can manage their disease with dietary changes alone. Others require medications or insulin replacement.

There is also a third type of diabetes called *gestational diabetes,* which affects about 4 percent of pregnant women. Although this type of diabetes usually disappears after the baby is born, research suggests that women who develop gestational diabetes have an increased risk of developing type 2 diabetes later in life.

The information in the rest of this chapter pertains only to type 2 diabetes. People with type 1 or gestational diabetes should consult a private nutritionist or trained diabetes educator for one-on-one dietary counseling.

WHAT AFFECTS TYPE 2 DIABETES?

Type 2 diabetes was once called *adult-onset diabetes,* but now we know that even young children can develop this disease. The number one risk factor—by far—is being overweight. Genetics, age, and lack of exercise also contribute to your personal risk, but body weight is the biggest contributor. The American Diabetes Association recommends that anyone who is overweight should talk with his or her physician to see if testing is appropriate. If your doctor believes you're at significant risk, she'll order blood tests to rule out a thyroid disorder, and to determine if you have diabetes or prediabetes. There are two tests used to check for diabetes:

A Fasting Plasma Glucose test (FPG) measures blood glucose after an overnight fast. It is quick, convenient, and inexpensive. Normal fasting blood sugar is below 100 mg/dL. If your blood glucose is 126 mg/dL or higher, the test will be repeated. Two readings of 126 mg/dL or higher means a diagnosis of diabetes. If your blood glucose is 100 to 125 mg/dL, your diagnosis is prediabetes. (Prediabetes used to be called *impaired glucose tolerance* or *impaired fasting glucose*.)

An Oral Glucose Tolerance Test (OGTT) measures blood glucose after an overnight fast, and again 2 hours after you drink a high-glucose liquid. This test is more sensitive than FPG, but it is inconvenient because of the 2-hour wait between blood draws. Normal 2-hour blood glucose is below 140 mg/dL. If your 2-hour blood glucose is 200 mg/dL or higher, the test will be repeated. Two readings of 200 mg/dL or higher means a diagnosis of diabetes. If your 2-hour blood glucose is 140 to 199 mg/dL, your diagnosis is prediabetes.

WHAT ARE THE DANGERS OF PREDIABETES?

It's probably obvious, but the greatest danger of prediabetes is that it can lead to diabetes. In fact, research shows that most people with prediabetes will develop diabetes within 10 years unless they lose weight (at least 5 percent of body weight), become more active, and make changes to their eating habits (like embracing the eating plan I'll tell you about later in this chapter).

Prediabetes is also one of the hallmarks of another disorder called *the metabolic syndrome*. The metabolic syndrome describes a cluster of risk factors that, when taken together, create a toxic environment in your blood vessels. Doctors diagnose metabolic syndrome in patients who have at least three of the following conditions: high blood pressure (130/85 mmHg or higher), high triglycerides (150 mg/dL or higher), low HDL cholesterol (below 50 mg/dL for women, below 40 mg/dL for men), large waist circumference (greater than 35" for women, greater than 40" for men), or fasting blood sugar higher than 110 mg/dL. The combination of any three is dangerous, even if the numbers are only slightly out of the normal range. People with the metabolic syndrome have an increased risk of heart attack and stroke. If you have been diagnosed with metabolic syndrome but have a normal fasting glucose level (below 100 mg/dL), follow the 4-step plan outlined in my cardiovascular disease chapter (page 147). If you have been diagnosed with metabolic syndrome and your fasting glucose level is elevated (higher than 110 mg/dL), follow the 4-step program outlined at the end of this chapter. You should also read the cardiovascular disease chapter to learn about the most beneficial foods to eat (and not!) in order to bring

FAQS

Is it safe for people with diabetes to drink coffee?

Coffee has a bad reputation, a largely undeserved one, especially when it comes to its effect on diabetes. Many studies have linked moderate coffee drinking with a lower risk of developing type 2 diabetes. A Swedish study found that people with diabetes and low glucose tolerance who regularly drank coffee had less glucose resistance and better beta cell function. Caffeinated or decaffeinated, instant or filtered coffee, all can lower diabetes risk. But of all the varieties, decaffeinated coffee seems to have the greatest effect. The Iowa Women's Health Study, which followed nearly 29,000 women for about 10 years, found that drinking decaffeinated coffee reduced the risk of developing diabetes by 33 percent, while coffee with caffeine reduced the risk by only about 21 percent. Because some other studies have shown that caffeine reduces insulin sensitivity, decaf is definitely the way to go.

down all other elevated numbers, such as blood pressure, LDL cholesterol, and triglycerides.

The good news is that prediabetes doesn't necessarily progress to diabetes. The Diabetes Prevention Program, which studied more than 3,000 people with prediabetes, showed that participants who changed their diets, lost weight, and started exercising reduced their risk of developing diabetes by an astounding 58 percent. That's slashing your risk of diabetes by more than half, without drugs! Treatment with the medication metformin reduced the risk of diabetes by 31 percent—still significant, but less than the combined effect of diet and exercise. Every step you take—and I mean that both literally and figuratively—can help prevent or delay the onset of disease. Every year you don't have to deal with the complications of diabetes is a blessing for your future health.

One of my clients is counting on those blessings. Dina, 49, went to her doctor for a routine checkup and blood work before her second marriage, and discovered that she had the metabolic syndrome. Her fasting blood sugar was 125—just shy of full-fledged diabetes. In addition, she had triglycerides of about 200, high blood pressure, and total cholesterol of 340—her "bad" LDL cholesterol was over 200! (Although LDL cholesterol is not a diagnostic marker for metabolic syndrome, optimal levels are less than 100.). At 5'5" and 163 pounds, Dina was also overweight and carried a significant amount of fat around her middle. She also had a family history heart disease—her brother had died of a heart attack in his late 30s. Until her test results came back, Dina had eaten whatever she wanted and didn't give a darn about exercise. Her doctor set her straight: "Those days are over. You're getting married and have a whole new adventure ahead of you. You have a lot to live for." He wrote her a prescription for a cholesterol-lowering medication and sent her to me.

After just two months following every point of my 4-Step Program for Diabetes, Dina lost 16 pounds and trimmed 4" off her waist. Her fasting blood sugar was down to 105—still too high, but a significant improvement. Her blood pressure was now in the normal range and her blood lipids were lower, too, thanks to medication and nutrition changes. Her triglycerides had fallen to 130 (now considered normal), and her total cholesterol had fallen to about 210 (the bad LDL cholesterol dropped below 130!). She drew her motivation from both fear and hope—fear of meeting the same early death as her brother, and hope for years of love and happiness she dreamed of sharing with her new husband. Hope, for many of us, blooms as we see the powerful effects making just a few changes can have on our overall health.

WHAT ARE THE DANGERS OF TYPE 2 DIABETES?

If you have diabetes, it is important to understand that it's a chronic condition. You can control the disease, but it will never go away. The best you can hope is that your disease will go into a form of remission—contained, but subject to return. You'll need to monitor your blood sugars daily, and your doctor will want to periodically check your progress, too. One of the most powerful medical tools is a blood test for glycosylated hemoglobin, more commonly called *HbA1C* or simply *A1C*. This test doesn't require fasting, and it estimates how well you've been controlling blood glucose over the past two to three months. So A1C captures more than your blood glucose level at the moment your doctor draws blood for the test—it is a measure of whether you're controlling your diabetes . . . or if your diabetes is controlling you.

High A1C levels mean a high risk of complications from diabetes. To put it bluntly, uncontrolled blood sugar is a poison. Because all cells need and use glucose, many different body systems are affected. The most common problems faced by people with diabetes are:

CARDIOVASCULAR PROBLEMS

Although a little extra blood sugar doesn't sound dangerous, it is toxic to your blood vessels. High levels of glucose form free radicals, unstable molecules that damage cellular membranes, including the delicate cell membranes of your blood vessels. Over the long-term, the damage may trigger the immune system to address the damage. Unfortunately the inflammatory chemicals sent to the site of the damage further assault the blood vessels. The process can lead to serious cardiovascular problems . . . which in turn may cause a heart attack or stroke. (For more information about the cardiovascular system, see page 127.)

EYE DISEASES

Diabetes increases your risk of cataracts, which cloud the lens, and glaucoma, which can lead to blindness from damage to the optic nerve. In addition, uncontrolled blood glucose damages the delicate blood vessels in the retina, leading to a condition called *diabetic retinopathy*. Diabetic retinopathy is the leading cause of blindness in America, but that doesn't mean it's in your future. Studies show that people can prevent retinopathy by keeping their blood sugar levels as close to normal as possible. Once retinopathy develops, careful blood sugar control can keep the disease from progressing.

NEUROPATHY

Uncontrolled diabetes exposes your nerves to something like a sugar bath, which leads to degeneration of nerve axons—the bodies of the nerve cells. In addition, the protective coating around the nerves—the myelin—may be stripped, slowing the speed at which nerves can transmit sensory messages. If the blood vessels that feed the nerves are damaged by diabetes, then those nerves can die.

Early nerve damage may not cause any discomfort. Mild symptoms can include tingling or numbness, particularly in the feet. Over time, neuropathy progresses and may cause pain or large areas of numbness. Scientists estimate that about 26 percent of people with type 2 diabetes have painful neuropathy. If nerves die, muscles of the feet or hands can whither. As the nerve damage becomes more extensive, it can cause impotence, dizziness, gastrointestinal problems, and general weakness.

Because the feet are usually affected first, good foot care is critically important. You may overlook a blister, sore, or cut if that part of your foot is numb. If your foot becomes infected, it could eventually spread internally to the bone. In some cases, an infection can become so severe that it becomes necessary to amputate the limb.

The longer you have uncontrolled diabetes, the greater your risk of neuropathy, and the greater the potential damage. But, as with eye diseases and other complications, studies have shown that neuropathy can be delayed and yes, even prevented if you control blood glucose level strictly.

HOW FOOD AFFECTS DIABETES

Let's talk about food on a grand scale for a minute. Regardless of whether you have prediabetes or diabetes, the best thing you can do for your health is to lose weight. I know, I know . . . that's what your doctor said, right? But did she tell you that you don't have to slim down to swimsuit shape to reap the benefits? Research has shown that losing even small amounts of weight—as little as 10 pounds over two years—can reduce the risk of developing diabetes by up to 30 percent. That's a small amount of weight to lose for such a large return on the quality of your life! And if you add more lifestyle changes, you'll reduce your risk even more. Among people with diabetes, weight loss improves insulin sensitivity and glycemic control, reduces triglycerides and LDL cholesterol, and lowers blood pressure. That is to say, losing a few pounds may very well save your life. (For more information on the basics of losing weight, see Weight Loss on page 19.)

But healthy eating for diabetes prevention or control is about more than weight loss . . . .

HIGH-QUALITY CARBOHYDRATES
VERSUS LOW-QUALITY CARBOHYDRATES

During digestion, carbohydrates break down to create glucose, which enters the blood stream, triggering a rise in insulin, which is necessary for the glucose to enter cells. In people with diabetes, this system is defective, so glucose stays in the blood. This is what you are checking when you test your blood sugar level.

You have no doubt heard about the concept of the *glycemic index* (GI). GI is a measure of how fast and how high a particular food will raise blood sugar. Foods with a high GI raise blood sugar faster and higher than foods with a low GI. It's a controversial topic in nutrition because when it comes right down to it, GI values simply aren't very user-friendly. One type of food can have many different GI values depending on ripeness (of a fruit or vegetable), method of preparation, and other factors. For example, a ripe banana has a higher GI than a green banana, and a baked potato has a different GI than a boiled potato. If you eat a high-GI food with a protein (and/or a food containing fat), the GI value goes down because protein and fat slow down the absorption of carbohydrate. Beyond that, a tomato grown in a North Carolina farm may have a different GI than a tomato grown in a Pennsylvania greenhouse. The myriad factors that influence GI values boggle the mind! There's an easier way to achieve low-glycemic eating without feeling like every meal is an exercise in advanced mathematics.

If you're looking for foods that raise blood sugar levels slowly and gently like rolling waves, choose high-quality carbohydrates (see list below) instead of low-quality carbs, and whenever possible, couple these carbs with protein and/or healthy fat. For example, eat brown rice and vegetables (high-quality carbs) together with grilled chicken or pork tenderloin (lean protein). High-quality carbs are full of vitamins, minerals, and fiber. They are found primarily in plant foods, including whole grain products, brown and wild rice, oats, vegetables, fruits and legumes. In addition, some of these high-quality carbs also contain soluble fiber, a component of plant cell walls. Soluble fiber slows the absorption of glucose from food in the stomach, which also helps keep blood sugar under control. Studies have shown that eating a diet rich in whole grains and high-fiber foods may reduce the risk of diabetes by between 35 and 42 percent.

BEST FOODS FOR HIGH-QUALITY CARBS: *Vegetables, fruits (fresh, frozen; unsweetened), beans, peas, lentils, brown rice, wild rice, barley, oatmeal, whole grain cereals, whole grain breads, whole grain crackers, quinoa, amaranth, wheat berries, millet*

BEST FOODS FOR SOLUBLE FIBER: *Psyllium seeds (ground), oat bran, rice bran, oatmeal, barley, lentils, Brussels sprouts, peas, beans (kidney, lima, black, navy, pinto), apples, blackberries, pears, oranges, grapefruit, cantaloupe, strawberries, bananas, peaches, broccoli, carrots, cauliflower, cabbage, spinach, sweet potatoes, yams, white potatoes, tomatoes, avocado, raspberries, corn, almonds, flaxseed (ground), sunflower seeds*

Low-quality carbs, on the other hand, have much less nutritional value. They are made primarily of sugar, including sugar itself, candy, soft drinks, syrup, honey, jam and jelly, cakes, and most other foods we typically think of as sweets or desserts. Refined starches—the "white" carbs, such as white rice and white bread—are also low-quality carbohydrates because they act very much like sugars once you begin to digest them. You should also avoid drinking fruit juice—all fruit juice, even 100% pure fruit, fruit juice. Although these beverages certainly provide better nutrition than soft drinks, they're concentrated in fruit sugar and raise blood sugars quickly. The same thing goes for dried fruit. Like fruit juice, dried fruit provides ample nutrition and fiber, but when the water content is removed from fresh fruit, the dried, dehydrated version becomes super concentrated in sugar and can cause a sharp rise in blood sugar. Clearly not worth the spike! Root vegetables—such as potatoes, carrots, beets, and turnips—have a higher glycemic index than other, non-root veggies, such as broccoli, peppers, and mushrooms. However, you can enjoy moderate amounts of root vegetables if you eat them with lean protein at meals (instead of eating them alone). For example, a balanced dinner might include grilled chicken, broccoli, and a small baked white or sweet potato topped with fat-free sour cream; lunch might include turkey breast in a whole wheat pita pocket with 1 cup crunchy baby carrots.

Your goal, then, is to choose high-quality carbohydrates whenever possible, and to limit or avoid most low-quality carbs.

MODERATE TOTAL CARBOHYDRATES, COUPLED WITH PROTEIN

If you stick with high-quality carbs, can you eat as much as you want? Unfortunately, NO. To best control your blood sugars, you have to *moderate* ALL carbs—even if they're the best of the best carbohydrates. Your total carb intake should be limited to about 40 percent of your daily food intake. That's why on my meal plan you'll notice things like "half a baked white or sweet potato" or "reduced-calorie, whole wheat bread." I've picked the best of the best carbs, but still had to limit the total amount.

To further slow or prevent a blood sugar rise, remember that, in general, carbs should be eaten together with high-quality protein. Some foods—such as lentils, beans, yogurts, milk, split peas, and soybeans—naturally contain both high-quality carbohydrate and lean protein. My food plan incorporates everything—moderate amounts of high-quality carbohydrate, coupled throughout the day with protein. If you like to have the plan laid out for you in detail, it's all there; if you like to add your own flair to meals, use it as a reference guide.

BEST FOODS FOR HIGH-QUALITY PROTEIN: *Turkey breast, chicken breast, seafood and fish, veal, pork tenderloin, lean ham, lean beef, egg whites, yogurt (fat-free, low-fat), milk*

CARB COUNTING AND THE EXCHANGE SYSTEM

People with diabetes are sometimes told they need to count carbs or follow a food exchange system to standardize their diets.

Counting carbs is particularly important for people who take insulin because their dosage is dependent on the amount of carbohydrate they need to offset. They determine the number of carbs they will eat in a particular meal, calculate the amount of insulin they will need to clear those carbs from their blood, then give themselves an injection (or program the amount into their insulin pump). Every "portion" of food in a carb-counting list is equal to 15 grams of carbohydrate—including grains, fruits, dairy products, and starchy vegetables. All you need to know is that every 15 grams of carbohydrate counts as 1 carb choice. For example, one medium apple = 15 grams of carbs = 1 portion. Some doctors and diabetes educators instruct their patients either to count total carb grams, or count the number of carb portions. If you are a carb counter, I have provided total carbohydrate grams after each of the meals and snacks in the 4-Step Program.

The Food Exchange System organizes food according to their nutritional content: Starch, Fruit, Vegetable, Fat-Free/Reduced-Fat Milk (including milk and yogurt), Very Lean Meat, Lean Meat, Medium-Fat Meat, High-Fat Meat, and Fat. If your doctor has instructed you to follow the exchange system, then follow those recommendations. I have included exchange information alongside carb grams after each of the meals in my 4-Step Program.

(fat-free, 1% reduced-fat), enriched/fortified soy milk, cheese (fat-free, reduced-fat), beans (lima, black, navy, white, pinto, garbanzo), lentils, split peas, tofu, tempeh, soybeans, nuts (soy nuts, peanuts, almonds), peanut butter

HEALTHY FATS VERSUS SATURATED AND TRANS FATS

All fats are not created equal—some can decrease your risk of diabetes and complications, while others are downright dangerous. Let's talk about the bad fats first.

Avoid Saturated Fats. Saturated fats are found in animal-based foods, including meats, butter, whole-milk dairy products (including regular yogurt, cheese, and ice cream), and poultry skin. They are also found in some high-fat plant foods, including palm oil. Some studies have shown that eating a diet with lots of saturated fats can lead to insulin resistance, and may increase the risk of diabetes by up to 20 percent. In addition, many studies confirm that saturated fats increase the risk of heart disease. Because people with diabetes already have an increased risk of heart disease, eating these unhealthy fats will push your risk even higher. By making a few simple changes, you can dramatically reduce the amount of saturated fats in your diet:

- Avoid: butter, cream cheese, lard, sour cream, doughnuts, cake, cookies, chocolate bars, chocolate chips, ice cream, fried foods, pizza, cream- or cheese-based salad dressing, cheese sauce, cream sauce, animal shortening, high-fat meats (including hamburgers, bologna, pepperoni, sausage, bacon, salami, pastrami, spareribs, and hot dogs), high-fat cuts of beef and pork, whole-milk dairy products. If a food label lists palm oil, and the saturated fat content is more than 2 grams per serving, put the package back on the shelf.
- Choose: lean meat only (including skinless chicken and turkey, lean beef, lean pork), fish, reduced-fat or fat-free dairy products.
- Always remove skin from poultry.
- Prepare foods by baking, roasting, broiling, boiling, poaching, steaming, grilling, or stir-frying. No deep-fat frying.

Avoid Trans Fats. Trans fats are worse than saturated fats for diabetes and its complications. Trans fats were developed in a laboratory to improve the shelf life of processed foods, and to turn oils solid. Most stick margarines contain trans fats, and trans fats are found in many packaged baked goods, crackers, potato chips, snack foods, fried foods, and fast food that use or create *hydrogenated oils*. (Good news for consumers—all food labels must now list the amount of trans fats, right after the amount of saturated fats.) By substituting vegetable oil for trans fats, you may be able to reduce your risk of diabetes by about 40 percent, and you can reduce your risk of heart disease by 53 percent. Whether you already have diabetes or are working to prevent it, there is no amount of trans fats you can safely incorporate into your diet, so try to keep them as far from your plate as possible.

Choose Omega-3 and Monounsaturated Fatty Acids. Polyunsaturated fatty acids (PUFAs) come in two varieties—omega-3 fatty acids and omega-6 fatty acids. Scientists believe that PUFAs have many beneficial effects, including improving insulin sensitivity by changing the composition of cell membranes and aiding in glucose metabolism. When it comes to food, omega-3 fats are the PUFAs you want to pay close attention to.

Studies have shown that omega-3s from fish oil may delay the development of glucose intolerance, but the effects are unclear when it comes people who already have diabetes. The studies are all over the place—some show worsening of glycemic control with increased intake of fish oil, others show improved insulin sensitivity, and yet others no benefit or harm at all. Because there is no clear consensus, if you have diabetes, I would not recommend taking fish oil supplements (unless instructed by your endocrinologist). However, food sources of omega-3s are a safe bet, especially if they replace other, more harmful fats in your diet. Omega-3s from food will definitely help reduce your risk of heart disease, so I highly recommended them for all my clients with diabetes.

BEST FOODS FOR OMEGA-3 FATTY ACIDS: *Wild salmon, herring, mackerel (not king), sardines (fresh, canned) , anchovies, rainbow trout, Pacific oysters, omega-3–fortified eggs, flaxseed (ground and oil), walnuts, butternuts (white walnuts), seaweed, walnut oil, canola oil, soybeans*

Monounsaturated fats, found in olive oil and some nuts, are generally considered among the healthiest of fats. Research into the effects of olive oil on diabetes has been limited, but one Danish study found that people who ate a diet high in monounsaturated fats and low in low-quality carbohydrates had lower fasting blood glucose, lower average glucose levels, and lower peak blood glucose responses. Consider using olive and canola oil for cooking, adding a thin slice of avocado on your next sandwich, tossing olives into your salad, and snacking on an ounce of healthy nuts instead of sweets.

BEST FOODS FOR MONOUNSATURATED FATS: *Olive oil, canola oil, avocado, macadamia nuts, hazelnuts, pecans, almonds, peanuts, cashews, Brazil nuts, pistachio nuts, pine nuts, peanut butter, olives*

OTHER VITAMINS AND MINERALS

Calcium and Vitamin D. According to the Nurses' Health Study, which followed more than 83,000 women for 20 years, both calcium and vitamin D may help prevent type 2 diabetes. Women who got at least 800 IU of total vitamin D daily from food and/or supplements had a 23 percent lower risk of developing diabetes compared with those who consumed less than 200 IU daily.

Women who got at least 1,200 milligrams total calcium daily from food and/or supplements had a 21 percent lower risk of developing diabetes compared with those who consumed less than 600 milligrams per day. Combining vitamin D and calcium was even better—women who got at least 800 IU vitamin D *and* 1,200 milligrams calcium reduced their risk of diabetes by 33 percent. Strive to add more vitamin D–rich foods to your diet. It can be difficult to get all the vitamin D you need from foods, so consider taking a supplement. (See Supplements section, page 205, for more information.)

Scientists are unclear about exactly what these nutrients do to reduce diabetes risk. It could be that vitamin D regulates the insulin-producing cells of the pancreas, and calcium may improve insulin sensitivity. Of course, the synergy between the two makes sense—the body can't absorb or use calcium without vitamin D. Improvements in insulin sensitivity are important for everyone with diabetes, but calcium also seems to help control blood pressure, which contributes to heart disease. So whether you have prediabetes or diabetes, calcium and vitamin D are wise food choices.

I recommend that women aim to eat at least three servings of calcium-rich foods daily, and to consider taking a calcium supplement if they can't reliably fit calcium into their meals. (See the Supplements section, page 205, for more information.) Men should eat no more than two or three servings of calcium-rich foods daily, and should never take a calcium supplement without approval from their doctors—some early research suggests that high calcium diets may increase the risk of prostate cancer.

FAQS

I've heard that vinegar can help lower blood glucose levels. Is it true?

There is some research evidence that taking vinegar before meals may reduce the rise in blood glucose and insulin that can occur after eating. A Swedish study published in 2005 found that vinegar dampened the body's metabolic responses after a meal. In addition, the researchers discovered that vinegar helped people feel full and satisfied longer, even two hours after eating. If you want to try vinegar, I recommend talking with your doctor first—if it really does work, you may need to change your treatment plan (and medications). In the research studies scientists gave participants a "cocktail" of 4 teaspoons vinegar mixed with 3 tablespoons water before each meal.

BEST FOODS FOR CALCIUM: *Yogurt (fat-free, low-fat), milk (fat-free, 1% reduced-fat), enriched/fortified soy milk, cheese (fat-free, reduced-fat), tofu with calcium, sardines (with bones), wild salmon (with bones), soybeans, calcium-fortified whole grain waffles, bok choy, kale, white beans, broccoli, almonds*

BEST FOODS FOR VITAMIN D: *Wild salmon (with bones), mackerel (not king), sardines (with bones), herring, fortified milk (fat-free, 1% reduced-fat), enriched/fortified soy milk, egg yolks, mushrooms (especially shiitake), vitamin D–fortified margarine (soft tub, trans fat–free), fortified whole grain cereals*

Magnesium. Scientists believe that magnesium works hand-in-hand with enzymes involved in carbohydrate metabolism. In laboratory animals, abnormally low blood levels of magnesium led to insulin resistance. Other research confirms the benefit of magnesium for people—the combined results from two large studies—the Health Professionals' Follow-up Study, which followed more than 42,000 men for 12 years, and the Nurses' Health Study. Compared with people who consumed very low amounts of magnesium (less than about 250 milligrams daily), high daily magnesium reduced the risk of developing diabetes by about 33 percent. The amounts that defined *high* were 377 milligrams daily for women, and 458 milligrams daily for men—both close to the RDA recommended amount of 400 milligrams per day. Strive to add more magnesium-rich foods to your diet. Because most people don't get enough magnesium from food alone, consider taking a supplement, as well. (See the Supplements section, page 205, for more information.)

> **BEST FOODS FOR MAGNESIUM:** *Pumpkin seeds, spinach, Swiss chard, amaranth, sunflower seeds, cashews, almonds, quinoa, tempeh, sweet potatoes, white potatoes, soybeans, millet, beans (black, white, navy, lima, pinto, kidney), artichoke hearts, peanuts, peanut butter, chickpeas (garbanzo beans), brown rice, whole grain bread, sesame seeds, wheat germ, flaxseed*

BONUS POINTS

- **Get your team together.** Diabetes is a life-long, whole-body problem. Although your primary care physician may have been the one to order blood glucose testing, you need a team of professionals to guide you through all the medical details. Ideally your team will include your primary care physician, an endocrinologist (a hormone specialist) who understands the intricacies of insulin, a registered dietitian to help you fine-tune your eating plan, an ophthalmologist (an eye specialist) who can look for diabetes-related signs of damage to the retina, a podiatrist (a foot health specialist) who can help prevent complications from diabetes-related nerve damage and skin sores, and a dentist to keep periodontal disease and other infections under control. Because people with diabetes have a high risk of heart disease, your primary care physician will also be your guide to preventing and/or managing high blood pressure and/or high cholesterol (or your primary care physician may refer you to a cardiologist).

- **Monitor your blood glucose levels every day.** Some people fight against checking their blood sugar levels, but daily monitoring really is the only way to know if they are under control. Foods, activity level, medications, illness, and even stress can affect blood glucose. Unless you check, you won't know whether your levels are holding steady or spiraling out of control. Your doctor will tell you how often you need to check. Some people only need to check once a day, others may need to check four or five times per day. In addition, you should ask—in advance—what to do if your blood glucose readings are abnormal.

- **If you have diabetes medication, take it as directed.** People who have head-splitting migraines remember to take their medications because pain is a terrific motivator. People who take medication for severe acne have no trouble remembering to take it, because they know if they miss a few doses, the consequences will be written all over their faces. But diabetes symptoms are silent, and thinking they won't pay the price for missed meds means far too many people "forget" or to decide against taking prescribed medications, despite the grave risks of heart disease, nerve damage, and other complications. Don't be one of them. Take medications or insulin as directed by your physician. If you have uncomfortable side effects or questions about your medication or treatment plan, talk with your doctor.

- **Exercise.** Next to weight control and medical treatment, exercise is the most important thing you can do to take control over diabetes. Exercise decreases body fat and promotes weight loss. But even if you don't lose weight as a result, exercise will improve blood sugar control and your body's response to insulin, and can even reduce triglycerides. So activity helps diabetes control directly, and also helps prevent heart disease.

  It is never too late to start a healthful program of exercise. There are virtually no risks, other than a few sore muscles at the beginning. Studies have reported significant improvements in blood sugar control after just eight weeks. A review of research discovered that all levels of activity were beneficial, from moderate-intensity walking to high-intensity resistance training with weights. The important thing is the activity, not how much weight you lose. Aim for at least 150 minutes of moderate-intensity exercise per week (that's just two and a half hours total for the week). For most people, that means planning to be active for 30 minutes, five days per week. Feel free to add-on—you might try low-intensity activities, such as tai chi, stretching, or yoga. For fighting the complications of diabetes, any kind of activity beats sitting on the couch. The key is to find something you enjoy doing—walking, swimming, cycling, dancing—and get moving.

- **Keep a food record.** As you get control over your weight and blood sugar, it can be helpful to keep a log that includes some specific information about your eating habits. Every time you eat, jot down 1) where you are; 2) what time it is; 3) how hungry you are before beginning to eat; 4) how hungry you are when you stop eating; 5) the foods and amounts eaten; and 6) your thoughts or feelings at the time. Over time, you'll start to see patterns that can help you learn to eat only when you are physically hungry, and not just as a way to relieve anxiety or stress. It can also help you to stay focused on new food habits. Some clients enjoy the process. They find that they feel empowered by it, and keep food records for months. Others just do it for a few weeks, stopping once they understand their personal eating patterns. I strongly recommend keeping the record for at least a week—you may be surprised at what you learn.

- **Learn the value of distraction.** Your food record will help you identify the times of day and situations in which you're mostly likely to make poor food choices and that's an important first step. Once you know the weak spots, you can plan new activities to take the place of unhealthy habits. One trick that many of my clients use is a combination of delay and distraction. If you get the urge to eat (you're not physically hungry and it isn't a mealtime), set a timer and wait 20 minutes. In that time, do something else to keep your mind off food—clean out a closet (or purse!), organize your email files, put on a fresh coat of nail polish, call a friend, schedule your outstanding appointments, pick up that knitting you've been meaning to finish . . . anything that keeps your hands busy and off food. If you still want to eat when the timer goes off, have a healthy snack. Most people discover, however, that their craving disappears.

- **If you smoke, quit.** Smoking increases the risk of developing diabetes. Once you have diabetes, smoking makes every problem and complication worse. Smoking raises blood glucose levels, constricts blood vessels, and causes inflammation. As a result, people who smoke have an increased risk of kidney disease, nerve damage, blood vessel damage, and foot and leg infections. One extra piece of advice: Many people gain weight after quitting smoking because they try to satisfy their nicotine cravings by eating more. NOT a good strategy for anyone, but it is particularly dangerous for people with diabetes. Talk with your doctor about the best ways to quit smoking without overeating.

- **Drink alcohol only in moderation . . . if at all.** Drinking between one-half and two alcoholic drinks per day has been shown to reduce the risk of developing type 2 diabetes by an average of 40 percent compared to nondrinkers or heavy drinkers. However, among people who already have diabetes, there is some question about the benefits of alcohol. A review of medical literature published in 2004 concluded that there doesn't seem to be any significant risk of moderate alcohol consumption for people with diabetes. *Moderate* typically means drinking no more than one serving of alcohol per day if you're a woman, and no more than two servings if you are a man. (A serving is 12 ounces of beer, 5 ounces of wine, or 1 ½ ounces of liquor.) If you have diabetes, I also recommend checking with your doctor to make sure that alcohol is safe for you, and that you understand how it might affect your blood glucose levels. If you don't already drink alcohol, don't start.

- **Brush and floss regularly.** Just as unregulated diabetes leads to high levels of glucose in your blood, it also leads to higher-than-usual levels of glucose in your saliva. This high-glucose environment in your mouth allows bacteria to multiply and live quite happily, raising the risk for dental decay. Plus, diabetes makes fighting infection harder, so that if gum disease develops, you'll have a more difficult time getting rid of it than someone without diabetes. Studies have born this out—among people with periodontal disease, those who also have diabetes have more severe gum disease than those without diabetes, with deeper gum "pockets" and a greater loss of attachment that could eventually mean tooth loss. On the flip side, getting treatment for gum disease may help with diabetes management. Research suggests that people with diabetes who gain control over their periodontal problems have *better* glycemic control after gum treatment than before. For healthy teeth and gums, dentists and nutritionists alike recommend that you see your dentist regularly, brush with a fluoride toothpaste at least twice a day, and remember to floss.

- **If you have sleep apnea or daytime sleepiness, seek treatment.** Excessive daytime sleepiness is often a sign of sleep apnea, a disorder that causes interruptions in breathing during sleep. Breathing stops for 10 seconds or more because of faulty signals from the brain, or because the soft tissue at the back the throat relaxes and blocks the airway (called *obstructive sleep apnea,* or OSA). This can happen several times per night. Each time, the sleeper will partially awaken, begin to breathe again, and then fall back asleep. Most people with sleep apnea don't know what is happening, or why they feel so tired after what seemed like a full night's rest. People with diabetes are more likely to have sleep apnea than people without diabetes. Even more intriguing is the possibility that sleep apnea may contribute to diabetes. OSA itself increases the risk of insulin resistance, and may be a roadblock to controlling your diabetes. If you have sleep apnea, or if you experience unusual sleepiness during the daytime, talk with your doctor. A full night's sleep is not just a luxury, it's a health necessity.

- **Be meticulous with your foot care.** The key words are *clean* and *dry*. Wash your feet daily in warm water, and dry with a clean soft towel. Do not soak your feet, or use hot water. Inspect your feet every day for sores, blisters, calluses, swelling, bruising, or breaks in the skin—talk with your doctor about how to treat them. Don't walk barefoot—always wear shoes or slippers, and wear clean, soft socks with your shoes. Talk with your podiatrist about other ways to keep your feet safe.

SUPPLEMENTS

For years, scientists have been hunting for a "magic bullet" to treat diabetes—one or more nutrients that could be taken in supplement form to improve glycemic control. As of now, the search is still on. Researchers have tested all logical possibilities, including antioxidants, vitamin E, and fish oil. Results are confusing and inconsistent, sometimes showing a benefit, and sometimes showing that taking a particular supplement actually makes blood sugar control worse.

The follow supplements are generally considered safe, and have quite a bit of supporting research. But diabetes management and blood glucose control can be tricky and tenuous. Before taking *any* supplement, talk with your endocrinologist, especially if you are already taking a hypoglycemic or insulin-sensitizing medication.

FAQS

I used to read a lot about chromium picolinate supplements. Are they valuable for people with diabetes?

Back in the 1990s, chromium picolinate was popular as a simple treatment that scientists thought might help improve glycemic control and insulin sensitivity. Most of the studies that supported that claim had been done on laboratory animals, which is never the same as investigating the effects of a treatment on people. More recently, the picture for chromium picolinate has turned much less optimistic. In 2006, scientists reported that they were unable to find any benefit of chromium picolinate supplements in people with type 2 diabetes, even when relatively high dosages were tested. A major review of all high-quality studies found that the data were ultimately inconclusive—no one can say with any degree of certainty whether chromium is helpful or not. More research will need to be done, but as of right now, I can't recommend chromium supplements for diabetes control.

1. **Multivitamin.** If you want to assure that you get your daily supply of all vitamins and minerals, consider taking a multivitamin. Look for a brand that contains 100% DV of most nutrients. If you are a man, or a women who is no longer menstruating, choose a "senior" formula, which doesn't contain iron. I cannot recommend taking high doses of any individual vitamins at this time.

2. **Calcium, with vitamin D$_3$ and magnesium.** In addition to taking a multivitamin, women may want to consider taking supplements of calcium with vitamin D$_3$ (cholecalciferol, the most potent form) and magnesium. Vitamin D$_3$ is important because it allows the body to absorb and use calcium. Magnesium is important because people seldom get enough of this important mineral through food or a multivitamin pill.

   Women should aim to get 1,000 to 1,200 milligrams calcium daily from food and supplements, plus a total of 800 IU vitamin D_3 and 400 milligrams magnesium per day. Because calcium is better absorbed when you take no more than 600 milligrams at a time, calcium supplements need to be taken twice a day, what is called a divided dose. Take half the day's dosage in the morning, and the other half later in the day (with food if it is a calcium carbonate).

Men should aim to get no more than 1,000 milligrams of calcium from food sources only (about two to three servings), because some research shows a possible link to increased calcium intake and prostate cancer. However, vitamin D and magnesium are just as important for men as they are for women—aim to get a total of 800 IU vitamin D_3, and 400 milligrams magnesium per day. (Although calcium supplements are not recommended, men can consider taking a separate vitamin D_3 and magnesium supplement—after checking with their endocrinologist.)

3. **Water-soluble cinnamon extract.** Perhaps the most promising new supplement for people with diabetes is *Cinnulin PF*, a capsule that contains a water-soluble cinnamon extract. Several studies have shown that cinnamon can increase the power of insulin, and may lower fasting glucose levels. Scientists are still investigating what substances give cinnamon its disease-fighting force, and more studies need to be completed before it becomes a common treatment, but if recent research holds up, fasting glucose can be reduced by up to 29 percent. From cinnamon! Sprinkling a little on your skim milk cocoa won't do the trick, though. New research reports that saliva harms some of the active ingredients in the spice so in order for it to work, you have to take it in capsule form. Cinnulin PF contains a water-soluble extract that has had the toxins removed while retaining the diabetes-fighting active ingredients. The manufacturer recommends taking 250 milligrams per day; I recommend talking with your doctor first.

JOY'S 4-STEP PROGRAM
FOR TYPE 2 DIABETES

Follow this program if you have diabetes or prediabetes.

STEP 1 ... START WITH THE BASICS

These are the first things you should do to regain control over your blood glucose and manage diabetes.

- Begin a program of exercise.

- If you smoke, quit.

- If you have diabetes, be a good patient—monitor your blood glucose levels, take your medications, and gather a great medical team.

- Start keeping a food log.

STEP 2 ... YOUR ULTIMATE GROCERY LIST

A diabetes food plan is about eating high-quality carbs instead of low-quality carbs, choosing healthy fats instead of trans fats or saturated fats, and eating plenty of foods rich in soluble fiber, vitamin D, calcium, and magnesium. I've also added some high-quality (lean) proteins you should choose instead of high-fat varieties, plus some foods used as ingredients in the meal plans and recipes. You don't have to purchase every item . . . but these foods should make up the bulk of what you eat for the week. If you find yourself getting bored, try some unfamiliar foods from these groups—they may become favorites.

FRUIT

ALL fresh fruit, but especially:	Apricots (fresh, not dried)	Berries (blackberries, raspberries, strawberries)	Grapefruit Oranges Peaches
Apples	Bananas	Cantaloupe	Pears

VEGETABLES

ALL vegetables, but especially:	Broccoli	Lentils	Potatoes, white
Artichoke hearts	Brussels sprouts	Mushrooms (especially shiitake)	Seaweed
Avocado	Cabbage		Soybeans (edamame)
Beans (black, kidney, lima, navy, pinto, white, garbanzo)	Carrots	Olives	Spinach
	Cauliflower	Onions	Swiss chard
	Chickpeas (garbanzo beans)	Peas	Tomatoes
		Peas, split	Yams
Beets	Corn	Peas, sugar snap	
Bok choy	Kale	Potatoes, sweet	

SEAFOOD

ALL seafood and fish, but especially:	Herring	Salmon, wild (with bones)	Trout, rainbow
Anchovies	Mackerel (not king)		
	Oysters, Pacific	Sardines (with bones)	

LEAN MEATS/EGGS/SOY FOODS

Beef, ground (lean only)	Eggs, omega-3–fortified	Tofu with calcium	Veal
	Ham, lean	Turkey bacon	Veggie burger
Beef, lean	Pork tenderloin	Turkey breast	
Chicken breast	Tempeh	Turkey burger	

NUTS AND SEEDS (PREFERABLY UNSALTED)

Almonds	Flaxseed, ground	Pecans	Sesame seeds
Brazil nuts	Hazelnuts	Pine nuts	Soy nuts
Butternuts (white walnuts)	Macadamia nuts	Pistachio nuts	Sunflower seeds
	Peanut butter	Psyllium seeds, ground	Walnuts
Cashews	Peanuts	Pumpkin seeds	

WHOLE GRAINS

Amaranth	Breads, whole grain (including English muffins, 70-calorie mini-pita, crackers)	Millet	Tempeh
Barley		Oat bran	Tortillas (tomato, whole grain, or spinach)
Bread, reduced-calorie whole wheat (45 calories or less per slice)		Oatmeal	
		Quinoa	Waffles, calcium-fortified whole grain
	Cereals, fortified whole grain	Rice (brown, wild)	
		Rice bran	Wheat berries
		Rice cakes	

DAIRY

Cheese (fat-free, reduced-fat)	Cheese, goat (preferably reduced-fat)	Margarine spread, vitamin D–fortified, reduced-fat soft tub, trans fat–free	Sour cream (reduced-fat, fat-free)
Cheese (for meal plan): fat-free or reduced-fat Cheddar, Swiss, mozzarella	Cheese, Parmesan or Romano		Soy milk, enriched/fortified
	Cream cheese (fat-free, reduced-fat)	Milk (fat-free, 1% reduced-fat)	Yogurt (fat-free, low-fat with artificial sweetener)

MISCELLANEOUS

Almond extract	Espresso powder, instant	Mayonnaise, reduced-fat	Popsicles, sugar-free
Baking powder			Salt substitute
Baking soda	Flour, all-purpose	Mustard, Dijon	Soy crisps
Broth, chicken, low-sodium, low-fat	Flour, whole wheat pastry	Nonstick cooking spray	Soy sauce, reduced-sodium
Cinnamon, ground	Garlic	Nutmeg	
Cocktail sauce	Garlic powder	Oil, canola	Steak sauce
Cocoa powder, unsweetened	Hummus	Oil, flaxseed	Sugar substitute (such as Equal or Splenda)
	Jell-O gelatin, sugar-free, low-calorie	Oil, olive	
Cornstarch		Oil, sesame	Vanilla extract
Dressing, salad, reduced-calorie (Caesar, vinaigrette)		Oil, walnut	Vinegar
	Ketchup	Onion powder	
	Maple extract	Paprika	
		Pepper, black	

STEP 3 ... GOING ABOVE AND BEYOND

If you want to do everything you can to prevent or control diabetes, here are some additional things you might try:

- Consider taking a multivitamin. Women may consider taking a calcium supplement with vitamin D_3 and magnesium built in. Men may consider taking vitamin D_3 and magnesium, without calcium.

- Talk with your doctor if you want to consider taking cinnamon supplements.

- Avoid eating foods high in saturated fats, including butter, ice cream, whole milk, cheese, and fatty meats. Also, avoid trans fats.

- Drink alcohol in moderation, if at all.

- Take extra care of your teeth and feet.

- Seek treatment for sleep apnea, or excessive daytime sleepiness.

DAYTIME SLEEPINESS

If you find yourself becoming sleepy during the day, don't automatically assume that it is due to insomnia from sleep apnea. I had a client who became unbearably sleepy every day around 3:00 p.m. His blood sugars, which he tested twice each day (once in the morning and once at night), were always well within normal, thanks to his combination of diet, exercise, and glucose-lowering medications. He sought help for sleep apnea and continued with a stellar eating plan, but weeks later, he was still crashing in the afternoon. Finally, he tested his blood sugar at 3:00 p.m. To everyone's surprise, his blood sugar was very low—below 60. His doctor adjusted his medication, and he regained his energy. If you find yourself losing the battle to stay awake in the middle of the day, test your blood sugar. If it is low, work with your physician to find a way to level it out. In my office, the mantra is: When in doubt, test your sugars.

STEP 4 ...MEAL PLANS

These sample menus include foods and specific food combinations that have been shown to help glycemic control. Each meal is perfectly balanced with the right mix of high-quality carbs, protein, fat, and calories to help keep your blood sugars under control. Some people find counting carbs helpful and necessary. Therefore, I provide the total calories and grams of carbohydrate for every meal and snack (each meal is 45 grams carb or less). And for people who are most comfortable using the food exchange system, I also present how each meal breaks down into various exchanges. Make sure you pay close attention to the carbohydrate portions with each meal—my numbers and your blood sugars will count on it. If your blood sugars test high on any particular day, choose the lower-carb meal options. Please note places where reduced-calorie breads are used. See Joy's Picks (page 447) for breads that are 45 calories or less per slice.

Every day, choose *one* option for each of the three meals—breakfast, lunch, and dinner. Then, one or two times per day, choose from a variety of my suggested snacks. Approximate calories have been provided to help adjust for your personal weight management goals. If you find yourself hungry (and if weight is not an issue), feel free to increase the portion sizes for protein and fat only—extra portions of carbohydrate may increase your blood sugar. Beverage calories are *not* included. If you'd prefer something other than water, stick with sugar-free beverages only.

BREAKFAST OPTIONS

(Approximately 300 to 400 calories, less than 45 grams carbohydrate)

Ham and Cheese Omelet with Toast

Beat 1 whole egg with 3 egg whites. Cook in heated pan coated with nonstick cooking spray. Add 2 ounces chopped lean ham. When bottom side is cooked, gently flip. Top with 2 tablespoons shredded fat-free cheese. Fold omelet over and cook until cheese melts and egg mixture is firm; season with salt substitute and ground black pepper. Enjoy with 1 toasted slice whole wheat bread (or 2 toasted slices reduced-calorie whole wheat bread) topped with 2 teaspoons reduced-fat soft tub, trans fat–free margarine spread.

319 calories, 16 g carbohydrate
Exchanges: 1 medium-fat meat, 4⅓ very lean meats, 1 starch, ¾ fat

Toast with Cream Cheese, Tomato, Onion, and Lox

2 slices reduced-calorie, whole wheat bread, toasted. Top each with 1 tablespoon fat-free or light cream cheese, sliced tomato, onion, and 2 ounces smoked salmon.

300 calories, 26 g carbohydrate
Exchanges: 2 lean meats, 1 starch, 1 vegetable, ½ fat

Cinnamon-Walnut Cottage Cheese with Apple Slices

1 cup fat-free or 1% reduced-fat cottage cheese mixed with optional cinnamon and topped with 1 tablespoon chopped walnuts and 1 tablespoon ground flaxseed. Enjoy with 1 sliced apple.

320 calories, 29 g carbohydrate
Exchanges: 4 very lean meats, 1 fruit, 2 fats

Scrambled Eggs with Turkey Bacon and Fruit

Beat 1 whole egg with 3 egg whites. Cook in heated pan coated with nonstick cooking spray, adding preferred chopped vegetables (onion, red and green peppers, tomato). Enjoy with 2 strips reduced-fat turkey bacon and 1 orange (or ½ grapefruit or ¼ cantaloupe).

320 calories, 30 g carbohydrate
Exchanges: 1 medium-fat meat, 2 lean meats, 1⅓ very lean meats, 1 vegetable, 1 fruit

Oatmeal with Berries, Flaxseed, and Nuts

½ cup dry oatmeal prepared with water; top with 2 tablespoons ground flaxseed (or wheat germ), 2 tablespoons chopped nuts (walnuts, pecans, soy nuts, or slivered almonds) and ½ cup berries (sliced strawberries, raspberries, and/or blackberries). Sweeten with optional sugar substitute.

350 calories, 43 g carbohydrate
Exchanges: 1 starch, 1 fruit, 4 fats

Cereal with Milk and a Hard-Boiled Egg

1 cup whole grain fortified cereal with 1 cup milk (fat-free, 1% reduced-fat, or enriched/fortified soy). Enjoy with 1 hard-boiled egg (or 2 strips reduced-fat turkey bacon).

320 calories, 43 g carbohydrate
Exchanges: 1 medium-fat meat, 1¼ starch, 1 fat-free milk

Strawberry-Banana Cottage Cheese with Almonds

1 cup fat-free or 1% reduced-fat cottage cheese mixed with ¼ sliced banana, ½ cup chopped strawberries, and 2 tablespoons slivered almonds.

332 calories, 27 g carbohydrate
Exchanges: 4 very lean meats, 1½ fruits, 2 fats

Breakfast Burrito

Beat 1 whole egg with 2 egg whites. Cook on heated griddle coated with nonstick cooking spray. Mix cooked eggs with ¼ cup black beans and 2 tablespoons fat-free or reduced-fat shredded cheese; wrap in 1 whole grain or spinach tortilla (150 calories or less), adding optional onions, peppers, salsa, and/or hot sauce.

380 calories, 35 g carbohydrate

Exchanges: 1 medium-fat meat, 1 lean meat, 1 very lean meat, 2¾ starch, optional 1 vegetable

Whole Grain Waffles with Yogurt and Nuts

2 frozen whole grain waffles, toasted and topped with 6 ounces fat-free flavored yogurt (any brand that uses artificial sweetener, 100 calories or less) and 1 tablespoon chopped nuts (walnuts, pecans, soy nuts, peanuts, or slivered almonds).

319 calories, 43 g carbohydrate

Exchanges: 2 starch, 1 fat, 1 fat-free milk

Vegetable Scramble with Toasted English Muffin

Sauté ½ cup each sliced mushrooms, chopped pepper, chopped onion, and broccoli florets in nonstick cooking spray until soft. Beat 1 whole egg with 2 to 3 egg whites and pour over vegetables. Add 2 tablespoons chopped tomato and continue to cook until eggs are cooked. Season with a pinch of salt and pepper. Enjoy with 1 toasted whole grain English muffin, dry or with optional 2 teaspoons reduced-fat soft tub, trans fat–free margarine. (For ½ of English muffin, you may substitute one of the following fruits: 1 orange, 1 plum, ½ cup berries, ½ grapefruit, or ¼ cantaloupe.)

363 calories, 43 g carbohydrate

Exchanges: 1 medium-fat meat, 1 very lean meat, 2 starch (or 1 starch and 1 fruit, optional ¾ fat), 2 vegetables

Rice Cakes with Cottage Cheese and Tomato

3 rice cakes topped with sliced tomato, onion, and 1 cup fat-free or 1% reduced-fat cottage cheese mixed with 2 tablespoons ground flaxseed.

330 calories, 33 g carbohydrate

Exchanges: 4 very lean meats, 1½ starch, 1 vegetable, 2 fats

Peanut Butter Pita and String Cheese

1 (70-calorie) whole grain pita bread (or 1 slice whole wheat bread) with 1 level tablespoon peanut butter. Enjoy with 1 or 2 reduced-fat string cheeses.

320 calories, 18 g carbohydrate

Exchanges: 1 to 2 medium-fat meats, 1 starch, 2 fats

LUNCH OPTIONS

(Approximately 400 to 500 calories, less than 45 grams carbohydrate)

Ham, Cheese, and Avocado Sandwich

4 ounces sliced lean ham (or turkey breast), 1 ounce reduced-fat Swiss cheese, 2 to 3 thin slices avocado, lettuce, tomato, and onion on 2 slices reduced-calorie whole wheat bread (45 calories or less per slice); add optional mustard, 2 teaspoons reduced-fat mayonnaise or hummus. Enjoy with 1 cup green, red, or yellow peppers sticks.

416 calories, 34 g carbohydrate

Exchanges: 1 lean meat, 4 very lean meats, 1 starch, 1 vegetable, 1¾ fats

Caesar Salad with Grilled Chicken or Shrimp

Unlimited Romaine lettuce leaves topped with 4 ounces grilled chicken (or cooked shrimp), 1 ounce gated Parmesan cheese (4 to 5 level tablespoons), and optional anchovies (4 fillets); tossed with 4 tablespoons reduced-calorie Caesar dressing (40 calories or less per tablespoon) or 2 tablespoons regular Caesar dressing.

413 calories, 22 g carbohydrate

Exchanges: 2 lean meats, 4 very lean meats, 4 fats

Open-Faced Tuna Melt

Mash 1 can (6 ounces) water-packed light tuna (or canned chicken breast or canned wild salmon) with 1 tablespoon reduced-fat mayonnaise, minced onion, and freshly ground black pepper; spread on 2 toasted slices reduced-calorie, whole grain bread (45 calories per slice). Top each open slice with thinly sliced tomato and 1 small slice (¾-ounce) fat-free or reduced-fat cheese (any variety, including Cheddar, Swiss, or American). Bake in 350°F oven until cheese melts. Enjoy with celery and red, yellow, and green pepper sticks.

453 calories, 31 g carbohydrate

Exchanges: ¾ lean meat, 6 very lean meats, 1 starch, 1 vegetable, 1 fat

Turkey Burger with Veggies

1 (5-ounce) lean turkey burger with lettuce, tomato, onion, and 2 tablespoons ketchup on ½ whole grain bun (or in one 70-calorie pita pocket). Enjoy with 1 cup steamed vegetables (broccoli, cauliflower, spinach, etc.) topped with optional 1 tablespoon grated Parmesan cheese.

416 calories, 37 g carbohydrate

Exchanges: ½ lean meat, 5 very lean meats, 2 vegetables

Edamame with Wild Salmon Dijonnaise

1 cup boiled edamame (soybeans in the pod). Enjoy with 5 ounces canned wild salmon with bones, drained, mashed, and mixed with 1 tablespoon reduced-calorie mayon-

naise, 1 to 2 teaspoons Dijon mustard, minced onion, and black pepper to taste. Serve on large bed of leafy greens (spinach, romaine, etc.) tossed with fresh lemon juice or 2 tablespoons low-calorie dressing.

400 calories, 18 g carbohydrate

Exchanges: 1 medium-fat meat, 5 lean meats, 1 starch, 1 vegetable, 1 to 2 fats

Spinach Salad with Beets, Goat Cheese, and Walnuts

A large bed of spinach leaves topped with ½ cup sliced beets, ½ cup sugar snap peas, 2 ounces goat cheese (preferably reduced-fat), and 2 tablespoons chopped walnuts. Toss with 2 teaspoons olive oil and unlimited vinegar or fresh lemon juice (or 2 to 4 tablespoons low-calorie dressing).

460 calories, 27 g carbohydrate

Exchanges: 2 medium-fat meats, 5 vegetables, 4 fats

Mushroom-Cheddar Omelet with Sweet Potato

Sauté ½ cup sliced mushrooms and ½ cup sliced onion in heated pan coated with non-stick cooking spray until soft. Beat 1 whole egg with 3 egg whites, pour over sautéed vegetables, and season with preferred herbs. When bottom is cooked, gently flip over and add 1 ounce reduced-fat or fat-free cheese. Fold omelet over and continue cooking until egg mixture firms and cheese melts. Enjoy with 2 thin slices avocado plus ½ medium baked sweet or white potato topped with 2 tablespoons fat-free or reduced-fat sour cream.

420 calories and 33 g carbohydrate

Exchanges: 1 medium-fat meat, 1 lean meat, 2⅓ very lean meats, 1 starch, 2 vegetables, 2 fats

Cottage Cheese with Cantaloupe and Almonds

½ cantaloupe filled with 1 cup fat-free or 1% reduced-fat cottage cheese and topped with 1 tablespoon slivered almonds (or sunflower seeds).

402 calories, 33 g carbohydrate

Exchanges: 4 very lean meats, 1 fruit, 1 fat

Grilled Chicken–Pepper Wrap with Avocado

5 ounces grilled chicken mixed with unlimited chopped onion and red, yellow, and green peppers sautéed in nonstick cooking spray or 1 teaspoon olive or canola oil. Wrap in 1 whole wheat spinach or tomato tortilla (100 calories or less). Enjoy with 3 thin slices avocado and unlimited sliced cucumber.

431 calories, 40 g carbohydrate

Exchanges: 5 very lean meats, 1 starch, 4 vegetables, 2 fats

Veggie Tuna Salad with Pita

Veggie Tuna Salad (page 274), served on a bed of romaine or spinach leaves. Enjoy with mini whole wheat pita bread (70 calories or less) and 1 cup baby carrots with 2 tablespoons low-calorie vinaigrette dressing.

404 calories, 37 g carbohydrate
Exchanges: 6 very lean meat, 6 vegetabless, 3 fats

Baked Fish with Green Beans and Potato

5 ounces grilled or baked fish (Easy! 3-Step Microwave Salmon, page 345, or any grilled fish). Serve with 1 cup steamed green beans and ½ baked potato topped with 2 tablespoons reduced-fat or fat-free sour cream.

475 calories, 31 g carbohydrate
Exchanges: 5 lean meats, 1 starch, 2 vegetables, 1 fat

Salad with the Works

Choose one of the following 4-ounce protein options: sardines (with bones), canned light tuna in water, wild salmon (with bones), chicken breast, turkey breast, ham, shrimp, lean roast beef, tofu, or fish. Place on large bed of leafy greens (i.e., lettuce, spinach, collard greens, endive) mixed with ½ chopped pepper (red, yellow, or green), 5 cherry tomatoes, and ¼ cup each sliced mushrooms, chopped cucumbers, sliced beets, chopped red onion, and artichoke hearts. Add 2 tablespoons chickpeas (garbanzo beans), 5 sliced olives, and ¼ chopped avocado. Toss with 2 teaspoons olive oil and 2 tablespoons vinegar or fresh lemon juice (or 2 to 4 tablespoons low-calorie dressing).

468 calories, 38 g carbohydrate
Exchanges: 4 very lean meats, 5 vegetables, 4 fats

DINNER OPTIONS
(Approximately 500 to 600 calories, 45 grams or less carbohydrate)

Turkey Meatballs in Red Pepper–Tomato Sauce

1 serving Turkey Meatballs in Red Pepper–Tomato Sauce (page 79). Enjoy with side salad of 2 cups chopped romaine lettuce, ½ chopped pepper, ¼ sliced onion, ½ cup sliced mushrooms, and ½ chopped cucumber, tossed with 2 teaspoons olive oil and 2 tablespoons vinegar (or 2 to 4 tablespoons low-calorie dressing).

553 calories, 42 g carbohydrate
Exchanges: 4 lean meats, 1 starch, 6 vegetables, 3 fats

Pesto Salmon with Roasted Artichoke Hearts and Potato

1 serving Pesto Salmon with Roasted Artichoke Hearts (page 157) or 5 ounces any grilled, baked, poached, or broiled fish with 1 cup steamed vegetables. Serve with

½ medium baked sweet potato topped with 1 tablespoon reduced-fat, soft tub trans fat–free margarine.

550 calories, 39 g carbohydrate
Exchanges: 5 lean meats, 1 starch, 2 vegetables, 2 fats

Sirloin Steak with Mozzarella and Tomato Salad

5 ounces grilled sirloin steak (trimmed of all fat) with optional 2 tablespoons steak sauce or ketchup. Enjoy with mozzarella and tomato salad: slice ½ red tomato and 1 ounce reduced-fat mozzarella cheese, line alternate slices of tomato and mozzarella on plate and drizzle with 2 tablespoon low-calorie balsamic vinaigrette. Serve with 12 steamed or grilled asparagus spears.

550 calories, 39 g carbohydrate
Exchanges: 1 medium-fat meat, 5 lean meats, 2 vegetables, 2 fats

Pork Tenderloin with Cauliflower Mashed Potatoes

5 ounces grilled, baked, or broiled lean pork tenderloin. Enjoy with 1 serving Cauliflower Mashed Potatoes (page 222) and a side salad of 2 cups chopped lettuce, ¼ cup each chopped pepper, onion, cucumber, mushrooms, and grated or chopped carrots. Toss with 1 to 2 teaspoons olive oil and 1 to 2 tablespoons vinegar or fresh lemon juice (or 2 to 4 tablespoons low-calorie salad dressing).

510 calories, 27 g carbohydrate
Exchanges: 5 lean meats, 1 very lean meat, 6 vegetables, 1 to 2 fats

Orange Pepper Beef Stir-Fry with Cucumber Slices

1 serving Orange Pepper Beef Stir-Fry (page 101). Enjoy with 1 sliced cucumber.

519 calories, 38 g carbohydrate
Exchanges: 4 lean meats, 1 starch, 4 vegetables, 1½ fats

Chopped Chicken Salad with Apples and Walnuts

1 serving Chopped Chicken Salad with Apples and Walnuts (page 325).

500 calories, 45 g carbohydrate
Exchanges: 4 very lean meats, 2 starch, 1 vegetable, ½ fruit, 3 fats

Turkey Tacos with Lettuce, Tomato, and Cheese

3 servings Turkey Tacos (page 250) with optional salsa and hot sauce.

513 calories, 30 g carbohydrate
Exchanges: 9 very lean meats, 2 starch, 1 vegetable, 1½ fats

Sweet and Sour Tofu-Veggie Stir-Fry with Edamame

1 serving Sweet and Sour Tofu-Veggie Stir-Fry (page 251). Serve with 1 cup boiled edamame (soybeans in the pod)—go light on salt or use salt substitute instead.

526 calories, 42 g carbohydrate

Exchanges: 1 medium-fat meat, 3 lean meats, 2 starch, 2 vegetables, 1 fat

Cheddar Burger with Baked Potato

1 (5-ounce) lean hamburger (or turkey or veggie burger) topped with 1 ounce melted reduced-fat Cheddar cheese, sliced tomato, onion, and optional 2 tablespoons ketchup (no bun). Serve on a bed of unlimited leafy greens tossed with 2 tablespoons low-calorie salad dressing. Enjoy with ½ medium plain baked potato topped with 1 tablespoon reduced-fat soft tub, trans fat–free margarine spread. (For the potato, you may substitute ½ hamburger bun, preferably whole wheat.)

520 calories, 42 g carbohydrate

Exchanges: 6 lean meats, 1 starch, 2 vegetables, 3 fats

Satay Chicken with Broccoli and Brown Rice

5 ounces chicken breast, grilled or pan-fried with 2 teaspoons canola or sesame oil, with satay dipping sauce (1 level tablespoon creamy smooth peanut butter mixed with 1 tablespoon reduced-sodium soy sauce and 1 teaspoon minced garlic). Serve with 1 cup steamed broccoli and ½ cup cooked brown rice.

502 calories, 38 g carbohydrate

Exchanges: 5 very lean meats, 1 starch, 2 vegetables, 4 fats

Shrimp Cocktail with Grilled Fish, Brussels Sprouts, and Brown Rice

5 large (3 ounces) shrimp with 1 tablespoon cocktail sauce. Serve with 5 ounces fish fillet (wild salmon, flounder, sole, tilapia, or trout), grilled with 1 teaspoon olive oil and preferred seasonings. Enjoy with 1 cup steamed Brussels sprouts and ½ cup cooked brown rice tossed with 1 tablespoon toasted, slivered almonds.

531 calories, 40 g carbohydrate

Exchanges: 8 very lean meats (if you choose salmon, 3 very lean meats and 5 lean meats), 1 starch, 2 vegetables, 2 fats

Hearty Turkey Meat Loaf with Cauliflower Mashed "Potatoes"

1 serving Hearty Turkey Meat Loaf (page 156). Enjoy with 1 serving Cauliflower Mashed "Potatoes" (page 222) or 1 cup steamed cauliflower topped with 1 to 2 tablespoons Parmesan or Romano cheese). Serve with 1 cup steamed green beans (or asparagus or broccoli) tossed with 1 tablespoon reduced-fat, soft tub trans fat–free margarine spread and 2 tablespoons toasted, slivered almonds.

500 calories, 42 g carbohydrate

Exchanges: 1 lean meat, 4 very lean meats, 1 starch, 5 vegetables, 3 fats

SNACK OPTIONS

100 calories or less

If a sugar-free food contains less than 20 calories or less than 5 grams of carbs per serving, it is a free food. Such foods should be limited to three per day and MUST be spread out throughout the day.

- Sugar Free Low-Calorie Jell-O Gelatin

  10 calories, 0 g carbohydrate

  Exchanges: free food

- Sugar-free popsicles (check labels, nutrition information varies from brand to brand)

  Exchanges: If the popsicle contains less than 20 calories or less than 5 grams of carb per serving it is a free food.

- 1 reduced-fat string cheese

  80 calories, 0 g carbohydrate

  Exchanges: 1 medium-fat meat

- 1 hard-boiled egg (or 3 hard-boiled egg whites)

  75 calories, 0 g carbohydrate

  Exchanges: 1 medium-fat meat (if egg whites are used, 1⅓ very lean meats)

- 2 ounces turkey or lean ham wrapped in lettuce leaves

  70 calories, 2 g carbohydrate

  Exchanges: 2 very lean meats

- 10 almonds, unsalted

  80 calories, 3 g carbohydrate

  Exchanges: 2 fats

- Celery sticks with 2 tablespoons fat-free cream cheese

  40 calories, 4 g carbohydrate

  Exchanges: 1 very lean meat

- 1 level tablespoon peanut butter with celery sticks

  100 calories, 4 g carbohydrate

  Exchanges: 2 fats

- 1 slice fat-free cheese on 1 plain rice cake

  70 calories, 10 g carbohydrate

  Exchanges: 1 very lean meat, ½ starch

- 8 baby carrots with 2 level tablespoons guacamole (substitute pepper sticks for the carrots and carbs drop to 6 grams)

  90 calories, 10 g carbohydrate

  Exchanges: 2 vegetables, 1 fat

- ½ apple, sliced, with 1 level teaspoon peanut butter

  70 calories, 10.5 g carbohydrate

  Exchanges: ½ fruit, 1 fat

- 8 baby carrots and 2 level tablespoons hummus (substitute pepper sticks for the carrots and carbs drop to 9 grams)

  85 calories, 13 g carbohydrate

  Exchanges: 1½ vegetables, 1 fat

- 6 ounces fat-free plain or flavored yogurt with artificial sweetener

  90 calories, 17 g carbohydrate

  Exchanges: 1 fat-free milk

100 to 200 calories

- 8 macadamia nuts

  150 calories, 3 g carbohydrate

  Exchanges: 3 fats

- ½ cup fat-free or 1% reduced-fat cottage cheese mixed with 1 tablespoon chopped nuts

  130 calories, 4 g carbohydrate

  Exchanges: 2 lean meats, 1 fat

- Whole nuts: 1 ounce (¼ cup) almonds, cashews, toasted pecans, soy nuts, walnuts, or peanuts

  180 to 200 calories, 5 g carbohydrate

  Exchanges: 4 fats

- ½ cup fat-free or 1% reduced-fat cottage cheese mixed with 2 tablespoons ground flaxseed

  140 calories, 7 g carbohydrate

  Exchanges: 2 lean meats, 2 fats

- ¼ cup pistachio nuts or sunflower seeds in the shell

  180 calories, 7 to 9 g carbohydrate

  Exchanges: 4 fats

- 8 baby carrots dipped in ½ cup fat-free or 1% reduced-fat cottage cheese

  110 calories, 10 g carbohydrate

  Exchanges: 2 lean meats, 1½ vegetables

- 1 bell pepper, cut up, with ¼ cup guacamole

  144 calories, 11 g carbohydrate

  Exchanges: 2 vegetables, 2 fats

- 1 cup edamame (boiled soybeans in the pod), lightly seasoned with salt substitute

  150 calories, 12 g carbohydrate

  Exchanges: 1 medium-fat meat, 1 starch

- 1 bell pepper, cut up, with ¼ cup hummus

  118 calories, 13 g carbohydrate

  Exchanges: 2 vegetables, 2 fats

- 10 almonds with 1 apple

    150 calories, 21 g carbohydrate

    Exchanges: 1 fruit, 2 fats

- 1 slice reduced-calorie, whole wheat toast with 1 level tablespoon peanut butter

    140 calories, 14 g carbohydrate

    Exchanges: ½ starch, 2 fats

- 6 ounces fat-free, plain or artificially flavored yogurt mixed with 2 tablespoons ground flaxseed (or 1 tablespoon chopped nuts)

    150 calories, 20 g carbohydrate

    Exchanges: 2 fats, 1 fat-free milk

- 1 apple, sliced, with 1 level tablespoon peanut butter

    166 calories, 22 g carbohydrate

    Exchanges: 1 fruit, 2 fats

- 1 ounce plain soy crisps (check labels, nutrition information will vary)

    Exchanges: 1 lean meat, 1 starch

SPECIAL SUGAR-FREE RECIPES

- Chocolate-Hazelnut Biscotti (page 223)

    40 calories, 6 g carbohydrate

    Exchanges: ½ starch

- Chocolate Angel Food Cake (page 226)

    70 calories, 15 g carbohydrate

    Exchanges: 1 starch

- Sour Cream Coffee Cake with Cinnamon and Walnuts (page 224)

    240 calories, 29 g carbohydrate

    Exchanges: 2 starch

CAULIFLOWER MASHED "POTATOES"

Whether you're watching your carbs or trying to lose weight, or if you simply love hot, creamy comfort food, this recipe is calling your name. It's very popular among my clients (and staff nutritionists!) and 1 serving provides only 78 calories and 9 grams of carbs.

Makes 4 servings, ¾ cup each

1	head cauliflower, cut into florets of roughly the same size
¾	cup low-sodium, low-fat chicken broth
1	tablespoon cornstarch
4	ounces fat-free cream cheese
2	tablespoons grated Romano or Parmesan cheese
½	teaspoon garlic powder
¼	teaspoon onion powder
¼	teaspoon paprika
	Salt
	Ground black pepper

1. Steam the cauliflower over boiling water for 15 to 20 minutes, until tender. Drain. Place the cauliflower in a food processor or blender along with ½ cup broth. Puree on high until smooth. Transfer the puree to a medium saucepan.

2. In a cup, dissolve the cornstarch in the remaining ¼ cup broth, and add to the cauliflower puree. Add the cream cheese, Romano or Parmesan cheese, garlic powder, onion powder, and paprika. Cook over medium heat, stirring, 2 to 3 minutes, until the puree begins to thicken. Season with salt and pepper to taste. Serve immediately.

PER SERVING
78 calories, 8 g protein, 9 g carbohydrate, 2.8 g total sugar, 1 g fat (1 g saturated), 0 mg cholesterol, 262 mg sodium, 3 g fiber

EXCHANGES
1 very lean meat, 2 vegetables

CHOCOLATE-HAZELNUT BISCOTTI

When it came time to test recipes, I knew biscotti had to be included—they are among my personal favorite desserts. I made two batches, one with white flour and one with whole wheat pastry flour, completely expecting the white flour version to taste better. But low and behold, they were equally fantastic! Spend the time to make a batch of these crunchy sugar-free cookies, they're well worth it.

Makes 20

1½	cups whole wheat pastry flour
1	cup sugar substitute
½	cup unsweetened cocoa powder, preferably Dutch-process
1½	tablespoons instant espresso powder
1	teaspoon baking soda
¼	teaspoon salt
2	eggs
2	egg whites
2	teaspoons vanilla extract
1	teaspoon almond extract
¼	cup hazelnuts, toasted and coarsely chopped

1. Preheat the oven to 300°F. Line a large baking sheet with parchment paper or waxed paper.

2. Sift the flour, sugar substitute, cocoa, espresso powder, baking soda, and salt onto a piece of waxed paper or foil. In a large bowl, combine the eggs, egg whites, vanilla, and almond extract. Beat with an electric mixer set on medium speed. Reduce the speed to low and gradually add the flour mixture until a stiff dough forms, adding the hazelnuts when the dough is about half mixed.

3. On a floured surface, divide the dough in half. Form each half into a 12"-long log, pressing down the top slightly to a 3" width. Transfer the logs to the prepared baking sheet, placing them an inch or two apart. Bake until almost firm to the touch, about 40 minutes. Remove from the oven and let cool for 10 minutes.

4. Using a spatula, carefully transfer the logs to a work surface. Using a serrated knife, cut logs on the diagonal into ½"- to ¾"-thick slices. Arrange the slices, cut side down, on the baking sheet. Return to the oven and bake 30 minutes longer, turning once halfway through. Cool completely on a wire rack. Store in an airtight container in the refrigerator for up to 2 weeks.

PER BISCOTTI
40 calories, 2 g protein, 6 g carbohydrate, 0 g total sugar, 1 g fat (0 g saturated), 14 mg cholesterol, 73 mg sodium, 1 g fiber

EXCHANGES
½ starch

SOUR CREAM COFFEE CAKE WITH CINNAMON AND WALNUTS

This is a perfect dessert to bake when you're looking to enjoy something special. It's a bit more caloric and carb-heavy than my other sugar-free, sweet treats . . . but it is undeniably lighter and safer for your diet than traditional sour cream coffee cake. The walnuts, eggs, and fat-free sour cream lend great taste and help slow the absorption of carbs in the blood. This cake is a *huge* hit with my family and friends!

Makes 8 servings

TOPPING

²⁄₃	cup all-purpose flour
¹⁄₃	cup sugar substitute
1	teaspoon ground cinnamon
¹⁄₂	teaspoon freshly grated nutmeg
¹⁄₄	cup reduced-fat, soft tub trans fat–free margarine spread, frozen for 15 minutes

CAKE

³⁄₄	cup all-purpose flour
³⁄₄	cup whole wheat pastry flour
1¹⁄₄	cups sugar substitute
1¹⁄₂	teaspoons baking powder
1	teaspoon baking soda
¹⁄₄	teaspoon salt
1	cup fat-free sour cream
2	eggs
¹⁄₄	cup canola oil
2	teaspoons vanilla extract
1	teaspoon maple extract
¹⁄₂	cup walnuts, coarsely chopped

1. Preheat the oven to 350°F. Grease a 9" round springform pan. Line the bottom with a round of parchment paper or coat with cooking spray.

2. To make the topping, in a small bowl, stir together the flour, sugar substitute, cinnamon, and nutmeg. Add the margarine and using a pastry cutter or your fingers quickly cut or rub in the margarine until coarse crumbs form. Cover and refrigerate.

3. To make the cake, on a piece of wax paper or aluminum foil, sift the all-purpose flour, whole wheat flour, sugar substitute, baking powder, baking soda, and salt. In a large bowl, whisk together the sour cream, eggs, oil, vanilla, and maple extract until well blended. Add the flour mixture. Using an electric mixer on medium speed or a wire whisk, beat until smooth and creamy, 1 to 2 minutes.

4. Spoon half of the batter into the prepared pan and spread evenly. Sprinkle evenly with half of the topping. Cover evenly with the remaining batter. Sprinkle evenly with the nuts, gently pressing them into the batter. Cover with the remaining topping.

5. Bake until the topping is golden brown and a toothpick inserted into the center of the cake comes out clean, 40 to 45 minutes. Transfer the pan to a wire rack and let cool for 20 minutes. Remove the sides of the springform pan. Serve the cake warm or at room temperature, cut into wedges.

PER SERVING
240 calories, 6 g protein, 29 g carbohydrate, 0 g total sugar, 12 g fat (1.5 g saturated), 45 mg cholesterol, 323 mg sodium, 2 g fiber

EXCHANGE
1 lean meat, 2 fats, 2 starch

CHOCOLATE ANGEL FOOD CAKE

You won't believe that there are just 70 calories in one slice of this light, airy cake—and with no sugar at all! Serve at your next dinner party, trust me, no one will know the difference.

Makes 8 servings

³⁄₄	cup whole wheat pastry flour
1½	cups sugar substitute
¼	cup unsweetened cocoa powder
2	teaspoons instant espresso powder
1½	cups egg whites (from about 10 eggs)
¼	teaspoon salt
2	teaspoons vanilla extract

1. Preheat the oven to 350°F. Line a 10" angel food cake pan with parchment paper or coat with cooking spray.
2. In a large bowl, sift the flour, sugar substitute, cocoa powder, and coffee *three times*. Set aside.
3. In a large metal bowl, beat the egg whites with the salt on high speed until they become stiff but not lumpy, 4 to 6 minutes. They should cling firmly to the side of the bowl when tilted. Add the vanilla, but do not mix.
4. With a spatula, gently fold one-third of the egg whites into the flour mixture. Repeat twice until all the egg whites are just combined, but not deflated.
5. Gently spread the batter into the prepared pan. Bake until the cake springs back when touched, 35 to 40 minutes. Remove from the oven and invert the pan onto its feet or the neck of a wine bottle. Let cool completely.
6. Gently run a long knife between the cake and the outer rim of the pan, pressing it firmly against the pan to prevent tearing the cake. Run the knife or a skewer around the inside of the tube. Invert the pan and remove the cake.

PER SERVING
70 calories, 7 g protein, 15 g carbohydrate, 0 g total sugar, 0 g fat, 0 mg cholesterol, 144 mg sodium, 2 g fiber

EXCHANGE
1 starch

CHAPTER 10

OSTEOPOROSIS

All too often, the first sign of osteoporosis is a broken bone. For my client Janice, it was her wrist. At age 64, her overall good health was the envy of more than one of her close friends—she felt good, looked younger than her age, and regularly saw her internist and gynecologist for routine checkups. Then she slipped and fell in the snow . . . and osteoporosis, which had been silently developing for years, made itself known.

Osteoporosis is defined by low bone mineral density (BMD), as measured by an x-ray bone density scan. If a scan shows your bone density is a bit low, your diagnosis is osteopenia, or pre-osteoporosis. If BMD is quite low, the diagnosis is osteoporosis. The results of bone density scans are expressed in terms of T scores. Scores ranging from –1.0 to –2.5 indicate osteopenia; less than –2.5 means osteoporosis.

Regardless of the cause, if you have low bone density you're facing a higher-than-average risk of breaking a bone. If you are lucky, your doctor will recognize some of the risk factors and send you for a bone density scan *before* you have to endure the pain and recovery of a break. Unfortunately for Janice, the first clue was that sickening crunch of her wrist breaking.

When I first saw Janice, she had just started taking osteoporosis medication, but her doctor wanted her to have an intensive nutrition intervention as well. During our first

FAQS

I know I need to get more calcium in my diet because my diet is pretty bad. I don't exercise much, and I've always been on the thin side, so I guess I could be at risk of osteoporosis. If I'm taking a multivitamin with calcium in it, do I really need to take a separate calcium supplement, too?

Calcium is bulky, so there is no way to fit a day's supply in a multivitamin. Most multivitamins have, at most, 100 to 200 milligrams of calcium—much less than the 1,000 to 1,200 milligrams you'll need. So yes, you really should be taking a separate calcium supplement. But if you radically change your diet, you may be able to get enough calcium from diet alone. Start counting your servings of high-calcium foods. If you consistently eat at least three servings of a high-calcium food every day, you're probably safe. But if your diet is erratic, then take 500 to 600 milligrams of calcium with D_3 once a day in the morning or afternoon. By the evening, think back to how you ate during the day. If you ate two or more servings of a high calcium food that day, then you can skip the evening dose. If not, take an additional 500 to 600 milligrams with a snack before bed. (However, if you have been diagnosed with osteoporosis or osteopenia, always take the second dose of calcium.)

meeting, I found out why she needed my help. She ate terribly, making meals from whatever food was on hand—generally lots of processed foods—without giving a thought to what nutrients she might be missing.

I rose to the challenge. For 90 minutes, I gave her a thorough lesson in osteoporosis, and a comprehensive meal plan filled with food choices rich in nutrients that would help her condition—more about these in the pages to follow. I also recommended that she start taking a calcium supplement with vitamin D_3 (cholecalciferol, the most potent form of vitamin D). I explained the benefits of exercise, and how to alternate strength training and weight-bearing exercises. I suggested that she walk on the treadmill five times per week, 40 minutes per session, at a speed of 3.5 miles per hour. By the time Janice left, I felt confident that she had all the tools she needed to turn a corner.

Two weeks later, Janice returned to the office with her food journal filled out and ready for my evaluation. She had done nothing! Well, next to nothing. She took the calcium supplements, but she didn't do any exercise, and, most distressing of all, she had made no changes in her diet.

Janice understood my instructions, but when it came time to implement them, she felt overwhelmed. Embracing a new way of eating meant overcoming the inertia of eating patterns she'd established decades ago. She'd never been that interested in planning and cooking meals anyway. To my eyes—brutal honesty alert!—her eating life was just so *boring*. Every day for breakfast Janice ate a toasted English muffin with peanut butter washed down with a cup of black coffee. Every morning. For years! The thing was, it didn't matter to her. She ate the same foods day in and day out because it was just easier that way. I have nothing against peanut butter or whole wheat English muffins—that's a fine quick breakfast—but it didn't supply her with essential nutrients we all need and it did nothing to help her fight low bone mineral density.

I learned an important lesson from Janice. I know I advised her well nutritionally, but there's a second, sometimes greater challenge to tackle beyond that—changing a lifetime of apparently harmless eating habits. Janice felt healthy. Janice looked terrific. But all the while, Janice's bones had quietly been losing mass, becoming thinner and thinner. Breaking her wrist was frightening and painful, but didn't mean she could instantly embrace a whole new way of eating.

I decided to take another tack. This time I gave Janice three specific goals to focus on.

First, I told her she that if she wanted to eat the same foods for breakfast day after day, fine, but she had to switch to foods that would specifically address her needs—namely cereal with skim milk, sliced banana, and a glass of calcium-fortified orange juice. Second, she could eat whatever she wanted for dinner, but she had to eat a high-calcium appetizer. She decided on pre-dinner salad of leafy greens topped with 1 ounce of feta or shredded cheddar cheese and, in signature Janice fashion, ate that every day. And third, before bed, I instructed her to eat a snack of yogurt. Those changes alone gave her four hits of high-calcium, bone-strengthening foods (plus potassium from the orange juice, dairy, and banana; vitamin C from orange juice; folic acid from fortified cereal, orange juice, and leafy greens; vitamin K from leafy greens; and vitamin D from the morning milk). In addition, Janice decided that instead of 40 minutes of treadmill walking, she would walk her dog for an additional 15 minutes per day and join Curves gym with a friend.

At the end of a year, these few changes (with medication) helped Janice do more than arrest bone loss—she actually *increased* bone density in her spine.

Initially Janice was one of the least compliant people I've ever seen in my practice. So why am I telling you her story? Because you don't have to be perfect right off the bat or at every meal to see real results. By the end of this chapter, you'll have all the tools you need to make your bones healthier. It's a lot of information. If you can't do it all right away, that's perfectly fine. Do one thing. Then do another. Eventually, all those little things add up. But you have to do something—your bones are too important to ignore.

WHAT AFFECTS OSTEOPOROSIS?

Children are taught that bones are like steel girders, the framework of the glorious structure that is the human body. The problem with that analogy is that girders are designed to last hundred of years without losing strength. In reality, bones are more like the interstate highway system—they fall apart, crack, get potholes, and then get patched up again so we can continue using them.

Nor are our bones uniformly dense. The outer layer is called *compact bone,* and it is relatively solid. But just under the compact bone is another layer called *spongy bone,* which isn't soft, but it is porous, with holes like a sponge or Swiss cheese. And because bone is live tissue, there are also nerves and blood vessels to feed the cells, as well as other structures. Bones also contain specialized cells that help form bone (*osteoblasts*) and break down or *resorb* bone (*osteoclasts*). Osteoclasts and osteoblasts work like little construction crews, constantly remodeling, working to keep the bones healthy and strong. If your overall health is good and you eat nutritionally sound meals, there is a balance—for every bit of bone lost, an equal amount of bone is created.

With osteoporosis, though, more bone is lost than formed. As you might imagine, the spongy bone—with all its holes and slender walls—becomes weak and compromised more quickly than compact bone. Breaks can occur anywhere, but the most common sites are the hip and wrist, which are more likely bear the impact of a fall. The bones of the back (vertebrae) are also affected, but they don't break . . . they are crushed. The weight of the body is enough to compress the back bones, causing a multitude of tiny fractures in the spongy bone. Over time people with osteoporosis can become shorter—they lose a little height each time a vertebra compresses.

No one knows definitively what causes some people to develop osteoporosis, but some factors are clear:

HORMONAL CHANGES

Estrogen and testosterone are important for bone health because they regulate bone loss, or resorption. Both these hormones seem to inhibit the formation of osteoclasts (the cells that break down bone), so when hormone levels are high, there are more bone-building cells than bone-destroying cells. If hormone levels fall, the balance shifts, and bone density is lost.

The question, then, is what causes levels of estrogen or testosterone to fall? The most common cause is aging. Men can develop osteoporosis when they get older as testosterone levels slowly decline. For women, menopause causes an extreme drop in estrogen, and their greatest bone loss occurs within the first ten years after menopause. That's why many physicians recommend that women get a bone density scan when they turn 50 or when they enter menopause, whichever comes first. That first test acts as a baseline. The scan should be repeated one or two years later to get a sense of the rate of bone loss.

Menopause isn't the only thing that triggers osteoporosis. Unfortunately, I've been seeing a lot of young women in my practice, women referred to me by their doctors because eating disorders have begun to ravage their bones. When a woman's weight drops too low, her hormones get out of whack, her estrogen levels fall, and she stops menstruating. In terms of bone health, a too-thin woman in her 20s looks a lot like a post-menopausal woman in her 60s. The only real cure is for the young woman to gain enough weight to start menstruating again, and then to maximize her bone density while she can—that is, until about age 30, when bone density reaches its peak.

CORTICOSTEROIDS

Corticosteroid medications are used to treat a number of common illnesses, including asthma and some autoimmune disorders. But steroids seem to inhibit the bone-building activity, and may also increase bone resorption. It has been estimated that up to half of all people who take steroids long-term will end up with osteoporosis. Significant bone loss can occur after even a relatively short course of corticosteroids—7.5 milligrams of prednisone for two to three months may require treatment to prevent bone loss.

BODY WEIGHT

Bones get stronger if they get more use. In the earlier stages of life, exercise helps build bone. And as much as it pains me to say it, weight builds bone. When it comes to osteoporosis, thin women have a greater risk than heavy women. Think about it—bones that support a 170-pound woman work harder than bones that carry a 110-pound woman. Studies have shown that lean muscle mass helps strengthen bone density more than fat, but overall weight still contributes to strong bones.

Of course, my advice is not for you to put on a few pounds for the sake of strengthening your bones! Being overweight puts you at greater risk for so many life-threatening diseases that it is never a wise choice. But women who diet excessively to keep their weight fashionably low are hurting their bones, now and in the future.

OTHER DISEASES

Any disorder that reduces the body's ability to absorb calcium and other nutrients can cause osteoporosis. The most common is celiac disease, an autoimmune disorder that causes the small intestines to lose their absorption capability. Previously thought to be a rare disease of childhood, celiac disease is now known to affect about 1 percent of Americans, and can strike at any age. (For more information, see Celiac Disease, page 417.)

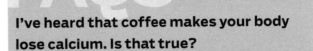

I've heard that coffee makes your body lose calcium. Is that true?

Well, it happens, but not significantly. *Does coffee affect absorption of calcium?* Yes, but hardly at all. A person can safely drink up to three cups of coffee a day without putting their stores of calcium at risk. Any shortfall can be recouped with just 2 tablespoons of milk per cup. Adding low-fat milk to your coffee should be plenty to keep your calcium levels in the black.

HOW FOOD AFFECTS OSTEOPOROSIS

Next to genetic predisposition, poor nutrition is the most common cause of osteoporosis. Making healthy food choices can help prevent dangerous bone loss, and food is one of the most important treatments recommended by physicians and nutritionists alike once osteoporosis is diagnosed.

GOOD FOODS TO CHOOSE

CALCIUM AND VITAMIN D

When it comes to osteoporosis prevention or treatment, the two most important nutrients are calcium and vitamin D.

Bone is made mostly of calcium. In addition, calcium fuels many other body functions, such as muscle movement, nerve operation, and immune activation. Typically, we get our daily dose of calcium from food. But if your diet isn't the greatest, your body will use your bones as a lending institution, borrowing the calcium it needs today from the abundant supply in your bones. This creates a kind of calcium debt to your bones. If you eat enough high-calcium foods to keep functioning, any excess will be used to pay back the debt. But if you eat poorly, the debt never gets repaid. While you can skate by for a few years, eventually the debt will catch up with you in the form of weakened, thinning bones.

As we physically develop, our bones get denser and denser if we supply them by eating calcium-rich foods. After about age 30, our bones are as dense as they will ever be. That's why it is so important for children and young adults to get enough calcium in their diets; if they later need to "borrow" calcium from their bones, strong dense bones are the equivalent of a high spending limit on a credit card. After menopause, all women lose bone density because of hormonal changes. A woman with dense bones will be able to lose some density without developing osteoporosis. After menopause, it is still important to get enough calcium so that you don't run up a calcium debt any larger than necessary.

On the other hand, it is possible to get too much of good thing. Most people struggle to get the recommended 1,000 to 1,500 milligrams of calcium daily. But some folks can't help but go overboard when they finally see the light about bone health—they change their diets and take supplements . . . lots of supplements. Unfortunately, you can't make up for lost calcium overnight. The upper recommended limit for calcium consumption is 2,500 milligrams per day—taking more can reduce the body's ability to absorb other minerals, and may lead to kidney stones.

One interesting note: Some foods—most notably spinach and rhubarb—contain lots of calcium, but they also contain oxalates, substances that bind to the calcium, making it unavailable to your body. My list of calcium-rich foods includes only the absolute best sources, so every serving serves your bones.

> **BEST FOODS FOR CALCIUM:** *Yogurt (fat-free, low-fat), milk (fat-free, 1% reduced-fat), enriched/fortified soy milk, calcium-fortified fruit juice, cheese (fat-free, reduced-fat), tofu with calcium, sardines (with bones), wild salmon (with bones), soybeans, frozen yogurt (fat-free, low-fat), low-fat ice cream, calcium-fortified whole grain waffles, bok choy, white beans, kale, broccoli, almonds*

Calcium is useless without vitamin D. Vitamin D allows calcium to move from the gastrointestinal tract to the parts of the body that need it—including the bones. Without enough vitamin D, a child's bones can become so weak that they bow under the body's own weight, a condition called *rickets*. In adults, lack of vitamin D means that the body borrows calcium from bones to feed the rest of the body's needs. Eventually osteoporosis will set in.

Vitamin D can be made in the body through a reaction of the skin and sunlight. Just 10 to 15 minutes of sun on the bare skin of the arms three or four times a week is enough to keep most of us healthy. Of course, too much sunlight causes skin damage and premature aging, and may lead to skin cancer. That's why I recommend getting vitamin D from food sources and supplements.

> **BEST FOODS FOR VITAMIN D:** *Wild salmon (with bones), mackerel (not king), sardines (with bones), herring, fortified milk (fat-free, 1% reduced-fat), enriched/fortified soy milk, egg yolks, mushrooms (especially shiitake), vitamin-D–fortified margarine (soft tub, trans fat–free), fortified whole grain cereals*

OTHER NUTRIENTS

Although calcium and vitamin D are the superstars of osteoporosis prevention and treatment, there are many other nutrients that play a supporting role, including:

Magnesium: You don't need a chemistry class to know that acids can be corrosive. The same is true for acids formed in your body during the process of metabolism. These metabolic acids need to be balanced and neutralized by alkaline compounds, otherwise they can cause bone loss. Magnesium can help neutralize these acids.

In addition, magnesium helps your body absorb calcium. For calcium to be absorbed in the body, it needs two things: vitamin D (as we already discussed) and parathyroid hormone (PTH). Because magnesium affects PTH, it indirectly—but very critically—affects how much calcium is available for building and maintaining bone.

In scientific research, dietary magnesium gets mixed reviews—some studies show little or no effect, while others show significant increases in bone density or decreases in fractures. Despite these conflicting findings, magnesium is necessary for health, and I believe it is impossible to properly treat osteoporosis without including magnesium.

FAQS

I've heard that calcium can be leeched from bones by the phosphorus in soft drinks. Is that true?

No, it's a fallacy. In reality, there is much more phosphorus naturally found in meat than there is in soda. The main problem with soft drinks is that they replace calcium and vitamin D–rich milk in the diet. Back in the "good old days," kids drank milk with lunch and dinner, and they often started the day with a bowl of cereal and milk. More recently, milk has fallen out of favor, and soda has become the drink of choice. Studies have shown that kids who drink soft drinks instead of milk often have less bone density than kids who get plenty of calcium in their diets. The same is true for adults. So while soft drinks are partly to blame for low bone density, it's not because of the phosphorus.

BEST FOODS FOR MAGNESIUM: *Pumpkin seeds, spinach, Swiss chard, amaranth, sunflower seeds, cashews, almonds, quinoa, tempeh, sweet potatoes, white potatoes, soybeans, millet, beans (black, white, navy, lima, pinto, kidney), artichoke hearts, peanuts, peanut butter, chickpeas (garbanzo beans), brown rice, whole grain bread, sesame seeds, wheat germ, flaxseed*

Potassium helps to increase bone formation, improves calcium balance, increases bone mineral density, and reduces bone resorption by neutralizing metabolic acids. Researchers from the United Kingdom looked at the effects of dietary potassium on bone mineral density of more than 3,000 pre- and postmenopausal women. For women who were still menstruating, eating lots of potassium-rich foods increased bone mineral density by 8 percent—a relatively modest gain, but one that the researchers estimated could translate into a 30 percent reduced risk of fracture in later years.

Of course, it is difficult to separate the effects of potassium specifically from the effects of fruits and vegetables in general. Fruits and veggies, many of which contain significant quantities of potassium, have a whole rainbow of nutrients that contribute to bone health. A few studies have shown that supplements of potassium salts can reduce the amount of calcium lost in urine, but no one has yet determined whether that translates into healthier bones. The important thing to take away from all this is that potassium-rich *foods* will help keep your bones as healthy and strong as possible.

FAQS

My kids won't drink milk, and I can't stand drinking it myself—should I worry about the amount of calcium we're getting?

Milk is an easy way to get calcium, but it is certainly not the only way. All dairy foods contain calcium, and many kids enjoy eating yogurt and string cheese. Whenever possible, substitute foods your kids already eat with calcium-fortified versions. For example, there are calcium-fortified waffles and orange juice. If they still don't get enough calcium, you can always try one of the candy-flavored chewable calcium supplements, such as Viactiv or Nature's Made brands. My experience has shown that most kids don't like the chocolate flavors that adults are drawn to—they may eat them for a couple days, but then the appeal wears off. Instead, choose one of the other flavors, such as orange, strawberry, or caramel. (Always be careful to store the supplements where your children can't get them—if they think of them as candy, you can bet they'll be looking for opportunities to sneak extras. Too much calcium can be dangerous.) Another sneaky—but effective!—way to ensure your children get the calcium and vitamin D they need, is to buy a pill crusher at your local pharmacy, and mix one crushed calcium pill with a few tablespoons of yogurt or low-fat pudding.

BEST FOODS FOR POTASSIUM: *White potatoes, yams, yogurt, soybeans, Swiss chard, snapper, sweet potatoes, avocado, cantaloupe, artichokes, bananas, spinach, lettuce (especially romaine), radicchio, arugula, endive, black cod (sablefish), honeydew melon, pumpkin, milk (fat-free, 1% reduced-fat), carrots, beans (white, black, navy, kidney, pinto), lentils, lima beans, apricots, papaya, split peas, pistachio nuts, winter squash (acorn, butternut), enriched/fortified soy milk, watermelon, beets, tomatoes (including sauce, juice), kale, mushrooms, raisins, peanuts, plums, almonds, sunflower seeds, prunes (and juice), chickpeas (garbanzo beans), oranges (and juice), broccoli*

Vitamin K is important for the formation of osteocalcin, a type of protein found only in bone. People who suffer from fractures tend to have low vitamin K levels . . . and those who have high blood levels of vitamin K also tend to have high bone density. In studies of people with vitamin K deficiencies, those who took vitamin K supplements had less bone loss and fewer fractures. Therefore I highly recommend loading up on foods rich in vitamin K. One caveat: vitamin K is a natural blood thinner, so people who are taking blood-thinning medication (such as warfarin) should talk with their doctors before eating vitamin K–rich foods.

BEST FOODS FOR VITAMIN K: *Kale, spinach, collard greens, Swiss chard, turnip greens, endive, escarole, mustard greens, lettuce (all varieties), parsley, broccoli, Brussels sprouts, watercress, asparagus, okra*

Folate: Homocysteine is an amino acid that is usually a marker for atherosclerosis and heart disease. But scientific research now suggests that homocysteine may also be a marker for osteoporosis. In a 2006 Norwegian study, women with high levels of homocysteine also had low bone mineral density. In addition, women with low bone density also had low levels of the B vitamin called folate, which is known to lower homocysteine levels. Although more research needs to be done to clarify the role of folate, the hope is that women can reduce their risk of osteoporosis by eating more folate-rich foods.

BEST FOODS FOR FOLATE: *Fortified whole grain cereals, lentils, black-eyed peas, soybeans, oatmeal, turnip greens, spinach, mustard greens, green peas, artichokes, okra, beets, parsnips, broccoli, broccoli raab, sunflower seeds, wheat germ, oranges (and juice), Brussels sprouts, papaya, seaweed, berries (boysenberries, blackberries, strawberries), beans (black,* *pinto, kidney, garbanzo, navy), cauliflower, Chinese cabbage, corn, whole grain bread, pasta (preferably whole wheat)*

Vitamin C is essential for the health of collagen and other connective tissue, including the connective tissue in bones. Without enough vitamin C, bone density loss accelerate. Some studies have shown that eating lots of foods high in vitamin C increases bone mineral density and results in fewer fractures.

BEST FOODS FOR VITAMIN C: *Guava, bell peppers (yellow, red, green), orange juice, hot chile pepper, oranges, grapefruit juice, strawberries, pineapple, kohlrabi, papaya, lemons, broccoli, kale, Brussels sprouts, kidney beans, kiwi, cantaloupe, cauliflower, red cabbage, mangos, grapefruit (pink, red), white potatoes (with skin), mustard greens, cherry tomatoes, sugar snap peas, snow peas, clementines, rutabagas, turnip greens, tomatoes, raspberries, Chinese cabbage, blackberries, green tomatoes, cabbage, watermelon, tangerines, lemon juice, okra, lychees, summer squash (all varieties), persimmons*

Soy protein: Soy foods contain natural chemicals called isoflavones, which are phytoestrogens—plant substances that mimic estrogen. Knowing that women lose bone density after menopause because of the loss of estrogen, some scientists believe that the plant estrogens in soy foods could help increase bone density. It's still not clear whether that's true. In laboratory rats, isoflavones helped preserve bone. But in people, the effects are more complicated. Scientists theorize that soy may only help women before menopause (when they lose estrogen receptors as well as estrogen), or it could be that only certain forms of soy protein may be beneficial after menopause. For example, a Japanese study of postmenopausal women found that bone mineral density was higher in women who ate fermented soybeans (natto), but not in women who ate tofu or other soy products. But other studies have shown that long-term addition of soy protein in the diet seems to reduce bone turnover and may prevent bone loss after menopause. Although the optimal amounts of soy protein haven't been determined, I recommend you try to incorporate high quality soy foods into your diet a few times each week. *Important caveat:* although the topic of soy intake and breast cancer remains controversial because of the estrogen-like activity, I do NOT recommend soy foods for women who have had breast cancer. Furthermore, I would never recommend isoflavone *supplements* for anybody (breast cancer or not) because they have not yet been proven safe at high doses.

BEST FOODS FOR SOY PROTEIN: *Tempeh, tofu, soybeans, natto (fermented soybeans), soy nuts, soy flour, soy cheese, enriched/fortified soy milk, soy yogurt, soy crisps*

Protein: For many years, conventional wisdom was that protein increased the risk of osteoporosis because people who ate large amounts of protein had a large amount of calcium in their urine. Scientists thought that protein was somehow leeching calcium from the bones, which then found its way out of the body through urine. Excessive amounts of protein may indeed pose a problem, However, more recent research suggests the bigger issue may be eating too little protein.

Protein is an important component of bone, and absolutely necessary for bone strength. Studies show that people who don't get enough protein may have reduced calcium absorption, reduced bone density, and higher rates of bone loss. People who eat relatively large amounts of protein have a reduced risk of fractures and higher bone mineral density. Although more research needs to be done to understand the biochemical mechanisms involved, it doesn't seem to matter whether you get your protein from animal sources or vegetable sources. But, as mentioned earlier, too much protein from any source may still be harmful, so don't go protein crazy: no high-protein/no-carb diets or excessive amounts of protein bars or shakes.

The bottom line is that you need to ensure that you're getting an appropriate amount of protein through lean meats, poultry, fish, eggs, legumes, dairy, and soy foods. What defines appropriate depends on your weight. Here's a simple rule of thumb—take your weight, divide it in half and that's approximately how many grams of protein you need to eat every day for good bone health. If you weigh 140 pounds, you need about 70 grams of protein. The following guide will give you a sense of whether you're eating enough. Of course, many more foods than those listed below provide protein—even some brands of bread and cereal. I encourage you to read labels, and tally your protein grams for a day or two to make sure you're on track.

FOOD	APPROXIMATE GRAMS OF PROTEIN
1 egg	6
1 cup milk (fat-free, reduced-fat)	8
1 ounce cheese (fat-free, reduced-fat)	7 to 8
½ cup cottage cheese (fat-free, 1% reduced-fat)	14
1 cup fat-free yogurt	8 to 14
½ cup beans	7 to 9
1 ounce almonds	6
1 ounce peanuts	8
1 ounce soy nuts	12
6 ounces tofu	14
1 ounce lean beef, poultry, or fish	7
5 ounces skinless chicken breast or fish fillet	35
3 ounces sirloin steak (size of a deck of cards)	21

Keep in mind that fattier cuts of beef will provide *less* protein ounce per ounce when compared to leaner cuts. That's because the fat content takes up space and displaces protein. Reduced-fat and fat-free milk, cheese, and yogurts provide *more* calcium ounce per ounce than their full-fat counterparts, for the same reason. When fat is removed, the lost volume is replaced with more calcium-rich, reduced-fat dairy. Double bonus—less fat, more calcium!

BEST FOODS FOR PROTEIN: *Turkey breast, chicken breast, seafood and fish, veal, pork tenderloin, lean ham, lean beef, egg whites, yogurt (fat-free, low-fat), milk (fat-free, 1% reduced-fat), enriched/fortified soy milk, cheese (fat-free, reduced-fat), beans (lima, black, navy, pinto, garbanzo), lentils, split peas, tofu, tempeh, soybeans, nuts (soy nuts, peanuts, almonds), peanut butter*

FOODS TO LIMIT

VITAMIN A

Too much vitamin A can harm bones, increasing the risk of fractures. Although more research needs to be done, it looks as though too much vitamin A may stop vitamin D from doing its job of making calcium available to bones. In food, vitamin A comes from two sources: beta carotene and retinol—and recent studies suggest that *only retinol* causes problems. To avoid overdosing on retinol, the troublesome form of vitamin A, do not regularly eat liver or foods that are fortified with vitamin A. Furthermore, don't take any supplement that contains more than 2,000 IU retinol, including your multivitamin. Your multivitamin should provide 100% DV for vitamin A, but at least 50% should come from beta carotene or mixed carotenoids. Look for this information on your bottle's nutrient listing, right next to vitamin A.

SALT

Salt causes the body to lose a little bit of calcium through what scientists call *renal excretion,* and what everyone else calls *peeing.* The actual amount is very small, but if you are already fighting a calcium deficiency, or if you have bone density problems, every little bit counts. In addition, salt seems to increase bone resorption. Limit your salt intake, and on those days when salt can't be avoided, just try to eat an extra serving of reduced-fat dairy to make up for it.

BONUS POINTS

- **Talk with your doctor about osteoporosis prevention.** Because every individual is different, it is important to start talking with your doctor about your particular risk for osteoporosis as soon as possible. Topics to discuss include whether you need to get a bone density scan, whether your history of disease and medication makes you more likely to develop osteoporosis in the future, and whether some of the new bone-building medications might be right for you.
- **Exercise.** When you're younger, exercise helps build and maintain strong bones by turning on bone-building activities. When you move your muscles (and, by extension, your bones), the action stimulates osteoblasts to create more bone. That's why it's critical for children and young adults to get plenty of exercise during their bone-building years. And although this bone-building action does not appear to continue as we age, exercise remains equally important for bone health. That's because regular

physical activity maintains muscle tone and strength surrounding the bone and will help prevent falls and injuries that could lead to breaks and fractures. Weight-bearing exercises—those that require your body to carry its own weight, such as walking—are very helpful. Even better, however, are resistance exercises that require use of resistance bands, dumbbells, free weights, or weight machines. These types of exercises build healthy lean muscle mass which in turn protects your precious bone tissue underneath.

- **Maintain a healthy weight.** Although many women believe that there is no such thing as "too thin," there is. Eating disorders, celiac disease, and other medical problems can cause weight to drop to levels that are unhealthy for bones. Check the chart on page 21 to see if you fall in the category called "underweight." If so, you might want to consider talking with your doctor about how to bring your weight up to a healthy level.

- **Stop smoking.** For more than 20 years, smoking has been linked with a higher risk of osteoporosis, but the reasons why aren't clear. It could be that people who smoke have other risk factors that make them more likely to have low bone density, such as lower body weight, infrequent exercise, or poor food choices. It could also be that cigarette smoke spurs changes in some body hormones that might trigger bone loss. Some research with laboratory animals suggests that nicotine may have a direct effect on bone, namely inhibiting the production of bone-building osteoblasts.

- **Encourage those you love to stop smoking.** You want the people you love to protect their health, but on a more selfish level, their smoking may be hurting *your* bones. Harvard researchers studied bone health in more than 14,000 people in China, and discovered that nonsmoking women who were exposed to second-hand smoke were three times more likely to develop osteoporosis as women who had no exposure to smoke. The theory is that cigarette smoke may affect levels of estrogen, a hormone that regulates bone turnover. If you can't persuade the smoker in your life to quit the habit, try to establish house rules that will minimize your exposure such as only smoking outdoors or by an open window.

- **Drink alcohol only in moderation.** Alcohol can be your bones' friend or foe, depending on how much you drink. Heavy drinking weakens bone, but light drinking may actually make bones stronger. In a study of hundreds of women ages 65 to 77, researchers discovered that women who did not drink alcohol at all had the lowest bone density of all. Bone density was highest in women who drank two to four alcoholic drinks per week (*not* per day!). Women who drank more than four alcoholic drinks per week had lower total body bone mineral density (although still higher than nondrinkers). Scientists believe that alcohol works by reducing bone breakdown, and perhaps by increasing levels of estrogen. If you don't already drink alcohol, I can't recommend starting. But if you do drink, moderate drinking is optimal for bone density—four drinks per week should be your max.

- **Yo-yo no more.** Even though thin women are generally more susceptible to osteoporosis than overweight women, women who are chronic dieters may also be at increased risk of weak bones *regardless of how much they weigh*. Researchers believe that years of dieting cause women to eat so poorly that they don't get the nutrients they needed to build bones up to a healthy, strong level. Dieting by severely restricting total food intake is never a good idea. If you want a better way to lose weight, see Weight Loss on page 19.

SUPPLEMENTS

If you are concerned about osteoporosis, or if you have been diagnosed with osteopenia, and want to consider supplements *in addition to* the food fixes, I recommend:

1. **Multivitamin.** Because so many micronutrients are important for bone health, I always recommend taking a multivitamin. Look for a brand that contains 400 IU vitamin D in the form of D_3 (cholecalciferol, the most potent form), and at least 50 milligrams of magnesium. Your multi should also provide 100% DV of vitamin A (with at least 50% coming from beta carotene or mixed carotenoids). In addition, your multi should have 100% DV for several other nutrients, including vitamin B_6, vitamin B_{12}, folate, zinc, copper, and manganese. Avoid iron in your supplement unless you are a premenopausal woman.

2. **Calcium with vitamin D (and optional magnesium).** In addition to taking a multivitamin, I encourage my female clients to take calcium supplements as safety net. In studies, calcium supplements (with vitamin D_3) reduced the risk of hip and spine fractures by about 25 percent. That's an amazing benefit for taking just two little pills each day. When buying supplements, remember that calcium is *worthless* without vitamin D_3. It's also a bonus to buy a supplement with added magnesium since most people seldom get enough of this important mineral through food and their multivitamin pill. It is important to note that supplements need to be continued indefinitely—once stopped, bone density falls again, and risk of fracture increases.

    Special note for men: Some research shows a possible link between increased calcium intake and prostate cancer. Men should aim to get no more than 1,000 milligrams of calcium from food sources daily—about two to three servings. Men with diagnosed bone density issues should follow their doctors' advice about supplementation.

    Because calcium is better absorbed when you take no more than 600 milligrams at a time, calcium supplements need to be taken twice a day, known as a divided dose. That means taking half the day's dosage early in the day, and the other half later in the day. I tell my clients to be religious about the time and place they take calcium supplements so that it becomes as automatic as brushing your teeth. Keep a bottle of supplements next to where you store your breakfast foods to jog your memory about the first dose of the day. You can keep a second bottle on your desk at work as a reminder to take one at lunch. (If you are a woman taking a multivitamin with iron, never take the multi at the same time as the calcium supplement—iron can keep the body from absorbing calcium properly.)

    There are two main types of calcium supplements for you to choose from, depending on your preferences and other health issues.

■ *Calcium carbonate.* This is the most common and least expensive form of calcium. It must be taken with food or drink. Look for brands that contain 500 to 600 milligrams of calcium, plus at least 200 IU vitamin D_3 per pill. Take 500 to 600 milligrams (one tablet) twice each day—once with breakfast or lunch, and a second time with dinner or an evening snack. (Aim to get a total 800 IU vitamin D_3 daily; at least 400 IU from your multivitamin plus at least 400 IU from your calcium supplements. If for some reason you cannot take a multivitamin and/or calcium supplement with added D_3, I strongly suggest a separate vitamin D_3 supplement.

■ *Calcium citrate* causes the least gastrointestinal problems, so this form of calcium is better tolerated by people with indigestion or more serious GI concerns. You do not have to take calcium citrate with food and it is also more easily absorbed by the body. However, it is bulkier, so if you are not a committed pill-popper, you won't do well with calcium citrate. Each pill contains just 200 to 300 milligrams of calcium so you have to take twice as many pills as people who get their calcium supplement from calcium carbonate pills. Take 500 to 600 milligrams (two or three tablets) twice each day. I recommend taking your calcium citrate once with breakfast or lunch, and a second time before you go to bed. Look for a brand that also provides a daily cumulative dose of at least 400 IU Vitamin D_3. If you choose a calcium supplement without vitamin D_3, I strongly recommend a separate dose. At the end of the day, ensure your daily Vitamin D_3 totals 800 IU.

JOY'S 4-STEP PROGRAM
FOR OSTEOPOROSIS

Follow this program if you have osteopenia or osteoporosis, or a family history of bone density problems.

STEP1 . . . START WITH THE BASICS

These are the first things you should do to help preserve bone density:

- See your doctor for advice about osteoporosis diagnosis or prevention if . . . you are a woman in menopause who has never had a bone density scan . . . you have ever had an eating disorder . . . you have taken corticosteroid medications for three or more months at any time in your life.

- Take a multivitamin. See guidelines on page 239.

- Begin taking calcium supplements with vitamin D_3 and optional magnesium. If you're a man, speak with you physician before taking calcium supplements.

- Start an exercise program.

- If you smoke, quit. Encourage people in your life to quit smoking, too.

STEP 2 ... YOUR ULTIMATE GROCERY LIST

A nutrition plan is only as good as the foods that you choose. This list contains foods with high levels of nutrients that help strengthen bones, plus some foods used as ingredients in the meal plans and recipes. You don't have to purchase every item . . . but these foods should make up the bulk of what you eat for the week. If you find yourself getting bored, try some unfamiliar foods from the list—they may become favorites.

FRUIT

Apricots	Clementines	Limes (and juice)	Pineapple
Bananas	Grapefruit and juice	Lychees	Plums
Berries (boysenberries,	(pink, red)	Mangos	Prunes (and juice)
blackberries,	Guava	Melon, honeydew	Raisins
raspberries,	Juice, calcium-fortified	Oranges (and juice)	Tangerines
strawberries)	Kiwi	Papaya	Watermelon
Cantaloupe	Lemons (and juice)	Persimmons	

VEGETABLES

Artichokes (including	Chickpeas (garbanzo	Okra	Spinach
hearts)	beans)	Parsley	Squash, summer
Arugula	Collard greens	Parsnips	(all varieties)
Asparagus	Corn	Peas (black-eyed, split)	Squash, winter (acorn,
Avocado	Corn (for meal plan):	Peas, green	butternut)
Beans (black, white,	baby corn or frozen	Peppers (hot; yellow/	Swiss chard
pinto, kidney,	kernels	red/green)	Tomatoes (including
lima, garbanzo,	Endive	Pepper, jalapeño	cherry tomatoes,
navy)	Escarole	Potatoes, sweet	green tomatoes;
Beets	Kale	Potatoes, white	tomato sauce, juice,
Bok choy	Kohlrabi	Pumpkin	paste)
Broccoli	Lentils	Radicchio	Tomatoes, canned,
Broccoli raab	Lettuce (all varieties,	Rutabagas	diced, no salt added
Brussels sprouts	especially	Seaweed	(for meal plan)
Cabbage (including	romaine)	Shallots	Turnip greens
Chinese, red)	Mushrooms (especially	Snow peas	Watercress
Carrots	shiitake)	Soybeans (including	Yams
Cauliflower	Mustard greens	edamame)	

SEAFOOD

ALL seafood and fish are good sources of protein	Black cod (sablefish) Herring	Mackerel (not king) Salmon, wild (with bones)	Sardines (with bones) Snapper

LEAN MEATS/EGGS/SOY FOODS

Beef, lean Chicken breast Eggs Ham, lean	Natto (fermented soybeans) Pork tenderloin Soy crisps	Tempeh Tofu, extra-firm (for meal plan) Tofu with calcium	Turkey breast Veal

NUTS AND SEEDS (PREFERABLY UNSALTED)

Almonds Cashews Flaxseed	Peanut butter Peanuts Pistachio nuts	Pumpkin seeds Sesame seeds Soy nuts	Sunflower seeds

WHOLE GRAINS

Amaranth Bread, whole grain Cereal, fortified whole grain	Millet Oatmeal Pasta, preferably whole wheat	Quinoa Rice, brown Waffles, calcium-fortified whole grain	Wheat germ

DAIRY

Cheese (fat-free, reduced-fat) Cheese (for meal plan): fat-free, reduced-fat, Cheddar,	feta, mozzarella, Parmesan, Swiss Cheese, soy Ice cream, low-fat	Milk (vitamin D–fortified fat-free, 1% reduced-fat, enriched/fortified soy)	Yogurt (fat-free, low-fat) Yogurt, frozen (fat-free, low-fat) Yogurt, soy

MISCELLANEOUS

Basil, fresh Bay leaves Bread crumbs, whole wheat Broth, chicken, fat-free, low-sodium Chocolate syrup, light Cinnamon, ground Cornstarch Dill, fresh Flour, all-purpose Flour, soy Garlic	Ginger, fresh Honey Hot cocoa, diet (less than 200 calories) Hot sauce Margarine, vitamin-D–fortified, soft tub, trans fat–free Mayonnaise, reduced-fat Mint, fresh Mustard, Dijon Nonstick cooking spray Nutmeg	Oil, canola Oil, sesame Oregano, dried Paprika Parsley, fresh Pepper, black Pepper, crushed red Rosemary, dried and fresh Salad dressing, reduced-calorie Salsa Soy crisps	Soy sauce, reduced-sodium Sugar Taco seasoning, mild or hot Taco shells, hard or soft Thyme, fresh Vinegar, apple cider Vinegar, balsamic

STEP3 ...GOING ABOVE AND BEYOND

If you want to do everything you can to prevent or control osteoporosis, here are some additional things you might try:

- Limit the amount of salt you eat.

- Limit alcohol consumption to no more than four drinks per week.

- If you need to diet for weight loss, do it in a way that is smart for your bones. See Weight Loss, page 19, for more information.

- If you are underweight, talk with your doctor to learn the healthiest ways to bring your weight up.

HOW TO PILE ON THE POUNDS

If you need to gain weight as part of your strategy to avoid bone loss, it is important to add healthy pounds, as opposed to ice cream and doughnut pounds. Aim to add about 500 calories each day, for a gain of about 1 pound per week. Start by substituting products that are higher in healthy fats. For example, sauté vegetables in olive oil instead of steaming them, use full-fat salad dressing instead of light varieties, and add avocado to salads and sandwiches. Incorporate two or three healthy mini-meals each day, in addition to breakfast, lunch, and dinner. Hummus, guacamole, sunflower seeds, nuts (and nut butters), trail mix, energy bars, dried fruit, fruit-yogurt smoothies, granola bars, and healthy homemade muffins add good calories to your daily count. If your appetite is poor, or if you cannot gain weight, talk with your doctor.

STEP4 ...MEAL PLANS

These sample menus include foods that have been shown to strengthen bones, specifically foods high in calcium, vitamin D, magnesium, vitamin K, potassium, protein, vitamin C, and other nutrients.

Every day, choose *one* option for each of the three meals—breakfast, lunch, and dinner. Then, one or two times per day, choose from a variety of my suggested snacks. Approximate calories have been provided to help adjust for your personal weight management goals. If you find yourself hungry (and weight is not an issue), feel free to increase the portion sizes for meals and snacks. Beverage calories are *not* included.

BREAKFAST OPTIONS

(Approximately 300 to 400 calories)

Strawberry-Nut Yogurt Parfait

Spoon ⅓ cup vanilla fat-free yogurt into a parfait glass. Top with 2 heaping tablespoons sliced strawberries (or raspberries or blackberries) and 1 tablespoon soy nuts (or sunflower seeds or slivered almonds). Repeat the three layers two times (yogurt, berries, and then nuts).

Cereal with Milk and Fruit

1 cup whole grain cereal (120 calories or less) mixed with 1 cup milk (fat-free, 1% reduced-fat, or enriched/fortified soy). Enjoy with 1 cup sliced pineapple (or watermelon, berries, or ½ grapefruit, ½ banana, ½ mango, 1 orange, or 1 kiwi).

Melon with Cottage Cheese and Sunflower Seeds

½ cantaloupe or ¼ honeydew melon (1 to 1½ cups cubed) mixed with 1 cup fat-free 1% reduced-fat cottage cheese and topped with 1 tablespoon sunflower seeds (or 2 tablespoons wheat germ).

Oatmeal with Milk and Fresh Berries

½ cup dry instant oatmeal prepared with 1 cup milk (fat-free, 1% reduced-fat, or enriched/fortified soy); sprinkled with 2 tablespoons wheat germ (or ground flaxseed) and ½ cup berries (sliced strawberries, raspberries, and/or blackberries). Sweeten with optional 1 teaspoon sugar, honey, or artificial sweetener.

Breakfast Potato and Yogurt

1 medium baked white or sweet potato with skin. Enjoy with ¾ cup plain or vanilla fat-free yogurt (or ½ cup fat-free or 1% reduced-fat cottage cheese) mixed with cinnamon and optional 1 teaspoon sugar (or artificial sweetener).

Scrambled Eggs with Broccoli and Cheese

Beat 1 whole egg and 2 egg whites. Cook in small skillet coated with nonstick cooking spray. When eggs are almost cooked, add 1 cup cooked broccoli florets and 1 ounce shredded fat-free or reduced-fat cheese. Enjoy with ½ grapefruit (or ½ banana or 1 orange).

Strawberry-Kiwi Smoothie with Peanut Butter Toast

1 serving (2 cups) Strawberry-Kiwi Smoothie (page 122) with 1 slice whole grain toast topped with 1 level tablespoon peanut butter (or 2 heaping tablespoons fat-free or 1% reduced-fat cottage cheese sprinkled with 1 tablespoon of slivered almonds and optional cinnamon).

LUNCH OPTIONS

(Approximately 400 to 500 calories)

Ham and Cheese Sandwich

4 or 5 ounces sliced ham (or turkey breast or grilled chicken breast), 1 slice (¾-ounce) fat-free or reduced-fat cheese, lettuce, tomato, and onion on 2 slices whole grain bread or pita. Spread with 2 teaspoons reduced-fat mayonnaise or hummus and optional mustard. Serve with large handful baby carrots or bell peppers sticks.

Artichoke Salad with Grilled Chicken and Feta Cheese

1 cup canned, drained artichoke hearts mixed with 2 to 3 cups leafy greens (spinach, romaine, arugula, mustard greens, etc.), ½ cup cherry tomatoes, 1 ounce (¼ cup) crumbled reduced-fat feta cheese, 2 ounces grilled chicken (or lean ham or turkey breast). Toss with 2 teaspoons olive oil and unlimited vinegar or fresh lemon juice and seasonings.

Baked Potato with Broccoli and Cheese

Baked potato topped with steamed or boiled chopped broccoli and 1 ounce shredded reduced-fat or fat-free cheese (or ½ cup fat-free or 1% reduced-fat cottage cheese). Serve with 1 cup vegetable soup or Vegetable Oatmeal Bisque (page 323).

Edamame with Wild Salmon Dijonnaise

1 cup boiled edamame (soybeans in the pod), lightly salted. Enjoy with 5 ounces canned wild salmon with bones, drained, mashed, and mixed with 1 tablespoon reduced–fat mayonnaise, 1 to 2 teaspoons Dijon mustard, minced onion, and black pepper. Serve salmon on large bed of leafy greens (spinach, romaine, etc.) tossed with fresh lemon juice or 2 tablespoons reduced-calorie dressing.

Broccoli-Cheese Soufflé with Cottage Cheese and Almonds

1 serving Broccoli-Cheese Soufflé (page 121) with ½ cup fat-free or 1% reduced-fat cottage cheese topped with 1 tablespoon slivered almonds (or sunflower seeds, soy nuts, or ground flaxseed).

Tomato-Cheese Omelet with Tropical Mango-Citrus Smoothie

Beat 1 whole egg with 2 to 3 egg whites and cook in heated small skillet coated with nonstick cooking spray. When bottom is cooked, gently flip and add 3 tablespoons chopped tomato, optional dried basil, plus 1 ounce reduced-fat or fat-free cheese. Fold omelet in half and continue cooking until egg mixture firms and cheese melts. Enjoy with 1 serving (2 cups) Tropical Mango-Citrus Smoothie (page 123).

Mixed Vegetable Salad with Sardines

4 ounces (about 8) sardines with bones (canned in oil or tomato sauce) tossed with unlimited leafy greens, chopped tomato, carrots, mushrooms, sweet pepper, onion, and ½ cup beans (choose from white, navy, chickpeas). Drizzle with 2 to 4 tablespoons reduced-calorie salad dressing (or 1 teaspoon olive oil and 1 to 2 tablespoons vinegar or fresh lemon juice). Season with salt and ground pepper to taste.

DINNER OPTIONS

(Approximately 500 to 600 calories)

Whole Wheat Pita Pizza with the Works

Toast 1 split whole wheat pita bread (or use 200 calories of whole wheat pizza crust). Top each half with 2 to 3 heaping tablespoons marinara sauce and ¼ cup reduced-fat ricotta cheese, plus ½ cup cooked peppers and unlimited chopped broccoli florets sautéed in nonstick cooking spray until soft. Top each half with 2 tablespoons shredded reduced-fat mozzarella cheese and optional crushed red pepper and oregano. Heat in 350°F oven until cheese melts and bubbles.

Turkey Chili with Cheese

1 serving (2 cups) Turkey Chili (page 367) topped with 1 ounce shredded fat-free Cheddar cheese. Serve with ½ cup cooked brown rice (or amaranth or quinoa) and a salad of leafy greens (optional peppers, carrots, and artichokes) tossed with 1 teaspoon olive oil and unlimited balsamic vinegar or fresh lemon juice.

Tofu Salad with Snow Peas, Almonds, and Mandarin Oranges

6 to 8 ounces extra-firm tofu, cubed and chilled, tossed with 2 to 3 cups baby spinach leaves, 1 cup steamed and chilled snow peas, ½ chopped tomato, and ½ cup mandarin

oranges (canned in light syrup). Drizzle with 1 to 2 teaspoons sesame oil and 1 tablespoon reduced-sodium soy sauce and top with 1 to 2 tablespoon slivered almonds.

Healthy Chicken Parmesan and Broccoli

1 serving Healthy Chicken Parmesan and Broccoli (page 252).

Sweet and Sour Tofu-Veggie Stir-Fry with Brown Rice

1 serving Sweet and Sour Tofu-Veggie Stir-Fry (page 251) with 1 cup cooked brown
rice (or plain medium baked white or sweet potato).

Red Snapper with Fresh Herbs and Brussels Sprouts

6 ounces red snapper fillet poached in ⅔ cup water and ⅓ cup chicken stock or wine.
Add in 2 tablespoons each fresh parsley, dill, thyme, and rosemary and drizzle with
fresh lemon or lime juice just before serving. (Or, season fish with kosher salt and
ground black pepper and *lightly* brush with olive oil; grill or pan roast on medium-high
for about 3 minutes on each side, or until golden brown. You may substitute any favorite fish, but cooking times will vary.) Serve with 1 cup steamed Brussels sprouts (or
Swiss chard or asparagus), and 1 medium baked sweet or white potato.

Turkey Tacos

3 servings Turkey Tacos (page 250) with optional salsa and hot sauce.

SNACK OPTIONS

100 calories or less

- *Best Vegetables:* 1 cup raw or cooked bell peppers (red, green, yellow), bok choy, broccoli, broccoli raab, kale, Brussels sprouts, cabbage, sugar snap peas, tomatoes, mushrooms, okra, zucchini, squash, carrots, lettuce, leafy greens, spinach, collards, Swiss
  chard, watercress, asparagus, kohlrabi, okra, artichokes, beets, cauliflower, seaweed

- *Best Fruits:* 1 orange, tangerine, persimmon, kiwi, or guava; 2 clementines or plums;
  ½ papaya, mango, grapefruit, or cantaloupe; 1 cup boysenberries, blackberries, raspberries, cherries, sliced strawberries, watermelon, honeydew, or pineapple; ½ cup
  lychees; 4 apricots or prunes; 20 strawberries; 2 tablespoons raisins

- 1 cup milk (fat-free)

- 1 reduced-fat string cheese, or 1 ounce fat-free or reduced-fat cheese

- 1 hard-boiled egg

- 8 to 10 ounces fat-free skim latte

- 12 ounces fat-free, skim cappuccino or café au lait

- 6 ounces fat-free plain or flavored yogurt

- ½ cup fat-free or 1% reduced-fat cottage cheese, mixed with optional cinnamon

- 1 cup diet hot cocoa (100 calories or less)

100 to 200 Calories

- 1 small bag soy crisps (200 calories or less)

- 8 ounces fat-free or low-fat yogurt (plain or flavored, 200 calories or less, milk- or soy-based)

- ½ cup low-fat or fat-free frozen yogurt or ice cream (200 calories or less)

- Low-fat ice cream pop (200 calories or less)

- 2 cups Tropical Mango-Citrus Smoothie (page 123)

- 2 cups Strawberry-Kiwi Smoothie (page 122)

- 1 cup fat-free or enriched/fortified soy milk with 2 tablespoons light chocolate syrup

- 1 ounce (about ¼ cup) soy nuts, almonds, cashews, or peanuts

- ¼ cup sunflower seeds or pistachio nuts in the shell

- 1 cup boiled edamame (soybeans in the pod), lightly salted

TURKEY TACOS

In my house, Turkey Tacos are a sure thing—they're nothing fancy, but we never have leftovers. They're even a hit with my kids' picky-eater friends. And nobody has ever suspected the low-calorie swaps: lean ground turkey meat and reduced-fat shredded cheese. If you have extra time, set up bowls with chopped peppers, carrots, and sweet corn that your kids and their friends can add on their own. Or pick your favorites—any vegetable can go into a taco.

Makes 7 servings

- 1   pound extra-lean ground turkey breast
- 1   packet (1.25 to 1.5 ounces) taco seasoning, mild or hot , plus water as indicated on package
- 2   cups chopped or shredded lettuce
- 1   large tomato, finely chopped
- 1   cup shredded reduced-fat Cheddar cheese
- 7   hard or soft taco shells
       Salsa and/or hot sauce (optional)

1. In a large skillet, cook the turkey over medium-high heat until browned. Drain the fat. Stir in the taco seasoning and water. Bring to a boil. Reduce the heat and simmer, stirring occasionally, 5 to 6 minutes.
2. Evenly divide the turkey mixture, lettuce, tomato, and cheese among the taco shells. Top with salsa and/or hot sauce if you like.

PER SERVING
171 calories, 21 g protein, 10 g carbohydrate, 5 g fat (1 g saturated), 29 mg cholesterol, 248 mg sodium, 2 g fiber; plus 106 mg calcium (10% DV)

SWEET AND SOUR TOFU-VEGGIE STIR-FRY

If you haven't tried tofu, or just assume you won't like it, this dish may surprise your taste buds. It's loaded with nearly every bone-strengthening ingredient known to nutritionists (except for vitamin D) and tastes just as good cold if you have leftovers! Serve over brown rice or whole wheat pasta.

Makes 4 servings (1½ cups per serving)

½	cup fat-free, low-sodium chicken broth
¼	cup apple cider vinegar or rice wine vinegar
¼	cup reduced-sodium soy sauce
2	tablespoons apple juice concentrate
1	tablespoon cornstarch
1	package (14 ounces) extra-firm tofu with calcium, drained
2	tablespoons canola oil
1	large red pepper, seeded and thinly sliced
1	cup shredded Chinese cabbage or red cabbage
¼	pound green beans, quartered
2	cloves garlic, minced
1	teaspoon minced fresh ginger
1	small jalapeño chile pepper, seeded and minced (wear plastic gloves when handling)
1	cup baby corn or frozen corn kernels, rinsed under hot water
1	cup frozen whole soybeans, shelled and rinsed under hot water

1. In a small bowl, combine the broth, vinegar, soy sauce, juice concentrate, and cornstarch. Mix well and set aside. Pat the tofu dry with a paper towel, and cut into 1-inch chunks.

2. Spray a large wok or a nonstick skillet with nonstick cooking spray. Place over high heat and add 1 tablespoon of the oil. When the oil shimmers, add the tofu and brown 3 to 4 minutes on one side, then turn and brown the opposite side for 3 to 4 minutes. Transfer to a plate.

3. Reduce the heat to medium and add the remaining 1 tablespoon oil to the wok. Add the red pepper, cabbage, and green beans. Cook, stirring occasionally, 4 to 5 minutes, until the vegetables begin to soften but are still crisp. Stir in the garlic, ginger, and jalapeño, and cook an additional minute, until the mixture becomes fragrant. Add the corn and soybeans, and cook 2 to 3 minutes longer. Reduce the heat to low, and add the broth mixture, stirring until it thickens, 1 to 2 minutes. Off the heat, return the tofu to the wok or skillet and stir gently to coat with the sauce.

PER SERVING
336 calories, 22 g protein, 27 g carbohydrate, 17 g fat (1 g saturated), 0 mg cholesterol, 669 mg sodium, 6 g fiber; plus 341 mg calcium (34% DV), 827 mg potassium (24% DV), 21 mcg vitamin K (27% DV), 120 mg magnesium (30% DV), 158 mcg folic acid (40% DV)

HEALTHY CHICKEN PARMESAN AND BROCCOLI

This is my husband's *absolute* favorite recipe in the book. My youngest daughter, Ayden Jane, agrees. If you need more reasons to dig in, one serving provides your bones with more than a third of your daily calcium requirements; more than 20 percent each of daily requirements of magnesium, folic acid, and potassium; plus, the entire day's worth of vitamin K. Great taste and stellar nutrition—home run!

Makes 4 servings

2	tablespoons extra-virgin olive oil
1	medium onion, chopped
3	cloves garlic, minced
1	bay leaf
1	can (28 ounces) no-salted-added diced tomatoes
¼	cup fresh basil leaves, torn, plus 1 whole sprig
	Salt
	Ground black pepper
1	large bunch broccoli, cut into florets
¼	cup all-purpose flour
2	egg whites
1	cup whole wheat bread crumbs
¼	teaspoon dried oregano
¼	teaspoon dried rosemary
3	tablespoons grated Parmesan cheese
4	large skinless chicken cutlets (6 ounces each), pounded very thin
	Nonstick cooking spray
1	cup grated reduced-fat mozzarella cheese

1. Coat a large skillet with nonstick cooking spray. Place over medium heat and add the olive oil. When the oil is hot, add the onion, two-thirds of the garlic, and bay leaf. Cook, stirring, for 6 to 7 minutes, until the onion begins to soften and become translucent. Reduce the heat to medium and add the tomatoes and sprig of basil. Cook, stirring occasionally, until the sauce starts to thicken, about 10 minutes. Season with salt and pepper. Cover and simmer on low heat while you prepare the broccoli and chicken.

2. Preheat the oven to 450°F. Cover a large baking sheet with aluminum foil or parchment paper. Sprinkle the remaining garlic over the broccoli, and season with salt and pepper. Wrap the broccoli tightly in aluminum foil. Set aside.

3. Place the flour on a piece of waxed paper or aluminum foil. In a shallow bowl, beat the egg whites. On another piece of waxed paper or aluminum foil, mix the bread crumbs with the oregano, rosemary, 2 tablespoons Parmesan, and season with a pinch of salt and pepper.

4. Sprinkle both sides of the chicken cutlets with salt and pepper. Lightly dredge the cutlets in the flour, then dip in the egg whites, shaking off any excess egg, then dredge in the bread crumb mixture. Coat both sides of each cutlet with nonstick cooking spray and place on the prepared baking sheet.

5. Bake the chicken and foil packet of broccoli until the cutlets are golden and the broccoli is tender, 8 to 10 minutes. Remove the broccoli and chicken from the oven.

6. Preheat the broiler. Sprinkle the cutlet with the mozzarella and remaining 1 tablespoon Parmesan. Place under the broiler for 1 to 2 minutes, until the cheese is golden. (Watch carefully—they can burn easily!) Transfer the chicken and broccoli to a platter. Remove the bay leaf from the tomato sauce and ladle the sauce around the chicken. Sprinkle with the torn basil and serve immediately.

PER SERVING
569 calories, 59 g protein, 41 g carbohydrate, 16 g fat (4 g saturated), 111 mg cholesterol, 670 mg sodium, 7 g fiber; plus 365 mg calcium (36% DV), 86 mg magnesium (22% DV), 97 mcg vitamin K (122% DV), 1,017 mg potassium (29% DV), 113 mcg folic acid (28% DV)

CHAPTER 11

CATARACTS AND MACULAR DEGENERATION

For more than 75 years, Nat was a glutton for the printed word. He would read anything—newspapers, magazines, even instruction manuals—but he loved books best. He was active, with plenty of friends and a terrific family, but he was happiest when he could relax with a good novel. So it was particularly devastating when Nat lost most of his sight to macular degeneration. Now, when he finally has all the leisure time in the world, he can't read much more than the large type of the newspaper headlines. Instead of reading novels, he settles for listening to television and radio. It breaks his family's heart. My heart, because I'm a part of Nat's family—he is my husband's grandfather.

Vision loss, and the resulting loss of quality of life, is all too common—cataracts affect about half of all Americans over age 80, and approximately 13 million Americans have macular degeneration. In the past decade, research has pointed to nutrition as one of the factors that might reduce the risk *and* slow the progression of these disorders. I wish that this information had been available back when Nat was still in his prime, when it might have helped to preserve at least some of his sight. I'm sure he would have

FAQS

I understand that there may be a risk to taking high doses of certain vitamins for macular degeneration. Plus, I can't stand popping extra pills. Should I still take a multivitamin?

Yes. High levels of vitamin E supplements can be problematic but a daily multivitamin with only 100% DV for vitamin E is fine (and it will provide—at the very least—100% DV for zinc and vitamin C, along with some beta carotene as well). As for the additional zinc, beta carotene, and vitamin C pills, skip them if you're not a fan. Instead, try making one of my Smooth-SEE recipes (pages 276 and 277). They are both chock-full of the best nutrients for eyes, and are healthy for everyone, not just those with macular degeneration. Just be sure to account for the calories, if weight is a personal concern.

embraced the changes I'll discuss in this chapter if it meant he could spend even one more quiet hour with the mysteries he loves so much.

WHAT AFFECTS CATARACT DEVELOPMENT?

Light enters the eye through the pupil, the round, black opening at the center of the iris. Behind the pupil is the lens, which catches the incoming light and focuses it onto the retina at the back of the eye.

A cataract is formed when protein fibers in the lens change shape and clump together, clouding the normally transparent lens. This is similar to the process that turns the protein in egg albumin from clear to white when cooked. In fact, most well-developed cataracts look milky white, although in some rare cases, the lens can turn yellow or brown instead.

Cataracts develop slowly, over a period of years. But even before a cataract can be seen from the outside, vision can become blurry or cloudy, like looking through a fogged windshield. Other possible symptoms include worsened night vision, faded color vision, and starburst or halo effects around bright lights. Because cataracts can be surgically removed, these symptoms are only temporary—after surgery you may need glasses to see detail, but your sight will be clear.

No one knows exactly what causes eye proteins to clump and create a cataract. Many scientists blame unstable molecules known as free radicals, which can wreak havoc throughout the body, causing destruction and disease wherever they go through a complex chemical process called *oxidative stress*. And what creates free radicals? Well . . . the single greatest cause is just being alive. Natural metabolic processes from normal body functions like breathing and digesting food generate lots of free radicals, and unless they are neutralized, they build up over time. That's why our bodies seem to deteriorate slowly with age—it's the accumulated damage from years of free radical attacks. Anytime there is a major change in the way our bodies work, there is a potential increase in the number of free radicals produced, which is why many metabolic disorders, especially diabetes, are considered risk factors. People with diabetes have a 40 percent increased risk of cataracts . . . and their cataracts develop faster and earlier than those in people without blood sugar problems.

Two other major causes of free radicals are smoking and ultraviolet radiation from sunlight. That's why all cataract prevention strategies must include a commitment to stop smoking and reduce exposure to sunlight. Cataracts can also be caused by surgery for other eye problems, traumatic eye injury, or long-term use of corticosteroids. In very rare circumstances, genetic anomalies can create cataracts in newborn babies or infants.

HOW FOOD AFFECTS CATARACTS

The ultimate prevention for cataracts is simple: Never grow old.

For those of you who can't stop time, nutrition and lifestyle changes are your best bets for preventing or slowing the development of cataracts. Although research has not absolutely, positively proved nutrition's role in cataract prevention, science provides ample circumstantial evidence that eating the right foods could help . . . and I know for certain it can't hurt!

For cataract prevention, the primary nutrients you want to pay attention to are antioxidants and the B vitamins.

ANTIOXIDANTS: VITAMIN C AND VITAMIN E

As the name suggests, anti*oxidants* fight the *oxidative* stress caused by free radicals. There is no single antioxidant—rather, it is a broad category that includes vitamin C, vitamin E, lutein, beta carotene, and any number of other substances that can neutralize free radicals. All vegetables and fruits contain antioxidants, so eating a diet rich in those foods should help prevent cataracts. The few research studies that have been conducted confirm it.

The Nurses' Health Study revealed that women who ate a very healthy diet full of all kinds of antioxidants from vegetables, fruits, and whole grains were *half as likely* to develop cataracts as women who did not eat such a healthy diet. Those benefits were from food alone—if the women took vitamin C supplements, they actually lost that protection and had the same risk of cataracts as women who ate unhealthy diets. Why? No one knows. The truth is, those results were unexpected. We know that vitamin C is a potent antioxidant. We know that people who get lots of vitamin C in their foods (as measured by blood levels of vitamin C) have a reduced risk of cataracts, and at least one earlier study had shown that people who took supplements were less likely to have cataracts. And finally, we know that when laboratory mice eat vitamin C supplements, they have a reduced risk of cataracts. So this finding that vitamin C supplements did not reduce the risk for people is confusing.

The story on vitamin E is equally confusing. Although some research has shown that taking vitamin E supplements reduces the risk of cataracts, others show that the supplements almost *doubled* the risk of cataracts. No one knows why the science is so conflicting, for both vitamins. Regardless of the reasons, *the big-picture message is clear:* Eating lots of fruits and vegetables, including those rich in vitamins C and E, may be your best protection against cataracts.

BEST FOODS FOR VITAMIN C: *Guava, bell peppers (red, yellow, green), orange juice, hot chile peppers, oranges, grapefruit juice, strawberries, pineapple, kohlrabi, papaya, lemons,*

BEST SOURCES OF FOOD ANTIOXIDANTS: TOP 20 FRUITS, VEGETABLES, AND NUTS (as measured by total antioxidant capacity per serving size)

RANK	FOOD ITEM	SERVING SIZE	TOTAL ANTIOXIDANT CAPACITY PER SERVING SIZE
1	Small Red Bean (dried)	Half cup	13727
2	Wild blueberry	1 cup	13427
3	Red kidney bean (dried)	Half cup	13259
4	Pinto bean	Half cup	11864
5	Blueberry (cultivated)	1 cup	9019
6	Cranberry	1 cup (whole)	8983
7	Artichoke (cooked)	1 cup (hearts)	7904
8	Blackberry	1 cup	7701
9	Prune	Half cup	7291
10	Raspberry	1 cup	6058
11	Strawberry	1 cup	5938
12	Red Delicious apple	One	5900
13	Granny Smith apple	One	5381
14	Pecan	1 ounce	5095
15	Sweet cherry	1 cup	4873
16	Black plum	One	4844
17	Russet potato (cooked)	One	4649
18	Black bean (dried)	Half cup	4181
19	Plum	One	4118
20	Gala apple	One	3903

Source: USDA; Journal of Agricultural and Food Chemistry, June 9, 2004

broccoli, kale, Brussels sprouts, kidney beans, kiwi, cantaloupe, cauliflower, red cabbage, mangos, grapefruit (pink, red), white potatoes (with skin), mustard greens, cherry tomatoes, sugar snap peas, snow peas, clementines, rutabagas, turnip greens, tomatoes, raspberries, Chinese cabbage, blackberries, green tomatoes, cabbage, watermelon, tangerines, lemon juice, okra, lychees, summer squash (all varieties), persimmons

BEST FOODS FOR VITAMIN E: *Wheat germ oil, fortified whole grain cereals, sunflower seeds, almonds, hazelnuts, peanut butter, wheat germ, avocado, pine nuts, tomato paste, flaxseed oil, red bell peppers, canola oil, kiwis, peanuts, olive oil, mangos, turnip greens, Brazil nuts, asparagus, peaches, papaya, radicchio, collard greens, broccoli, Swiss chard, spinach*

ANTIOXIDANT: LUTEIN

Lutein is another antioxidant of tremendous interest to eye health researchers. Like all antioxidants, lutein can defuse potentially damaging free radicals. In addition, lutein may also prevent the development of some free radicals because it absorbs blue light—part of the short-wave spectrum of cataract-causing sunlight.

The Beaver Dam Eye study, which followed nearly 5,000 people to see what factors affected aging-related vision disorders, showed that people who ate large amounts of lutein-rich foods had a 20 percent reduced risk of cataracts compared with people who got very little lutein in their diets. Similar results were reported from the Nurses' Health Study and the U.S. Male Health Professionals Study. I don't recommend lutein supplements, however. No one knows everything there is to know about the effects of individual nutrients. It could be, for example, that lutein works best only when paired with other antioxidants, or with certain vitamins and minerals. Right now, the only solid information we have supports eating a diet full of lutein-rich leafy green vegetables, *plus* an abundance of other antioxidant-rich vegetables and fruits.

BEST FOODS FOR LUTEIN: *Kale, spinach, turnip greens, mustard greens, Swiss chard, radicchio, collard greens, summer squash (all varieties), watercress, green peas, persimmons, Brussels sprouts, broccoli, pumpkin, corn, lettuce (butterhead, Boston, Bibb, romaine), asparagus, green beans, okra, artichokes, green bell peppers, scallions, carrots*

B VITAMINS

There is strong evidence that two of the B vitamins—riboflavin (vitamin B_2) and niacin (vitamin B_3)—may help prevent cataracts, and early research suggests that thiamin (vitamin B_1) may also contribute to eye health.

Although these vitamins are not antioxidants, they contribute to antioxidant activity by providing some of the building blocks necessary to help the body make antioxidant compounds. So without enough riboflavin and niacin, the risk of cataracts increases. Indeed, several scientific studies have shown that people who eat a diet with plenty of foods rich in riboflavin and niacin can slash their risk of cataracts by about half compared with people who eat a diet with very little of those vitamins.

As with antioxidants, the information about the benefits of B vitamin supplements is less clear. The Blue Mountain Eye Study, the large Australian study with about 2,900 participants, found that those who took riboflavin supplements had a 20 percent lower risk of cataracts compared with people who didn't take supplements. Niacin supplements lowered risk by 30 percent, and supplements of other B vitamins—thiamin, folate, and vitamin B_{12}—also seemed to show some benefit. Combining these vitamins may have an even great effect. A large study conducted by the National Eye Institute in Bethesda, Maryland, showed that people who took a dual supplement containing both riboflavin and niacin reduced their risk of cataracts by 44 percent. Even general multivitamins providing 100% DV for these B vitamins seem to decrease risk by more than 30 percent. As promising as these results sound, the jury is still out on exactly how much of which types of B vitamins is necessary or optimal for cataract prevention. I can only recommend food sources, not pills (with the exception of a multivitamin providing 100% DV for riboflavin and niacin).

BEST FOODS FOR RIBOFLAVIN: *Liver, lean beef, venison, fortified whole grain cereals, yogurt (fat-free, low-fat), milk (fat-free, 1% reduced-fat), eggs, mushrooms (portobello, white), almonds, coffee*

BEST FOODS FOR NIACIN: *Fortified whole grain cereals, tuna (canned light), chicken breast, lean beef, veal, lean pork, mackerel (not king), turkey breast, wild salmon (fresh, canned), anchovies, kidney beans, peanut butter, peanuts, mushrooms, sunflower seeds*

TEA

Tea contains powerful antioxidants, and some research suggests that drinking relatively large amounts of tea—the equivalent of about five cups daily—may help prevent or delay cataract development. But antioxidants may tell only part of the story. While investigating the effects of tea on blood sugar in diabetic laboratory rats, researchers from the University of Scranton discovered that the animals that drank tea had lower blood sugar than those that did not drink tea. But there was also a side benefit—drinking tea reduced the level of glucose in the eye lens, *and* there was a lower incidence of cataracts. In fact, the tea-drinking rats had about half the risk of cataracts as non-tea-drinkers. Both green tea and regular black tea had the same effects, so feel free to choose the type you enjoy most. Or mix it up: green tea has about half as much caffeine, so it makes a soothing drink in the later afternoon or when you want to relax.

WHAT AFFECTS MACULAR DEGENERATION?

The retina is the part of the eye that receives light and images from the world and sends them to the optic nerve to be processed in the brain. The macula is the center, most sensitive part of the retina. It fine-tunes focus at the center of our visual field, the part that allows us to recognize faces, read words on a page, and discern detail in anything we look at. Macular degeneration, then, is a deterioration of the macula, gradually leading to central blindness. Peripheral vision remains clear, so it isn't a total lack of sight, but the loss of detailed vision. As Nat's story demonstrated, it's a life-altering change all the same.

There are two types of macular degeneration: Dry (also called *atrophic*), caused by a gradual breakdown of light receptors; and wet (also called *exudative*), caused by leaks in the blood vessels of the retina, which in turn cause scarring and tissue death. With both types, people usually notice vision distortions first, such as straight lines appearing wavy, along with difficulty reading and recognizing faces. As more and more receptors die, central vision disappears. In its early stages, wet macular degeneration can be treated with laser surgery to seal off the leaking vessels. There is no medical treatment for dry macular degeneration.

Macular degeneration happens most often in people over age 70, primarily women. Although it can run in families, no one knows what causes macular degeneration, or how to stop it once it begins.

HOW FOOD AFFECTS MACULAR DEGENERATION

The Age-Related Eye Disease Study (AREDS), a research project conducted by the National Eye Institute, has given us some clues about how nutrition might help prevent macular degeneration, or at least delay the progression to blindness. AREDS results showed that certain antioxidant vitamins and zinc helped to slow the progression of advanced macular degeneration by about 25 percent over a six-year period. The antioxidants—vitamins C and E, and beta carotene—are thought to prevent damage caused by free radicals, and the mineral zinc is important for the health of all body tissues, but is found in unusually high concentrations in tissues of the retina.

The results of AREDS were so impressive that in the wake of the study's publication, several supplement manufacturers created special macular degeneration–fighting formulas. However, a 2006 study by researchers from Harvard Medical School linked high levels of vitamin E with *increases* in a measure of inflammation called C-reactive protein (CRP) . . . and high levels of CRP has been linked to a greater risk of macular degeneration. Could it be that high levels of vitamin E could somehow increase your risk? It is too soon to know. But this conflicting information caused a seismic shift in how eye doctors advised their patients—vitamin supplements can no longer be considered purely beneficial. For this reason, I cannot recommend high doses of vitamin E from supplements, even when they are part of a special macular degeneration formulation. However, I definitely recommend food sources of vitamin E, and/or a multivitamin that *only* provides 100% DV for vitamin E.

BETA CAROTENE, VITAMIN C, VITAMIN E

A study led by researchers from Erasmus Medical Centre in Rotterdam, the Netherlands, followed a group of more than 4,000 people to see how diet affected the risk of developing macular degeneration. After eight years, the scientists compared the diets of people who developed the condition with the diets of those who did not. The results were encouraging: People who ate a diet rich in beta carotene, vitamin C, vitamin E, and zinc had a 35 percent reduced risk of developing macular degeneration compared with people who ate an average diet. And those who ate worse-than-normal diets, with low levels of those nutrients, actually had a 20 percent *increased* risk of disease. I highly recommend that anyone with a family history of macular degeneration follow the food plan for high-antioxidant, high-zinc foods to reduce their risk. For an easy way to get a large dose of all the nutrients, try one of my Smooth-SEE recipes (pages 276 and 277).

BEST FOODS FOR BETA CAROTENE: *Sweet potatoes, carrots, kale, winter squash (especially butternut), turnip greens, pumpkin, mustard greens, cantaloupe, red bell pepper, apricots, Chinese cabbage, spinach, lettuce (romaine, green leaf, red leaf, butterhead), collard greens, Swiss chard, watercress, grapefruit, watermelon, cherries, mangos, red ripe tomatoes, guava, asparagus, red cabbage*

BEST FOODS FOR VITAMIN C: *Guava, bell peppers (red, yellow, green), orange juice, hot chile peppers, grapefruit juice, strawberries, pineapple, kohlrabi, papaya, lemons, broccoli,*

FAQS

My doctor suggested that I cut down on sugary foods to try to prevent cataracts. I've never heard that before—is it good advice?

Cutting back on sugary foods is always a good idea. Whether it will help prevent cataracts is a hot research topic right now. Some scientists from Tufts University analyzed data from AREDS and discovered that eating lots of low-quality carbohydrates increased the risk of cataracts by up to 50 percent. Low-quality carbohydrates are defined as sugary foods, white rice, and anything made with refined white flour, including crackers, breads, rolls, muffins, pasta, and other baked goods. The theory is that these foods quickly raise blood sugars to very high levels and that there's a cumulative effect. In other words, the more low quality carbs you eat, the more you expose the lens of your eye to potentially dangerous levels of sugar. So if you want another fabulous reason to eat healthier foods—including more fruits, vegetables, and high-quality carbohydrates, such as whole grain food and brown rice—there it is.

kale, Brussels sprouts, kidney beans, kiwi, cantaloupe, cauliflower, red cabbage, mangos, grapefruit (pink, red), white potatoes (with skin), mustard greens, cherry tomatoes, sugar snap peas, snow peas, clementines, rutabagas, turnip greens, tomatoes, raspberries, Chinese cabbage, blackberries, green tomatoes, cabbage, watermelon, tangerines, lemon juice, okra, lychees, summer squash (all varieties), persimmons

BEST FOODS FOR VITAMIN E: *Wheat germ oil, fortified whole grain cereals, sunflower seeds, almonds, hazelnuts, peanut butter, wheat germ, avocado, pine nuts, tomato paste, flaxseed oil, red bell pepper, canola oil, kiwis, peanuts, olive oil, mangos, turnip greens, Brazil nuts, asparagus, peaches, papaya, radicchio, collard greens, broccoli, Swiss chard, spinach*

ZINC

AREDS and the Rotterdam study confirmed zinc's role in eye health. Zinc is found in the retina, and helps the functioning of enzymes responsible for eye health. In people with macular degeneration, levels of zinc in the retina can be very low, so eating zinc-rich foods is a logical first step for preventing and treating macular degeneration.

BEST FOODS FOR ZINC: *Oysters, lean beef, crab, ostrich, pork tenderloin, peanut butter, wheat germ, turkey, veal, pumpkin seeds, chicken, chickpeas (garbanzo beans), fat-free yogurt, fortified whole grain cereals, pine nuts, cashews, sunflower seeds, lima beans, lentils, pecans, cheese (fat-free, reduced-fat), fat-free milk, almonds, walnuts, peanuts, black-eyed peas, green peas*

LUTEIN AND ZEAXANTHIN

Lutein and zeaxanthin are a matched pair of antioxidants—almost without exception, foods that contain one also contain the other. And they are found in high concentrations in the tissue of the macula. Because they absorb 40 to 90 percent of blue light intensity, these nutrients act like sunscreen for your eyes. Studies have shown that eating foods rich in lutein and zeaxanthin can *increase* the pigment density in the macula—and greater pigment density means better retina protection, and a lower risk of macular degeneration. At least one study has confirmed that eating foods with high amounts of these antioxidants seems to reduce the risk of developing macular degeneration.

BEST FOODS FOR LUTEIN AND ZEAXANTHIN: *Kale, spinach, turnip greens, mustard greens, Swiss chard, radicchio, collard greens, summer squash (all varieties), watercress,* *green peas, persimmons, Brussels sprouts, broccoli, pumpkin, corn, lettuce (butterhead, Boston, Bibb, romaine), asparagus, green beans, okra, artichokes, green bell peppers, scallions, carrots*

OMEGA-3 FATTY ACIDS

Retinal pigment cells contain a type of omega-3 called docosahexaenoic acid (DHA), which helps protect light receptor cells in the eye from damage by sunlight and free radicals. In 2006, scientists speculated that fish oil and other sources of omega-3 fatty acids could be natural protection against age-related macular degeneration. If you want to take advantage of this research, I recommend eating two to three servings of fatty fish each week, and strive to incorporate the other omega-rich foods into your daily diet, too.

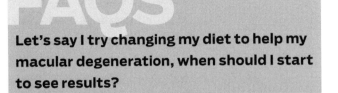

Let's say I try changing my diet to help my macular degeneration, when should I start to see results?

It varies from person to person. Some people might see a dramatic change after just one month, while others may only notice subtle changes, and still others may have to wait for their next ophthalmologist appointment when they are surprised to discover that they do better on the eye exam. But don't lose faith—all those eye-healthy vitamins and minerals are also helping to keep the rest of you healthy, too!

BEST FOODS FOR OMEGA-3 FATTY ACIDS: *Wild salmon (fresh, canned), herring, mackerel (not king), sardines, anchovies, rainbow trout, Pacific oysters, omega-3–fortified eggs, flaxseed (ground and oil), walnuts, butternuts (white walnuts), seaweed, walnut oil, canola oil, soybeans*

BONUS POINTS

- **Get regular eye exams.** It is important to get a regular comprehensive checkup by an optometrist or ophthalmologist—at least once a year if you're over age 60. Be sure that the exam includes eye dilation so that any change in your lens or retina can be spotted easily and early.

- **Protect your eyes from the sun.** One of the top causes of cataracts is radiation from the sun. Take steps to protect your eyes by wearing sunglasses and a hat with a brim whenever you are out in bright daylight.

- **Stop smoking.** Smoking increases your risk of both cataracts and macular degeneration, in part because it creates free radicals, and in part because smoking decreases the amount of oxygen to the eye.

- **If you smoke, don't drink alcohol or take beta carotene supplements.** I strongly encourage you to stop s moking, but if you haven't yet quit entirely, you have a couple other guidelines. Although alcohol alone doesn't increase the risk for cataracts, smokers who drink alcohol have a greater risk than smokers who don't drink. And beta carotene supplements may increase the risk of lung cancer in smokers, so that's a dangerous combination.

- **Maintain a healthy weight.** People with early-stage macular degeneration who are also overweight have double the risk of moving on to the advanced stage, so losing weight may help keep the disease from progressing. Plus, people who are overweight have a greater risk of developing type 2 diabetes, which increases the risk of cataracts. (See Weight Loss on page 19 for more information.)

- **Avoid eating foods high in saturated and trans fats.** Butter, stick margarine, cream, whole milk, ice cream, lard, cheese, beef fat, products made with hydrogenated oil, and other damaging fats can cause a buildup of plaque in blood vessels which can choke off blood flow—including blood flow to the eye. Any decrease in oxygen can harm the eye and promote tissue damage.

SUPPLEMENTS

FOR CATARACTS

If you are concerned about cataracts and want to consider supplements *in addition to* the food fixes, my only recommendation is for:

- **Multivitamin.** It is important to get the necessary amounts of the cataract-fighting B vitamins, along with a basic amount of vitamin C and E. Look for a standard multivitamin that contains 100 percent of vitamins C and E. Too much vitamin C from supplemental doses might actually increase the risk of cataracts . . . and too much vitamin E from supplemental doses might increase the risk of macular degeneration. Supplements with "mega" doses of any vitamin or mineral are not recommended.

FOR MACULAR DEGENERATION ONLY

For people who have been diagnosed with macular degeneration, the following supplements may help slow progression of the disease. Among the best studied are daily dosages of the following supplements:

I RECOMMEND THAT EVERYONE TAKE

- Multivitamin that provides *only* 100% DV for Vitamin E.

AND SPEAK WITH YOUR DOCTOR ABOUT THESE ADDITIONAL SUPPLEMENTS

- 500 milligrams vitamin C.
- 15 milligrams beta carotene. Smokers shouldn't take beta carotene because it may increase the risk of cancer (in smokers only).
- 80 milligrams zinc, with 2 milligrams copper to balance out the effect of such high levels of zinc, which can depress the immune system and block copper's availability in the body.

JOY'S 4-STEP PROGRAM
FOR CATARACTS AND MACULAR DEGENERATION

Follow this program if you have macular degeneration or cataracts, or a family history of these diseases.

STEP 1 ... START WITH THE BASICS

These are the first things you should do to address eye problems:

- See an optometrist or ophthalmologist for a comprehensive eye exam. If you are over age 60, have an exam every two years. If you notice any vision changes, see a doctor immediately—don't wait for your next appointment.

- If you have macular degeneration, talk with your physician about whether you are a good candidate to take the AREDS supplements, and whether you need to avoid zinc or beta carotene.

- If you smoke, quit.

- Protect your eyes from the sun by wearing a brimmed hat and sunglasses whenever possible.

STEP 2 ...YOUR ULTIMATE GROCERY LIST

A nutrition plan is only as good as the foods that you choose. This list contains foods with high levels of nutrients that contribute to eye health, plus some foods used as ingredients in the meal plans and recipes. You don't have to purchase every item . . . but these foods should make up the bulk of what you eat for the week. If you find yourself getting bored, try adding a food from the list that's new to you. My practice is full of people who are passionate fans of foods they've only recently started eating.

FRUIT

Apples (especially Red Delicious, Granny Smith, Gala)	Cantaloupe	Lemons	Pineapple
	Cherries	Limes	Plums (especially black)
	Clementines	Lychees	Prunes
Apricots	Cranberries, fresh and dried (and juice)	Mangos	Tangerines
Berries (blackberries, blueberries, raspberries, strawberries)	Grapefruit (and juice)	Oranges (and juice)	Watermelon
	Guava	Papaya	
	Kiwi	Peaches	
		Persimmons	

VEGETABLES

Artichoke hearts	Collard greens	Peas (green, sugar snap)	Squash, summer (all varieties)
Asparagus	Corn	Peas, black-eyed	Squash, winter (especially butternut)
Avocado	Green beans	Peppers (hot; yellow/ red/green bell)	Swiss chard
Beans (red, kidney, pinto, black, garbanzo, lima)	Kale	Potatoes, sweet	Tomatoes (including green tomatoes, red ripe tomatoes, cherry tomatoes, and tomato paste)
	Kohlrabi	Potatoes, white (including russet)	
	Lentils	Pumpkin	
Broccoli	Lettuce (romaine, green leaf, red leaf, butterhead, Boston, Bibb)	Radicchio	
Brussels sprouts		Rutabagas	Turnip greens
Cabbage (including Chinese, red)		Scallions	Watercress
Carrots	Mushrooms (including portobello, white)	Seaweed	
Cauliflower		Snow peas	
Celery	Mustard greens	Soybeans (edamame)	
Chickpeas (garbanzo beans)	Okra	Spinach	
	Onions		

SEAFOOD

Anchovies	Mackerel (not king)	Salmon, wild (fresh, canned)	Trout, rainbow
Crab	Oysters (including Pacific)		Tuna (canned light)
Herring		Sardines	

LEAN MEATS/EGGS

Beef, lean	Ham,	Pork (lean cuts,	Veal
Chicken	lean	including	Venison
Eggs (especially omega-3–fortified)	Liver	tenderloin)	
	Ostrich	Turkey	

NUTS AND SEEDS (PREFERABLY UNSALTED)

Almonds	Cashews	Peanuts	Sunflower seeds
Brazil nuts	Flaxseed, ground	Pecans	Walnuts
Butternuts (white walnuts)	Hazelnuts	Pine nuts	
	Peanut butter	Pumpkin seeds	

WHOLE GRAINS

Breads, whole wheat (including pita and crackers)	Cereal, fortified whole grain	Couscous, whole wheat	Wheat germ
		Pasta, whole wheat	

DAIRY

Cheese (fat-free, reduced-fat)	Cottage cheese (nonfat, 1% reduced-fat)	Milk (fat-free, 1% reduced-fat)	Yogurt (fat-free, low-fat)

MISCELLANEOUS

Chili, canned vegetarian, low-fat	Margarine spread, soft tub trans fat–free	Oil, walnut	Soup, canned split pea, low-fat
Coffee	Mayonnaise, reduced-fat	Parsley, fresh	Sugar
Dressing, salad, reduced-fat	Nonstick cooking spray	Pepper, black	Tea (green, black)
Guacamole	Oil, canola	Salt	Vinegar, balsamic or red wine
Horseradish (prepared)	Oil, flaxseed	Soup, canned butternut squash, low-fat	Worcestershire sauce
Hummus	Oil, olive	Soup, canned pumpkin, low-fat	

STEP3 ...GOING ABOVE AND BEYOND

If you want to do everything you can for eye health, here are some additional things you might try:

- If you like, feel free to take a multivitamin with 100% DV for B vitamins and folic acid. Look for a supplement that contains no more than 100% DV of any nutrient, especially vitamins C and E.

- If you specifically have macular degeneration (not cataracts), consider supplements of vitamin C, beta carotene, and zinc with copper, in the dosages recommended on page 264. At the very least, make sure your multivitamin provides 100% DV for beta carotene, zinc, and copper. If you smoke, cross beta carotene off your list. These are treatment-level dosages—if you do not have macular degeneration, do not take these supplements.

- Avoid eating foods high in saturated and trans fats, including butter, stick margarine, ice cream, whole milk, cheese, and products made with hydrogenated oils.

SUNGLASSES

Your choice of sunglasses makes a fashion statement, but please don't let that statement include the words *eye damage*. Not all designer models protect the eyes. Don't be fooled into thinking that large or dark lenses necessarily protect against radiation. The American Academy of Ophthalmology recommends choosing sunglasses that are certified to block 99 to 100 percent of UVA and UVB radiation. Glasses should fit well so they don't slide down your nose. If possible, look for models that wrap all the way around to your temples. Wear your sunglasses every time you go outside, even on cloudy days— radiation is still there even if the sun is hidden. If you wear contact lenses with UV protection, it is still important to wear sunglasses because contacts cover only a tiny portion of your eyes.

STEP4...MEAL PLANS

These sample menus include foods high in nutrients that have been shown to be protective against cataracts and macular degeneration, specifically antioxidants, beta carotene, vitamins C and E, zinc, B vitamins, and lutein.

Every day, choose *one* option for each of the three meals—breakfast, lunch, and dinner. Then, one or two times per day, choose from a variety of my suggested snacks. Approximate calories have been provided to help adjust for your personal weight management goals. If you find yourself hungry (and if weight is not an issue), feel free to increase the portion sizes for meals and snacks. Beverage calories are *not* included.

BREAKFAST OPTIONS

(Approximately 300 to 400 calories)

Cottage Cheese and Cantaloupe

½ cantaloupe filled with 1 cup fat-free or 1% reduced-fat or cottage cheese and topped with 1 tablespoon sunflower seeds and 1 tablespoon slivered almonds (or chopped walnuts).

Cereal with Milk and Fruit

1 cup whole grain fortified cereal (any brand 120 calories or less per serving) with 1 cup fat-free or enriched/fortified soy milk, topped with 1 tablespoon wheat germ. Enjoy with ½ pink grapefruit (or 1 orange).

Peanut Butter Pita

Whole wheat pita bread split and toasted, each half topped with 1 level tablespoon peanut butter.

Scrambled Eggs with Peppers, Mushrooms, and Onion

Sauté ½ cup each sliced onion, mushrooms, and red or yellow peppers in a skillet coated with nonstick cooking spray (or 1 to 2 teaspoons canola oil) until soft. Beat 1 whole egg with 2 egg whites. Add to vegetables and cook, stirring, until eggs are cooked. Serve with 1 slice whole wheat bread, toasted, with optional 1 teaspoon soft tub, trans-fat–free margarine.

Yogurt with Chopped Mango and Berries

1 cup fat-free or low-fat vanilla yogurt mixed with ½ chopped mango, ½ cup berries, and 1 to 2 tablespoons wheat germ (or chopped walnuts, almonds, pecans, or sunflower seeds).

LUNCH OPTIONS

(Approximately 400 to 500 calories)

Turkey Sandwich with Baby Carrots

4 ounces sliced turkey breast (or lean ham) and unlimited romaine lettuce and sliced tomato on 2 slices whole grain bread; add optional 2 thin slices avocado and/or 2 teaspoons reduced-fat mayonnaise. Enjoy with a large handful baby carrots.

Pumpkin Soup with Mixed Vegetables and Salad

3 cups pumpkin, butternut squash, or split-pea soup (canned, no cream or whole milk used in preparation). Enjoy with large mixed vegetable salad of unlimited leafy greens, tomato, pepper, onion, carrots, cucumber, mushrooms, etc., tossed with 1 teaspoon olive oil and unlimited vinegar or fresh lemon juice (or 2 tablespoons reduced-calorie salad dressing).

Grilled Chicken Salad

5 ounces skinless chicken breast on large bed of mixed greens (romaine lettuce, spinach, mustard greens, collard greens) and topped with ½ cup cherry tomatoes, 1 chopped bell pepper (red, yellow, green), artichoke hearts, and ½ cup chickpeas (garbanzo beans). Toss with 2 teaspoons olive oil and unlimited vinegar or fresh lemon juice.

Veggie Tuna Salad with Fresh Fruit

1 serving Veggie Tuna Salad (page 274). Enjoy with 150 calories of whole wheat pita bread or whole grain crackers and 1 orange or kiwi, or ½ mango.

Spinach Omelet and Sweet Potato

Beat 1 whole egg with 2 to 3 egg whites. Cook in heated skillet coated with nonstick cooking spray. When bottom is cooked, gently flip over. Top with unlimited spinach (raw or pre-sautéed) and optional 1 ounce reduced-fat cheese. Fold omelet over and cook until egg mixture is firm and cheese melts. Enjoy with a plain baked sweet potato (or 2 cups hearty vegetable soup).

DINNER OPTIONS

(Approximately 500 to 600 calories)

Pork Tenderloin with Cranberry Couscous

5 ounces baked, grilled, or broiled pork tenderloin (or veal, turkey, chicken breast, wild salmon, cod, tilapia, shrimp, or tofu). Enjoy with 1 cup cooked whole wheat couscous mixed with 2 tablespoons dried cranberries and 1 cup steamed Brussels sprouts.

Pasta with Chicken and Broccoli

1 serving (2 cups) Whole Wheat Penne with Chicken and Broccoli (page 368). Enjoy with a salad of leafy greens, tomatoes, peppers, carrots, and 1 tablespoon chopped walnuts tossed with 2 teaspoons olive oil and unlimited balsamic vinegar or fresh lemon juice.

Ostrich with Veggies and Sweet Potato

1 serving Caribbean Ostrich Steaks (page 273) or 5 ounces ostrich burger (or turkey burger). Enjoy with 1 cup steamed broccoli or asparagus and 1 plain baked sweet potato.

Vegetarian Chili and Salad

2 cups vegetarian chili. Enjoy with large salad of dark leafy greens, peppers, tomato, artichokes, and carrots tossed with 2 teaspoons olive oil and unlimited vinegar or fresh lemon juice.

Beef Tenderloin with Sautéed Spinach and Butternut Squash

5 ounces grilled beef tenderloin (or any other lean beef). Enjoy with 1 cup sautéed spinach in 1 teaspoon olive oil and garlic, and ½ cup baked butternut squash.

SNACK OPTIONS

100 calories or less

- *Best vegetables:* 1 cup raw or cooked spinach, kale, red/yellow/green peppers, broccoli, cauliflower, asparagus, carrots, green beans, sugar snap peas, Brussels sprouts, mustard greens, cabbage, or artichokes
- *Best fruits:* 1 guava, apple, peach, orange, or persimmon; 2 plums, kiwis, clementines, or tangerines; 4 prunes or apricots; 1 cup blueberries, blackberries, raspberries, sliced strawberries, cherries, watermelon, or pineapple; 20 strawberries; ½ mango, papaya, or grapefruit
- 1 level tablespoon peanut butter with celery sticks
- 10 almonds, unsalted
- 3 Brazil nuts
- 1 ounce reduced-fat cheese

100 to 200 calories

- ¼ cup toasted pecans
- 20 raw almonds (about 3 tablespoons)

- ½ cup fat-free or 1% reduced-fat cottage cheese mixed with 1 tablespoon chopped pecans (or almonds, wheat germ, or sunflower seeds)

- ¼ cup sunflower seeds in the shell

- 1 slice whole grain toast with 1 level tablespoon peanut butter

- Red/yellow/green pepper sticks with 2 tablespoons hummus or guacamole

- 1 cup fortified whole grain cereal

- 1 ounce peanuts (about 25 nuts)

- 1 cup plain fat-free yogurt mixed with ½ cup berries and 1 tablespoon wheat germ (or chopped walnuts)

- ½ cup chickpeas (garbanzo beans)

- 1 sliced apple with 1 level tablespoon peanut butter (or 1 ounce reduced-fat cheese)

200 calories or more

- Vision Mix (page 275)

CARIBBEAN OSTRICH STEAKS

Ostrich is a healthy and delicious lean substitute for any red or white meat—including beef, chicken, turkey, pork, and lamb—in any of your favorite recipes. It is loaded with zinc—one of the key ingredients for maintaining healthy eyes—plus, it absorbs seasonings, so it is highly versatile. Look for ostrich steak in Whole Foods stores, specialty stores, or order online (www.ostrich.com). If you have difficulty finding ostrich, you can also enjoy this recipe with boneless turkey breast cutlets.

Makes 6 servings

$\frac{1}{2}$	cup olive oil
$\frac{1}{2}$	cup orange juice
$\frac{1}{2}$	cup lime juice
2	scallions, chopped
1	tablespoon chopped fresh parsley
$\frac{1}{2}$	jalapeño chile pepper, seeded and minced (wear plastic gloves when handling)
	Coarse ground black pepper
2	pounds ostrich steak, cut into 6 slices
1	lime, sliced

1. Combine the oil, orange juice, lime juice, scallions, parsley, jalapeño, and black pepper to taste in a large zip-top bag. Add the ostrich and seal the bag, pressing out excess air. Marinate in the refrigerator for 2 to 3 hours.
2. Preheat a grill. Drain the steaks (discard the marinade). Grill the steaks over high heat for 2 to 3 minutes on each side, until browned. (You can also cook the steaks in a heavy skillet over high heat.) If you like, cut the steaks at an angle into thin slices. Garnish with lime slices.

PER SERVING
250 calories, 35 g protein, 2 g carbohydrate, 12 g fat (3 g saturated), 143 mg cholesterol, 110 mg sodium, 0 g fiber; plus 3 mg zinc (20% DV)

VEGGIE TUNA SALAD

Use *light* instead of albacore *white* canned tuna to get all the nutrition without too much mercury. Chopped peppers and carrots add beta carotene and vitamin C. Serve it on a bed of fresh spinach leaves for an added blast of lutein.

Makes 1 serving

1	can (6 ounces) chunk light tuna in water, drained
½	carrot, peeled and diced
½	celery stalk, diced
¼	red pepper, diced
¼	yellow pepper, diced
½	scallion, minced
1	tablespoon reduced-fat mayonnaise
½	teaspoon lemon juice
3	cups spinach leaves
4	medium-thick slices red tomato

1. In a medium bowl, flake the tuna into small pieces with fork. Add the carrot, celery, red and yellow pepper, scallion, mayonnaise, and lemon juice, and mix well with a fork.
2. Line a plate with the spinach and place the tuna mixture on top. Arrange the tomato slices around the tuna.

PER SERVING
227 calories, 40 g protein, 9 g carbohydrate, 4 g fat (1 g saturated), 43 mg cholesterol, 755 mg sodium, 9 g fiber; plus 100 mg vitamin C (150+% DV), 20 mg niacin (100% DV), 114 mcg selenium (150+% DV)

VISION MIX

This packable snack provides more than 90 percent of your daily requirement for vitamin E. For more antioxidants, try adding ½ cup dried cranberries, blueberries, or cherries. But be sure to watch portions—calories can add up quickly with this snack.

Makes 6 servings

4	cups whole grain cereal
½	cup raw almonds
½	cup unsalted oil-roasted peanuts
¼	cup unsalted sunflower seeds

In a large bowl, combine the cereal, almonds, peanuts, and sunflower seeds, and mix thoroughly. Divide evenly among 6 zip-top bags.

PER SERVING
237 calories, 8 g protein, 21 g carbohydrate, 14.5 g fat (1.5 g saturated), 0 mg cholesterol, 198 mg sodium, 4.5 g fiber

GREEN SMOOTH-SEE

My smoothies each provide a great big BLAST of eye-fighting nutrients—vitamins C and E, zinc, lutein, and beta carotene. They're the perfect concoctions for people who want to go that extra mile, as well as people who aren't interested in popping extra supplemental pills.

Calories always count, so remember to factor these smoothies into your plan's total calories. If weight is an issue, split into two servings and enjoy as a snack . . . or, count one full serving as your breakfast—either way the math is a snap. If weight is not an issue, enjoy a daily serving whenever you wish.

Makes 1 serving (about 1¼ cups)

1	medium carrot, peeled and grated
2	medium kiwis, skin removed
1	cup spinach leaves
½	cup watercress
½	cup plain, fat-free yogurt
¼	cup avocado, mashed (3 tablespoons)
2	tablespoons wheat germ
2	tablespoons water
1	tablespoon fresh lemon juice
1	teaspoon Worcestershire sauce
¼	teaspoon prepared horseradish
	Pinch of salt

In a blender or food processor, combine the carrot, kiwis, spinach, watercress, yogurt, avocado, wheat germ, water, lemon juice, Worcestershire, horseradish, and salt. Blend until smooth.

PER SERVING
323 calories, 16 g protein, 50 g carbohydrate, 9 g fat (1 g saturated), 0 mg cholesterol, 254 mg sodium, 14 g fiber; plus 172 mg vitamin C (287% DV), 8 IU vitamin E (26% DV), 4,118 mcg beta carotene, 1,520 mcg lutein + zeaxanthin, 4 mg zinc (29% DV)

CITRUS SMOOTH-SEE

As with the recipe at left, you'll need to factor the caloric value of this smoothie into your plan's total calories. That said, the math is a breeze. If weight is an issue, split into two servings and enjoy as a snack . . . . or, count one entire serving as your breakfast. If weight is not an issue, enjoy a daily serving whenever you wish.

Makes 1 serving (about 1¾ cups)

1	orange, zested, then peeled and cut into sections
½	medium pink grapefruit, peeled and cut into sections
1	carrot, peeled and grated
½	cup plain, fat-free yogurt
¼	cup raspberries
¼	cup cubed papaya
2	tablespoons wheat germ
1	tablespoon fresh lemon juice
1	tablespoon granulated sugar

In a blender or food processor, combine the orange zest and sections, grapefruit, carrot, yogurt, raspberries, papaya, wheat germ, lemon juice, and sugar. Blend until smooth.

PER SERVING
340 calories, 15 g protein, 71 g carbohydrate, 2 g fat (0 g saturated), 0 mg cholesterol, 138 mg sodium, 12 g fiber; plus 150 mg vitamin C (251% DV), 6 IU vitamin E (18% DV), 4,568 mcg beta carotene, 482 mcg lutein + zeaxanthin, 4 mg zinc (27% DV)

CHAPTER 12

MEMORY

No one has ever come to me specifically looking for nutritional help for a memory problem, but the topic comes up more often than you might think. For example, a client who has trouble recalling what she ate for breakfast the day she comes to see me might mention that she's been noticing more and more memory lapses. Or sometimes, while making conversation in the course of session, a client will tell me about a "funny thing" that happened. Like the guy who couldn't remember to put gas in his car and had to call AAA roadside assistance three times in a single month. Or the woman who was forever losing her cell phone, only relocating it when the ringing led her to the pantry . . . or the refrigerator . . . or the laundry hamper . . . or a basket of bathroom cleaning supplies.

Of course, memory changes aren't always so obvious. They can be subtle, hardly worth mentioning . . . except when they interrupt the rhythm and flow of our daily lives. We waste valuable time looking for keys, the cat, or a matching pair of socks—or even questioning our skills and ability to function at work. Memory problems can infuriate and frustrate us when that elusive thought is on the tip of the tongue—or the tip of the brain, in this case—but we just can't access it. And if we've seen a friend or family member descend into dementia, our own memory problems might trigger fear for our own future.

My absentminded clients are thrilled when they learn that there are nutritional and lifestyle strategies that may keep them from sliding down the slippery slope of memory loss. Every single suggestion listed here will also help improve overall health, so it's win/win, with no downside. Better memory, and better health.

WHAT AFFECTS MEMORY?

Memory is a tricky thing. So many factors can affect how it functions, and on top of that, how well your memory works on any given day is purely subjective. *You* know when "brain freeze" happens, but with very few exceptions, there are no physical signs that doctors can look for to pinpoint the cause. Even the memory disorder people fear most—Alzheimer's disease—can't be definitely diagnosed except at autopsy after death (for more on Alzheimer's disease, see page 283). For the most part, physicians make educated guesses about the cause of memory loss based on your medical history, physical examination results, and lifestyle.

Memory is carried in a network of brain cells called *neurons*. These cells are generally shaped like the roots, trunk, and branches of an oak tree—a long central *axon* (like the trunk of a tree) with smaller branches called *dendrites* on both ends. Each of these branches connects with other neurons, which in turn connect with more neurons, and so on and so on. Memory depends on your total number of brain cells and their connections, the smooth flow of communication between neurons, and the health of all those cells. That means that it is relatively easy for something somewhere in the brain to go on the fritz. Among the biggest factors that can affect memory are:

VASCULAR HEALTH

Every cell in your body needs a steady supply of oxygen and nutrients in order to stay alive and work properly but brain cells are especially needy, like hungry infants that need to eat regularly and often. Because oxygen and nutrients are carried in the blood stream, anything that impedes blood flow will starve those all-important memory cells. The plain truth is that a healthy heart makes for a healthy brain.

When clients ask me about memory, the first thing I do is review their medical history. Specifically, I look for the following signs that they might have a blood flow problem:

High blood pressure (hypertension). Physicians recommend that you maintain blood pressure at or below 120/80 mmHg. If your numbers are significantly higher than that, your health is generally at risk and your memory can suffer. High blood pressure damages the delicate lining of blood vessels and triggers the formation of plaque. Over time, plaque builds up on the inside of the vessels like leaves in a rain gutter, choking the blood supply everywhere in the body—especially the brain.

An ingenious study by researchers at the University of Pittsburgh showed how hypertension affects memory. The scientists compared people who had normal blood pressure with people who had high blood pressure on two different measures of memory. Verbal memory was tested by having the participants remember words, and spatial memory was tested by having the participants remember the position of items on a computer screen. While they were performing the tasks, the participants had their brains scanned to see where the blood was flowing. The results were surprising: the participants with hypertension had less blood flowing to the parts of the brain that controlled these types of memory *even though they performed equally as well on the tests* as the participants with normal blood pressure. The researchers predicted that, over time, too many neurons would be damaged and memory would be severely compromised. The lesson is that high blood pressure starts doing its damage even before you realize it, so it is hugely important to take action early.

High LDL, low HDL cholesterol. Cholesterol comes in two main varieties—the "bad" variety known as low-density lipoprotein (LDL) cholesterol, and the "good" kind known as high-density lipoprotein (HDL) cholesterol. LDL cholesterol is one of the components of blood vessel plaque—the higher your LDL cholesterol, the greater the chance your blood vessels are becoming narrowed. The optimal level of LDL cholesterol is below 100 mg/dL.

HDL cholesterol, on the other hand, acts almost like a plaque magnet, picking up the vessel-clogging cholesterol and carrying it away to the liver. So the higher your HDL levels, the better and healthier your blood vessels—and by extension, your memory—will be. HDL levels below 40 mg/dL are considered too low to be healthy.

High homocysteine levels. This role of this natural amino acid in heart health is still unclear. Some experts believe that homocysteine damages the blood vessel lining and encourages blood clots. We know that high blood levels of homocysteine (anything over 10 micromol/L) could be a sign of an increased risk of heart attack and stroke. For these reasons, lowering homocysteine levels is considered critical for health. Although no one knows yet whether lowering homocysteine levels will improve blood flow to the brain, the "fix" is so simple that it would be crazy not to take advantage of it. The best treatment for lowering homocysteine is not a new drug, but folic acid, vitamin B$_6$, and vitamin B$_{12}$ from food or supplements.

(For more on heart health, see Cardiovascular Disease, page 127.)

AGING

Almost everyone over age 40 has experienced memory problems. Part of the reason has to do with changes in our general health. As we get older, more things can and do go wrong with our bodies. Heart and blood flow problems, type 2 diabetes or prediabetes (glucose intolerance), and some autoimmune disorders can cause memory to decline. But there are other possible reasons for age-related memory loss. Beginning in our twenties, we typically

FAQS

Ever since I went through menopause, I can't seem to remember anything. Will changing my diet help?

Despite everything you might be experiencing, studies overwhelmingly show that there is no correlation between menopause and memory problems.

FAQS

I'm dieting to lose weight . . . and now my memory is shot. Did I diet away my brain cells?

No, no, a thousand times no. Your brain cells are all still there. However, it's not surprising that you're noticing changes. Dieting does two things. First, it is a preoccupying change. When you diet, you have to change the way you shop for food, prepare food, and think about food. British psychologists from the University of Bristol found that diet-related thoughts took over dieters' brains, effectively pushing out all other thoughts. Second, some people can go overboard when they diet. They think that they should eat as little as humanly possible, sometimes skipping meals. This can leave them feeling fuzzy-headed and forgetful. It's simply lack of enough energy getting to brain cells. My advice is to eat controlled portions of healthy foods every four to five hours to keep your blood sugar levels as close to steady as possible.

begin to lose brain cells, which means that we lose the very structures that hold our memories. In addition, older brains make less of certain brain chemicals necessary for memory encoding, so no matter how hard we try to commit something to memory, it may not stick. It would be like putting your keys in a briefcase that had a big hole in the bottom—you may think your keys are safe, but your storage system is leaky.

Some memory experts believe that older brains store information in a qualitatively different way than younger brains. Older brains have been around a lot longer and have built up a complex network of information and memories. Every new piece of information has to get wired into the existing network, and sometimes random bits of trivia get lost. This isn't necessarily a bad thing—it may mean that we get better at distinguishing between relevant and irrelevant information—but it does tend to make it more difficult for older people to recall specific pieces of information, such as names or appointments. (See there, it's not just you!)

Other big factors in age-related memory loss are exercise and nutrition. Good nutrition and an active lifestyle can protect your brain from aging the same way they can protect your body from looking dumpy before its time. Even though it sounds basic, a healthy diet goes a long way to putting the brakes on memory loss in middle and old age. Researchers at the University of California, Los Angeles, investigated whether adopting a healthy lifestyle can keep brains more youthful. Participants ate a more memory-healthy diet, exercised for cardiovascular training, learned relaxation strategies, and challenged their brains with memory games. After just two weeks, brain scans showed that their minds were working with greater efficiency, allowing them to remember with less effort. It's not a far stretch to imagine that these same lifestyle changes could, over the long term, make our 60- or 70-year-old brains more like our 20- or 30-year-old brains.

STRESS

These days, stress seems like an unpleasant but inescapable part of life. Until stress causes insomnia, overeating, or illness, most of us don't give it much thought, much less to its possible effects on memory. When you're stressed, your brain releases a steroid hormone called *cortisol,* which can damage your brain. It doesn't take long—just a week or so of ongoing stress can be toxic.

Chronic stress can also make you feel depressed or anxious, and these feelings can interfere with the way your brain processes memories. Every emotion, positive or negative, causes a shift in brain chemicals. For example, happiness is usually associated with increased levels of serotonin, and depression is associated with decreased levels of serotonin. Any time you change the chemical soup in your brain, you risk changing the way memories are encoded and retrieved. But the damage may be even more serious, leading to permanent memory disorders. For example, people who are clinically depressed throughout their lives have a greater risk of developing Alzheimer's disease. (For more information on mood and stress, see Mood on page 303.)

But these related factors can also affect memory for a much simpler reason—distraction. Stress, anxiety, and depression can take over your life, push all other thoughts out of your mind, and make everything seem less important. And whatever you don't consider important, you won't remember.

COULD IT BE ALZHEIMER'S DISEASE?

The horror of Alzheimer's disease (AD) is that it slowly strips away everything that makes us who we are. A lifetime of memories can disappear, leaving a mother unable to recognize her own children, a brother convinced he's never met his own twin. Day-to-day moments, those little kindnesses and conversations that make relationships possible, are gossamer fragile. Walk out of a room, and the room no longer exists.

When memory problems start becoming obvious, the first thing many of my clients wonder is if they have the beginnings of AD. It is impossible to know for certain.

Most cases of AD begin in people over age 60, and the risk increases as we get older. Estimates suggest that about 5 percent of people under age 75 have AD, but up to 50 percent of those older than age 85 may have it. These numbers can only be considered educated guesses because age-related dementia can look very similar to the symptoms of AD. The only way to get a definitive, 100 percent accurate diagnosis of AD is to examine the brain after death for the abnormal tell-tale signs of the disease: waxy-looking chunks called *amyloid plaques* and knotted clumps of fibers called *neurofibrillary tangles*.

Doctors may make a tentative diagnosis of AD after ruling out other problems, including blood vessel disease, depression, drug interactions, and brain tumors. Although it begins with mild memory difficulties, it usually progresses to more profound problems. People in the middle stages of AD can forget how to perform simple, routine tasks, such as opening a window or tying their shoes. So the time to worry isn't necessarily when you keep losing your cell phone, but when you forget what the cell phone is used for.

People suspected of having AD can take medications to slow the progression of the disease, but I think some of the most exciting research focuses on risk reduction. All of the dietary and lifestyle changes recommended in this chapter to help improve general memory function also seem to help prevent or delay the worst symptoms of AD. For example, scientists have discovered links between AD and heart disease. People with high levels of homocysteine have an increased risk of heart disease, and double the usual risk of AD. High blood pressure, high cholesterol, and uncontrolled type 2 diabetes all damage blood vessels, and all increase the risks of cardiovascular disease and AD. Cholesterol medications called *statins* also slow the progression of AD. And from a nutrition perspective, regular exercise, antioxidants in fruits and vegetables, omega-3 fatty acids in fish, and folic acid have all have been shown to decrease the risks of heart disease, memory loss, and AD.

If you are worried about AD, see your doctor. But you can also help yourself by following the nutritional advice in this chapter and in the chapter covering heart disease, page 127.

FAQS

My mom, my sister, my friends . . . they all say that their memories were great until menopause, and then POOF— big memory problems.

Well, as I mentioned earlier, memory generally declines with age, and menopause usually takes place when a woman is middle aged, so you shouldn't expect to have the same memory you did as when you were a teenager. But middle aged is still not "old." In fact, expecting memory problems to develop with age could actually be at the root of them. In 2006, researchers tested the recall abilities of middle-aged men and women. The study participants who took the memory test thinking that they were being compared with "old" people remembered fewer words than those who thought they were being compared with "young" adults or who didn't think there was any comparison group at all. The participants who were more anxious about age-related memory loss had the worst performances of all—but only when they thought they were being compared with seniors. The scientists believe that this deficit was possibly due to a kind of stereotyping: If we identify as "old," then we will behave as we think "old people" should, bad memory and all. This study lends scientific credence to the old adage that you're only as old as you think you are! There are other factors that also come into play. Women often notice a change in their memory function because menopause is a time of great change—physically, emotionally, socially, and familially, and they're carefully watching their every twitch. Menopause can also coincide with milestones that cause a certain amount of stress, a known cause of memory problems. If you have children, they are probably getting ready to go off on their own, just as your own parents may be experiencing health problems. You may feel that you are being pulled in several different directions at once. (See Mood on page 303 for more stress-busting advice.)

FATIGUE

Sleep is necessary for the body to recuperate after the physical and mental activities of the day. And recent studies have discovered that sleep is critically important for learning and memory. European researchers found that during sleep, we organize and consolidate our memories—the brain equivalent of burning a memory DVD. Without enough sleep, our memories don't settle in as well, so we are more likely to forget.

HOW FOOD AFFECTS MEMORY

A woman I know told me that when she was growing up, whenever she would balk at eating her vegetables, her mother would command, "Eat it—it's brain food." I told my friend to call her mom and thank her, because she's absolutely right. Vegetables, fruits, whole-grain foods, and fish can all be considered brain food. And not just because mom says so . . . memory experts say so, too!

GOOD FOODS TO CHOOSE

Here are nutrients that are important to memory:

ANTIOXIDANTS

The color of fruits and vegetables—red apples, purple blackberries, green broccoli—is caused by natural compounds called phytochemicals. There are thousands of phytochemicals in the world, and each fruit or vegetable can contain more than a hundred of them. You know about the importance of vitamins and minerals, right? Well, phytochemicals are a whole new class of nutrients that deserves your respect.

Many phytochemicals are antioxidants, which nourish and defend body cells—including neurons—against damage, called *oxidative stress,* caused during oxygen metabolism. Antioxidants also help prevent the buildup of plaque in the arteries, so there is good, strong blood flow to the brain. Overall, general studies of the effects of phytochemicals on memory suggest that the more you eat, the better. For example, a 25-year Harvard Medical School study of more than 13,000 women showed that the participants who ate relatively high amounts of vegetables over the years had less age-related decline in memory. Cruciferous vegetables and leafy green vegetables (including spinach and mustard greens) had the biggest effect on helping women retain their memory during the course of the study.

BEST CRUCIFEROUS VEGETABLES: *Broccoli, broccoli raab, Brussels sprouts, cabbage, Chinese cabbage, Chinese broccoli, cauliflower, collard greens, daikon, kale, kohlrabi, mustard (seeds and greens), rutabaga, turnips, bok choy, arugula, horseradish, radishes, Swiss chard, wasabi (Japanese horseradish), watercress and cress*

Certain phytochemicals have been specifically shown to help improve memory, or to prevent memory loss. The phytochemicals anthocyanin and quercetin actually *reversed* some of the age-related memory deficits in laboratory rats. Although it isn't possible to test the effects of nutrients with such specificity in people, it is possible that these same foods could work to reverse our own memory loss.

BEST FOODS FOR ANTHOCYANIN: *Blackberries, black currants, blueberries, eggplant, elderberries, raspberries, cherries, boysenberries, red/black grapes, strawberries, plums, cranberries, rhubarb, red wine, red onion, apples, peaches, red/purple cabbage, red beets, blood orange (fruit and juice)*

BEST FOODS FOR QUERCETIN: *Onions (red, yellow, white), kale, leeks, cherry tomatoes, broccoli, blueberries, black currants, elderberries, lingonberries, cocoa powder (unsweetened), apricots, apple with skin (especially Red Delicious), grapes (black, red, purple), tomatoes, tea (green or black), red wine, green beans, white beans, lettuce (butterhead, Boston, iceberg, Bibb), peppers (ancho, hot chile, green, yellow wax), celery, chives, red cabbage, lemons, grapefruit, horseradish root*

FOLIC ACID AND OTHER B VITAMINS

The closest thing we have to a magic bullet for fixing memory problems is folic acid (also known as *folate*). As I mentioned earlier, this nutrient may just be the single best way to lower blood levels of homocysteine, which is thought to damage blood vessels. In addition, folic acid seems to have a direct effect on memory. A study conducted at Tufts University in Boston followed about 320 men for three years. Those who had high blood levels of homocysteine showed memory decline, but if the men ate foods rich in folic acid, their memories were protected. This same study also showed that men who were deficient in vitamins B_6 and B_{12} showed a more rapid decline of memory than those who had adequate blood levels of those vitamins.

BEST FOODS FOR FOLIC ACID: *Fortified whole grain breakfast cereals, lentils, black-eyed peas, soybeans, oatmeal, turnip greens, spinach, mustard greens, green peas, artichokes,*

FAQS

What about ginkgo? I've seen it in teas and in supplements, and it seems to be everywhere. Is it helpful for memory?

The scientific evidence is mixed. Depending on which studies you look at, it helps memory or it doesn't, or it only helps for some kinds of memory . . . or not. The study outcomes haven't been consistent enough for me to have confidence in this particular supplement. If ginkgo were totally safe, I would say it couldn't hurt to try it, but there are reports of people developing spontaneous internal bleeding. And some extracts or whole-leaf ginkgo may contain relatively high amounts of natural toxins called *ginkgolic acids*. Plus, ginkgo can affect insulin release in people with diabetes, and can have dangerous interactions with some prescription medications. Overall, I can't recommend ginkgo for memory.

okra, beets, parsnips, broccoli, broccoli raab, sunflower seeds, wheat germ, oranges and orange juice, Brussels sprouts, papayas, seaweed, berries (boysenberries, blackberries, strawberries), beans (black, pinto, kidney, garbanzo, navy), cauliflower, Chinese cabbage, corn, whole grain bread, pasta (preferably whole wheat)

BEST FOODS FOR VITAMIN B$_6$: *Fortified whole grain breakfast cereal, garbanzo beans, wild salmon (fresh or canned), beef (extra-lean), pork tenderloin, chicken breast, white potatoes (with skin), oatmeal, banana, pistachio nuts (unsalted), lentils, tomato paste, barley, rice (brown, wild), peppers, sweet potatoes, squash (winter, acorn), broccoli, broccoli raab, carrots, Brussels sprouts, peanut butter, eggs, shrimp, tofu, apricots, watermelon, avocado, strawberries, whole grain bread*

BEST FOODS FOR VITAMIN B$_{12}$: *Shellfish (clams, oysters, crab), wild salmon (fresh or canned), fortified whole grain breakfast cereal, enriched/fortified soy milk, trout (rainbow, wild), tuna (canned light), lean beef, veggie burgers, cottage cheese (fat-free or 1% reduced-fat), yogurt (fat-free, low-fat), milk (fat-free, skim plus, 1% reduced-fat), eggs, cheese (fat-free, reduced-fat)*

An Australian study found that eating plenty of foods rich in folic acid was associated with faster information processing and memory recall. After taking B vitamin supplements for only five weeks, the women in the study showed overall improvements in memory. And in a Dutch study, older people who took 800 micrograms of folic acid for three years had a 25 percent lower level of homocysteine compared with a similar group that did not take folic acid. Most importantly, the people who took the supplement had the memory skills of people five years younger!

No one knows exactly how folic acid works to protect memory, but some experts suggest that, in addition to protecting blood vessels, it may affect the brain chemicals that allow neurons to communicate with one another.

OMEGA-3 FATTY ACIDS

There are good fats and bad fats, and omega-3 fatty acids fall solidly on the side of good. Omega-3s are found primarily in fatty fish, certain nuts and seeds, and fortified foods. A study conducted by researchers at the Rush University Medical Center in Chicago followed more than 3,000 men and women for six years to see how diet affected memory. People who ate fish at least once a week had a 10 percent slower decline compared with those who did not eat fish, a difference that gave them the memory and thinking ability of a person three years younger.

BEST FOODS FOR OMEGA-3s: *Wild salmon (fresh or canned), herring, mackerel (not king), sardines, anchovies, rainbow trout, Pacific oysters, omega-3–fortified eggs, flaxseeds (ground and oil), walnuts, butternuts (white walnuts), seaweed, walnut oil, canola oil, soybeans*

COFFEE

Any coffee lover can tell you they think more clearly after a good, strong cup of caffeinated coffee. Now, they have proof. Researchers from the University of Innsbruck in Austria used functional magnetic resonance imaging (fMRI) to examine the brain activity of people working on a memory task. The volunteers were tested twice, once after receiving the caffeine equivalent of about 2 cups of coffee, and once without any caffeine. Caffeine improved the memory skills and reactions times of the volunteers. In addition, caffeine increased brain activity in two locations—the memory-rich frontal lobe and the attention-controlling anterior cingulum. Without caffeine, there was no increase in brain activity. So if memory problems are a major concern for you, and if you don't have a medical condition that precludes caffeine, feel free to indulge in a cup or two in the morning to jump-start your brain. NOTE: If you have elevated low-density lipoprotein (LDL) cholesterol, you should limit your caffeine fix to plain brewed coffee or tea. There is some evidence that *unfiltered* coffee (the kind used to make espresso, cappuccino, and latte) may raise cholesterol levels, especially in people who are already battling high cholesterol. To be safe, skip the fancy brews and stick with a regular cup of joe, using skim or 1% reduced-fat milk, of course.

BEST SOURCES OF CAFFEINE: *Coffee, espresso, skim latte, skim cappuccino, skim café au lait, tea. Be cautious and moderate with added sugar!*

FAQS

I don't think dieting is a good idea for me. I feel like I'm walking around in a fog all the time.

Don't give up yet. You may be trying to lose weight too quickly, and not eating enough to get you through the day. Read about weight loss (page 19) to make sure you follow a sensible plan. If eating every four to five hours doesn't keep you clear-headed, try eating every two to three hours—in case you are experiencing true hypoglycemia. If low blood sugar is the problem, your between-meal snacks should be very small, ideally containing a mix of protein and high quality carbohydrate. For example, try a handful of walnuts and a banana, or a half-cup of low-fat cottage cheese with a quarter-wedge of cantaloupe, or 6 ounces of low-fat yogurt with 1 tablespoon slivered almonds, or an apple with a slice of low-fat cheese.

FOODS TO AVOID

Researchers at the University of Toronto fed laboratory rats either standard chow or an unhealthy high-fat diet for three months, and then tested them to see if there were any effects on memory. It probably won't surprise you to learn that the rats that ate unhealthy high-fat food did worse on all aspects of the memory test. This and other studies suggest that if you want to improve your memory, stay away from saturated fats and fried foods, including donuts, hamburgers, potato chips, cheese, and ice cream. These foods clog the blood vessels that deliver key nutrients to your brain, plus they can crowd out healthier foods in your diet.

BONUS POINTS

- **Move your body.** Because your brain only functions well when it has a steady supply of oxygen, anything that improves blood flow is good for your memory. Regular physical activity has been shown to decrease the risk of dementia and Alzheimer's disease by about half. Half! That's a huge benefit for doing any leisure activity you enjoy. So take a walk after dinner, go bowling, do some gardening, ride your bicycle, or take advantage of the new equipment at your local gym. If you get 30 minutes of activity per day, you'll be one step closer to a lifetime of better memory.

- **Flex your mental muscle.** Memory is thought to be related to the number of brain cells (neurons) we have and the connections between those cells. For decades, scientists held fast to the belief that new brain cells could only be formed in childhood—a neuron lost was gone forever. But in recent years, experiments have revealed that all mammals, including people, can form new brain cells well into adulthood. These new cells can become integrated into the brain's vast network, forming more and more pathways that can encode and hold our memories. How can we increase the number of brain cells? The most documented and efficient way is by exercising your brain. "Use it or lose it" is certainly true, but so is "nourish and flourish." That is to say, the more active the brain, the better your memory will be. The trick is to keep your mind active and challenged. Learn new skills, such as playing a musical instrument, speaking a foreign language, or—best of all—cooking healthier meals. Socializing, volunteering in the community, or taking a part-time job will give you mental skills you can't accomplish on your own. Reading; playing chess, bridge, or other games of strategy; starting a new hobby; or taking classes at a local college will also help keep your memory sharper longer.

- **Turn off the TV.** Zoning out in front of the television is the absolute opposite of a challenging brain activity. In 2005, researchers at the University of Washington in Seattle found that when very young children are exposed to television, they can show problems with thinking ability and memory years later. Adults who spend too much time watching TV miss out on brain-boosting activities. If you watch more than two hours of television a day, begin to cut down and substitute a more challenging project to fill your valuable time.

- **Eat breakfast.** You probably know that decades of studies have demonstrated that children learn and remember more at school if they eat breakfast. The first meal of the day is just as important for you. If you tend to skip breakfast or make do with just a cup of coffee, listen up. Eating within 90 minutes of waking up will help jump-start your brain and improve your daily memory.

- **Don't smoke.** Just as smoking increases risk of heart disease, it can also decrease blood flow to the brain and do serious damage to memory. As if all the other reasons for quitting weren't enough, add that to the list.

- **Give yourself a break.** Seek out ways to de-stress your life. Set aside a few minutes just for yourself—breathe deeply and relax. Meditate for a few minutes. Look for ways to simplify your life by taking on fewer projects and learning to say "no" to things you don't want to do. Exercise regularly, get enough sleep, and learn to go a little easier on yourself.

SUPPLEMENTS

Scientific studies have investigated various supplements and herbal remedies for memory improvement. Although I strongly believe that vitamins and minerals from food are your best defense against memory loss, if you want to consider supplements *in addition to* the food recommendations in this chapter, here is what research has to say about the most popular supplements:

1. **Multivitamin.** At least one study found that people over age 65 who took a multivitamin every day for a year had significant improvements in short-term memory. Look for brands that offer 100 percent of the Daily Value (%DV) for the B-vitamins: thiamin (B_1), riboflavin (B_2), niacin (B_3), B_6, B_{12}, and folic acid.

2. **Huperzine A.** Although this chemical was originally made from a Chinese moss called *Huperzia serrata,* modern huperzine A formulations are either made from purified moss or synthesized in a laboratory. Huperzine A works by increasing the level of a brain chemical called *acetylcholine,* and by protecting brain cells through its antioxidant properties. If you would like to try this supplement, I recommend taking 50 micrograms once or twice daily. Always check with your physician first. *Notes and cautions:* Huperzine A can decrease heart rate, and therefore shouldn't be used by people with heart problems. Consult your doctor before taking huperzine A if you have a gastrointestinal or urinary obstruction, peptic ulcer disease, asthma, or chronic obstructive pulmonary disease. Because of its effects on acetylcholine, consult your doctor before taking huperzine A if you are taking an anticholinergic medication (such as atropine, Cogentin, Akineton, Kemadrin, or Artane), or a cholinergic medication or acetylcholinesterase inhibitor (such as Aricept, Urecholine, phospholine iodine, Enlon, Reversol, Tensilon, Prostigmin, Antilirium, Mestinon, Anectine, Regonol, Quelicin, or Cognex).

3. **Ginseng.** For generations, people around the world have used this herb (also known as *Panax ginseng* or *Panax quinquefolius*) to improve memory. Study results are mixed— some show a benefit, others don't. But some of my clients firmly believe that ginseng helps them stay sharp mentally. Look for an extract standardized to contain 4 to 7 percent ginsenosides. Take 200 milligrams daily for two weeks, followed by one week of "rest." If you feel it was helpful, continue the two-weeks-on/one-week-off prescription. *Notes and cautions:* Although side effects are very rare, talk with your doctor if you experience increased breast tenderness, postmenpausal vaginal bleeding, or menstrual abnormalities. Other possible side effects include insomnia, raised blood pressure and/or heart rate, and nervousness. Women who are pregnant or nursing should not take ginseng. And because ginseng seems to stimulate the growth of breast cancer cells, people with breast cancer, and women with a strong family history of

breast cancer should avoid ginseng. Because of possible drug interactions, consult your doctor before taking ginseng if you are taking an antidepressant, digoxin, insulin or oral diabetes medications, or a blood thinning medication.

4. **Phosphatidylserine (PS).** Although PS isn't widely known in the United States, it is very popular in Europe as a treatment both for dementia and for ordinary age-related memory loss. PS is a natural component of cell membranes—especially brain cells. Years ago, PS supplements were made from the PS found in cow brains. Of course, mad cow disease put an end to that. Now, supplements are made mostly from soybeans. Nearly all the evidence showing that PS can improve memory was based on the cow-brain supplements. No one knows whether the current formulations from soy will work as well, but because most people can take PS with no problems, I sometimes suggest it for my clients who want to try everything possible to improve their memories. The usual dose for memory improvement is 100 milligrams once or twice a day. *Notes and cautions:* PS is a mild blood thinner, so consult your doctor before trying PS if you are currently taking regular doses of other blood-thinning drugs or supplement, including warfarin, aspirin, heparin, Trental, Plavix, Ticlid, garlic, or ginkgo.

JOY'S 4-STEP PROGRAM FOR MEMORY

Follow this program if you feel that your memory has been "slipping" lately.

STEP 1 ... START WITH THE BASICS

These are the first things you should do to start improving your memory.

- See your primary care physician for a physical examination. Your doctor will check your blood pressure to make sure it is within normal range (120/80 or less mmHg). Blood tests may be done to check for high cholesterol or high homocysteine, which could indicate the possibility of vascular disease.

- Quit smoking.

- Decrease stress. Relax. Be good to yourself.

- Try to get adequate amounts of sleep.

STEP2 ... YOUR ULTIMATE GROCERY LIST

A nutrition plan is only as good as the foods that you choose. This list contains foods with high levels of nutrients that might help improve memory, plus some foods used as ingredients in the meal plans and recipes. You don't have to purchase every item . . . but these foods should make up the bulk of what you eat for the week. If you find yourself getting bored, try some unfamiliar foods from these groups—they may become favorites.

FRUIT

Apples	blackberries,	Cranberries	Papayas
Applesauce,	blueberries,	Currants, black	Peaches
unsweetened	elderberries,	Grapefruit	Plums
Apricots	lingonberries,	Grapes (red, black,	Tangerines
Bananas	raspberries,	purple)	Watermelon
Berries	strawberries)	Lemons (and juice)	
(boysenberries,	Cherries	Oranges (and juice)	

VEGETABLES

Artichokes	Celery	Lettuce (butterhead,	Radishes
Arugula	Chickpeas (garbanzo	Boston, iceberg,	Rhubarb
Avocado	beans)	Bibb)	Rutabaga
Beans (black, pinto,	Chives	Mustard greens and	Seaweed
kidney, garbanzo,	Collard greens	seeds	Soybeans
navy, white)	Corn	Okra	Spinach
Beets	Daikon	Onions (red, yellow,	Squash (winter, acorn)
Bok choy	Eggplant	white)	Swiss chard
Broccoli	Green beans	Parsnips	Tomatoes (especially
Broccoli, Chinese	Horseradish	Peas, black-eyed	cherry tomatoes)
Broccoli raab	(including	Peas, green	Tomato paste and sauce
Brussels sprouts	horseradish root)	Peppers (ancho, hot	Turnip greens
Cabbage (red, purple,	Kale	chile, green, yellow	Turnips
Chinese)	Kohlrabi	wax)	Vegetable juice
Carrots	Leeks	Potatoes, sweet	Watercress (and other
Cauliflower	Lentils	Potatoes, white	varieties of cress)

SEAFOOD

Anchovies	Oysters, Pacific	Sardines	Trout (rainbow, wild)
Herring	Salmon, wild (fresh or	Shellfish (shrimp,	Tuna (canned light)
Mackerel (not king)	canned)	clams, oysters, crab)	

LEAN MEATS/EGGS/SOY FOODS

Beef, lean	Eggs (especially omega-3–fortified)	Pork tenderloin	Turkey, lean ground
Chicken breast		Tofu	Veggie burgers

DAIRY

Cheese (fat-free, reduced-fat)	Cheese, reduced-fat mozzarella (for meal plan)	Cottage cheese (fat-free, 1% reduced-fat)	Soy milk, enriched/fortified
Cheese, Parmesan		Milk (fat-free, 1% reduced-fat)	Yogurt (fat-free, low-fat)

NUTS AND SEEDS (PREFERABLY UNSALTED)

Butternuts (white walnuts)	Flaxseed, ground	Peanuts	Sunflower seeds
	Peanut butter	Pistachio nuts	Walnuts

WHOLE GRAINS

Barley	Cereal, fortified whole grain	Pasta, spinach	
Bread, whole grain (including crackers, buns, pitas, English muffins)	Oatmeal	Rice (brown, wild)	
	Pasta, preferably whole wheat	Wheat germ	

MISCELLANEOUS

Baking powder	Garlic	Oil, canola	Tea (black, green)
Baking soda	Hummus	Oil, flaxseed	Vinegar, balsamic or red wine
Cinnamon	Mayonnaise, reduced-fat	Oil, olive	Wasabi (Japanese horseradish)
Cocoa powder, unsweetened	Mustard, Dijon	Oil, walnut	Wine, red
Flour, all-purpose	Nonstick cooking spray	Soy sauce, reduced-sodium	

STEP3 ...GOING ABOVE AND BEYOND

If you want to do everything you can for your memory, here are some additional things you might try:

- Take a daily multivitamin with 100% DV of folic acid, vitamin B_6, and vitamin B_{12}.

- Although I can't personally recommend these supplements because of their potential for side effects in some people, some scientists believe that hupersine A, ginseng, and phosphatidylserine might help improve memory. Talk with your doctor before trying these potent supplements.

- Increase physical activity. Strive for at least 30 minutes daily of any activity that gets you moving.

- Increase mental challenges. Start doing the crossword puzzle, learn a musical instrument, take classes at a local college—anything that makes you think.

KEEP YOUR BRAIN FIT

Community colleges, churches, and recreational centers offer a wide range of classes to challenge your mind. You can find something for just about any interest . . . at little or no cost. Looking for inspiration? Here are some classes I found listed around the country: CPR and First Aid Training; Interior Decorating; Flight Instruction; Television Production; Art of Bonsai Gardening; Secrets of Animal Training; Genealogy; Web Site Development; Flower Arranging; Scrapbooking; Acting for Beginners; Philosophy of Plato; Religions of the World; Creative Writing; Firefighting Tactics and Strategies; Surfing for Seniors; Principles of Tax Accounting; and—my personal favorite—Kitchen Chemistry.

STEP 4...MEAL PLANS

These sample menus include the best memory foods, plus other nutrients related to vascular health.

Every day, choose *one* option for each of the three meals—breakfast, lunch, and dinner. Then, one to two times per day, choose from a variety of my suggested snacks. Approximate calories have been provided to help adjust for your personal weight-management goals. If you find yourself hungry (and if weight is not an issue), feel free to increase the portion sizes for meals and snacks. Beverage calories are *not* included. (Remember: If you have high cholesterol, choose tea or filtered coffee instead of an espresso-based beverage. If your doctor has instructed you to avoid caffeine, choose a decaffeinated variety.)

BREAKFAST OPTIONS

(Approximately 300 to 400 calories)

Oatmeal with Berries and Nuts

½ cup dry traditional oatmeal cooked with ½ cup water and ½ cup fat-free milk (or 1 cup fat-free milk); top with 1 cup mixed berries and 1 tablespoon chopped walnuts.

Yogurt Berry Pancakes with Applesauce

2 Yogurt Berry Pancakes (page 299), topped with 1 cup natural unsweetened applesauce and ½ cup blueberries.

Whole Grain Cereal with Milk and Fresh Fruit

1 cup whole grain cereal (no more than 150 calories per cup and at least 3 grams fiber) with 1 cup fat-free milk or enriched/fortified soy milk. Serve with 1 cup fresh fruit salad made from oranges, strawberries, grapefruit, and red or black grapes.

Peanut Butter Toast with Fruit

2 slices whole grain toast with 2 level tablespoons peanut butter. Serve with your choice of ½ banana (or 1 orange, 1 tangerine, ½ pink grapefruit, or ½ cup berries).

Scrambled Eggs, Tomatoes, Onions, and Spinach

1 omega-3–fortified whole egg plus 2 or 3 egg whites, 2 tablespoons chopped tomatoes, 2 tablespoons chopped onion, and unlimited spinach, (pre-sautéed in non-stick cooking spray) scrambled and cooked with nonstick cooking spray or 1 teaspoon canola oil. Enjoy with a toasted whole grain English muffin, dry (or skip the muffin and have 1 cup mixed berries or cherries).

LUNCH OPTIONS

(Approximately 400 to 500 calories)

Grilled Chicken Pita with Tomato and Avocado

5 ounces skinless chicken breast, grilled, with unlimited lettuce and tomato slices, 2 thin slices avocado, and mustard in a whole grain pita. Enjoy with ½ cup berries.

Spinach–Three Bean Salad with Fruit

Large bowl of fresh spinach leaves topped with a variety of unlimited cut-up vegetables (including beets) and three-bean combination (¼ cup each chickpeas, white beans, and kidney beans), tossed with 2 teaspoons olive oil and unlimited balsamic vinegar or fresh lemon juice. Serve with 1 apple.

Lentil Soup with Whole Grain Crackers

2 cups lentil soup—if store-bought, any variety 300 calories or less per 2-cup serving; 150 calories of whole grain crackers.

Salmon Salad Sandwich with Tomato and Onion

Salmon salad (5 ounces canned or fresh wild salmon mixed with 1 to 2 teaspoons reduced-fat mayonnaise and preferred seasonings) with unlimited lettuce, tomato, and onion slices on 2 slices whole grain bread or 1 whole grain pita.

Spinach-Cheese Omelet with Salad

Cook 1 omega-3 fortified egg plus 2 or 3 egg whites in heated pan coated with 1 teaspoon canola oil or nonstick cooking spray. Add unlimited raw or cooked spinach and 1 ounce grated reduced-fat mozzarella cheese. When bottom is cooked, gently flip over. Fold over and cook until egg mixture is firm. Enjoy with a mixed green salad topped with 1 tablespoon sunflower seeds (or chopped walnuts), 2 teaspoons olive oil, and unlimited balsamic vinegar or fresh lemon juice.

DINNER OPTIONS

(Approximately 500 to 600 calories)

Grilled Asian Salmon with Broccoli and Potato

1 serving Grilled Asian Salmon (page 300) with plain baked sweet or white potato. Serve with unlimited steamed broccoli or cauliflower.

Vegetarian Chili with Brown Rice and Steamed Spinach

2 cups vegetarian chili with 1 cup cooked brown rice or 1 cup black-eyed peas. Serve with 1 cup steamed spinach, kale, or Brussels sprouts.

Turkey Burger with Vegetable Salad

One 5-ounce lean turkey burger on whole grain bun (or pita) with mixed green salad loaded with lettuce, tomatoes, carrots, beets, onions, peppers, and artichokes and tossed in 2 teaspoons olive oil and balsamic vinegar or fresh lemon juice. Or skip the bun and instead enjoy 1 cup black-eyed peas.

Pasta with Turkey Meat Sauce and Vegetables

1 cup cooked whole wheat or spinach pasta tossed with turkey meat sauce (5 ounces sautéed extra-lean ground turkey meat cooked with tomato sauce and your choice of seasonings), topped with 2 tablespoons grated Parmesan cheese. Serve with 1 cup steamed cauliflower, kale, broccoli, broccoli raab, cabbage, Brussels sprouts, spinach, or bok choy.

Chicken and Vegetable Stir-Fry over Brown Rice

Stir-fry 5 ounces skinless white-meat chicken with unlimited strips of onion and tri-colored peppers (red, yellow, green) in 2 teaspoons olive oil and 2 to 3 teaspoons low-sodium soy sauce. Add additional veggies if you like. Serve over ½ cup cooked brown rice; enjoy with a mixed green salad tossed with 2 tablespoons low-calorie dressing (or 2 teaspoons olive oil and unlimited vinegar or fresh lemon juice).

SNACK OPTIONS

100 calories or less

- *Best Vegetables:* 1 cup raw or cooked veggies such as broccoli, broccoli raab, cauliflower, green beans, spinach, kale, Brussels sprouts, mustard greens, cabbage, bok choy, rhubarb, beets, artichokes, or seaweed

- *Best Fruit:* 1 apple or orange; 2 plums or tangerines; ½ grapefruit; 15 to 20 red or black grapes; 20 strawberries; 1 cup cherries, black currants, blueberries, blackberries, raspberries, boysenberries, or chopped strawberries

- 1 cup vegetable juice

- Celery sticks with 1 level tablespoon peanut butter

100 to 200 calories

- 1 ounce unsalted peanuts (about 25 nuts) or 1 ounce raw, unsalted walnuts (about ¼ cup or 14 walnuts)

- 1 cup fat-free plain yogurt mixed with ½ cup blueberries and 1 tablespoon wheat germ (or chopped walnuts)

- ¼ cup unsalted sunflower seeds in the shell

- 3 tablespoons hummus with celery or peppers

- 1 sliced apple with one level tablespoon peanut butter

- 1 cup dry whole grain cereal

- 1 cup boiled soybeans in the pod (edamame)

BLUEBERRY PANCAKES

This pancake recipe may look complicated, but it is fabulously easy and delicious—perfect for guests or a casual family breakfast.

Makes 4 servings, 2 pancakes each

1	large egg
1	cup plain, fat-free yogurt
1	tablespoon canola oil
1	cup all-purpose flour
1	tablespoon sugar
1	teaspoon baking powder
$\frac{1}{2}$	teaspoon baking soda
$\frac{1}{4}$	teaspoon cinnamon
	Pinch of salt
$\frac{1}{2}$	cup fresh or frozen blueberries

1. In a blender, combine the egg, yogurt, and oil. Blend until smooth. Transfer to a large bowl.
2. Sift together the flour, sugar, baking powder, baking soda, cinnamon, and salt. Sift into the yogurt mixture and blend well.
3. Spray a griddle with nonstick cooking spray and heat over medium-high heat. In batches, using about one-eighth of the batter for each pancake, ladle the batter onto the griddle. Sprinkle each with some blueberries and cook for about 30 seconds (or until bubbles form in the middle of pancake). Flip over and cook until golden.

PER SERVING
219 calories, 9 g protein, 35 g carbohydrate, 5 g fat (1 g saturated), 54 mg cholesterol, 295 mg sodium, 2 g fiber

GRILLED ASIAN SALMON

With only 270 calories per serving, this mouthwatering entrée is low-fat, easy to make, and bursting with brain-friendly omega-3 fats.

Makes 4 servings

4	(6-ounce) wild salmon steaks
½	cup reduced-sodium soy sauce
¼	cup orange juice
2	tablespoons chopped garlic
2	teaspoons Dijon mustard
2	teaspoons tomato paste
	Juice of ½ lemon

1. Place the salmon in a zip-top bag. Mix the soy sauce, orange juice, garlic, mustard, tomato paste, and lemon juice in a bowl. Pour into the bag with the salmon. Seal the bag, pressing out excess air. Refrigerate to marinate 4 to 6 hours.

2. Prepare a grill. Remove the salmon from the bag, reserving the marinade. Place the salmon on the grill and cook, turning once, for about 5 minutes on each side, or longer for well done. For extra flavor, lightly drizzle a few tablespoons of the marinade on salmon during grilling. Discard leftover marinade.

PER SERVING
270 calories, 37 g protein, 2 g carbohydrate, 11 g fat (2 g saturated), 100 mg cholesterol, 400 mg sodium, 0 g fiber

PART FIVE

FEELING GOOD

CHAPTER 13

MOOD

When Melissa came to see me with the goal of losing about 40 pounds, I quickly recognized how she got where she was, weight-wise. She had the kind of unfortunate habits I see in so many of my clients: Erratic eating schedule, sometimes skipping meals, sometimes bingeing, and settling for ready-to-eat, grab-and-go foods. Constantly busy and overextended, Melissa often found herself feeling angry and resentful because she felt that there was no time she could call her own. Everything took priority over her—the kids, the car pools, her husband, work, boss, friends . . . absolutely everything got a slice of Melissa's time except Melissa.

One side effect of Melissa's hectic lifestyle was a chronic bad mood. Her day was ruined by things most of us would shrug off, like if the morning newspaper didn't arrive at the exact time she expected it . . . or if her kids were assigned an extra helping of homework . . . or if the grocery store was out of her favorite brand of anything. She complained about the amount of time her husband spent on the golf course, but she also complained about him hanging around the house and getting underfoot. She was irritated by coworkers and supervisors alike. She barked at the people she loved, sniped at the people she worked with, and hated herself for being so explosive. The other side of Melissa's personality was weepy—during our first meeting, she cried twice. That was my first clue that Melissa needed help with her moods as much as she needed to lose weight . . . and she couldn't agree with me more!

I did three things for Melissa: First, I put her on a schedule so she would eat meals more regularly—this would help regulate her blood sugars and her moods every waking moment. Second, I gave her a calorie-controlled program for weight loss, which would help raise her self-esteem. And third, I drew her a food "road map," which showed her the direction she needed to take her diet in order to get the right combination of foods, vitamins, and minerals specifically shown to help improve mood.

After the first week on her new food program, Melissa lost 4 pounds, just the boost she needed. Over the next several weeks, her weight loss was steady, if a bit less dramatic. The next time I saw her, Melissa had lost 20 pounds and was halfway to her weight-loss goal. She looked fantastic, but that wasn't the best part—Melissa felt better than she had in years. She was level-headed, not as quick to react. As time went on, I saw Melissa morph from an uncertain, overbooked, overwrought slave to her raw emotions into a calm, beautiful, competent woman. She was slimmer. She ate better. And best of all, she was happy! She still had moments when she snapped or cried, but emotions didn't overwhelm her or rule her life. For the first time in a long time, Melissa didn't feel out of control.

Weight loss also bolstered Melissa's self-esteem and improved her moods. Mood-enhancing foods helped calm her inner turmoil. The covert part of this plan no doubt amplified it's effectiveness: In order to diligently follow her weight-loss and mood program, Melissa needed to make time for herself, something she hadn't done in years. Like so many of us, Melissa rushed through her life, doing everything for other people, but nothing for herself. If this sounds like you, hear this: It's critical for your physical health, your emotional well-being, and your moods that you learn to focus on your needs at least for some small portion of every day. I've found that taking time to shop for and prepare nutritious (and delicious!) meals can be the start of a new habit of caring for the self. How much you pamper yourself after that is entirely up to you.

Over the years, I've worked with many clients who suffered with clinical depression and postpartum depression and, much more often, people like Melissa who struggled with chronic bad moods. As successful as I've been with this mood program, it is not a cure-all. Even if you follow the advice in this chapter to the letter, you won't be happy every minute of every day, and you will still sometimes lose your cool. That's life. But if you are feeling battered by your moods, this program should help you feel significantly better—perhaps even within the first week.

WHAT AFFECTS MOOD?

If moods were merely psychological, if they were truly "all in the head," they wouldn't make us so miserable. Very few people would choose to remain in a pit of depression or keep their flashpoint anger if they could simply change their state of mind. But we don't always have control over how our feelings affect our lives because, for many of us, mood is as physical as a broken bone or acid reflux.

Scientists believe that mood is caused by changes in the production or availability of brain chemicals called *neurotransmitters*. The three main neurotransmitters—norepinephrine, dopamine, and serotonin—work together to balance mood. If there is a decrease in one or all of these chemicals, we will feel differently, even if we don't know exactly why. For example, neurotransmitters are responsible for feelings of anger, anxiety, motivation, irritability, happiness, impulsiveness, and depression. They can even affect general energy levels.

The reason you feel a particular way on a particular day is usually a complex combination of genetic susceptibility, life events and circumstances, and your body's general physical state. You may have noticed, for example, that your moods feel more intense at certain times of day . . . or if you are feeling tired . . . or during an illness . . . or in times of stress. Some women experience depression and irritability related to their monthly hormone fluctuations (see Premenstrual Syndrome, page 351, for more on PMS). And quite a few people are pushed over the emotional cliff by food-related issues, including what they eat, when they eat, and why they eat.

Nutrition-related mood problems can stem from long- and short-term roots. Poor eating habits can, over time, lead to deficiencies in some of the vitamins, minerals, and other nutrients that contribute to good mood. For example, the neurotransmitters that regulate mood are built from amino acids, which are found in protein-rich foods. If you don't get enough of a variety of different proteins in your diet, your brain chemistry will eventually suffer. Furthermore, the amino acid tryptophan can only be converted in the brain to serotonin—a mood calming neurotransmitter—when adequate carbohydrate is present. Eating patterns can even affect your moods from hour to hour—the proverbial "mid-morning slump" and many cases of flaring irritability can be caused by a dip in blood sugar from eating the wrong foods at the wrong time of day, or from not eating often enough.

For most people, a mood is a temporary state—we feel it, react to it, and after an hour or a day, we forget about it. But sometimes, a mood settles in and stays. Of all conditions seen in general medical practice, one of the most common is depression. Many people think of depression as extreme sadness, but that's just a partial description. Symptoms of depression also include feelings of hopelessness or helplessness, irritability, sleeping more or less than usual, difficulty concentrating or making decisions, weight gain or weight loss, and loss of energy. Of course, depression is only one possible cause of these problems, but

FAQS

My neighbor started taking something called DHEA [dehydroepiandrosterone]. He says it makes him feel fabulous, happier, and full of energy. Is this something I should consider?

I can't recommend DHEA for moods . . . or anything else, for that matter. DHEA is a powerful steroid hormone, which is metabolized in the body to androgens and estrogens. Although its effects are still not entirely known, some are potentially dangerous—for example, DHEA can cause growth of hormone-sensitive cancers, including prostate cancer and certain breast cancers. Until we know more about all the potential effects, I'd stay clear of DHEA.

if you experience any or all of these symptoms for longer than two weeks, it is important to see a doctor. Moods that persist require medical attention—they can be signs of a serious medical problem, so you'll want to make sure you get checked out. And if you do receive a diagnosis of depression, your doctor can prescribe medications to speed the time to feeling better.

HOW FOOD AFFECTS MOOD

No matter where your moods came from or how long they have lasted, eating the right foods can help you feel more energetic and less like you're riding an emotional rollercoaster built for one. Here are some of the main guideposts on your mood-food road map:

HIGH-QUALITY CARBOHYDRATES AND PROTEIN

There are two general categories of carbohydrates: high-quality and low-quality. High-quality carbs are full of vitamins, minerals, phytochemicals, and fiber. They are found primarily in plant foods, including whole grain products, oats, legumes, vegetables, fresh fruit, brown and wild rice, and potatoes. Low-quality carbs, on the other hand, have much less nutritional value. These less-than-stellar carbs (also called *simple sugars*) are foods that are made primarily of sugar, including sugar itself, as well as candy, soft drinks, syrup, jam and jelly, cakes, and most other foods we typically think of as sweets or desserts. Refined starches—the "white" carbs, such as white rice and white bread—are also low-quality carbohydrates because our digestive process quickly breaks them down. In other words, they act like simple sugars in the body.

Like all foods, carbohydrates affect body chemistry, and the type of carbohydrate you eat makes a big difference in determining metabolism, energy, and overall well-being. All carbohydrates provide energy to the body in the form of glucose—the *blood sugar* that feeds our cells. When blood sugar is up, we feel good; when blood sugar goes down, mood can plunge, too. So ideally, we want to eat the types of foods that give us a steady level of energy so that we can go through the day feeling great from start to finish. The goal, then, is to find the right combination of foods that allow blood sugar levels to rise gently, stay even over a long period of time, and then fall off slowly.

> **BEST FOODS FOR HIGH-QUALITY CARBS:** *Vegetables, fruits (fresh or frozen, unsweetened), beans, peas, lentils, brown and wild rice, barley, oatmeal, whole grain cereals, whole grain breads, whole grain crackers, quinoa, amaranth, wheat berries, millet*

All carbohydrates cause a rise in blood sugar that typically lasts about two hours before returning to baseline. With high-quality carbohydrates, blood sugar levels rise slowly and don't get very high. In addition, some of these high-quality carbs contain soluble fiber, a component of plant cell walls. Soluble fiber slows the absorption of glucose from food in the stomach, which also helps put a lid on blood sugar.

BEST FOODS FOR SOLUBLE FIBER: *Psyllium seeds (ground), oat and rice bran, oatmeal, barley, lentils, Brussels sprouts, peas, beans (kidney, lima, black, navy, pinto), apples, blackberries, pears, raisins, oranges, grapefruit, dates, figs, prunes, apricots, cantaloupe, strawberries, bananas, peaches, broccoli, carrots, cauliflower, cabbage, spinach, sweet potatoes, yams, white potatoes, tomatoes, avocado, raspberries, corn, almonds, ground flaxseed, sunflower seeds*

Low-quality carbs, on the other hand, cause an intense spike in blood sugar—it's quick and dramatic. These carbs trigger the highest highs, the Mount Everests of glucose levels. It is a long way down from the dizzying peak of surging blood sugar to your normal baseline. The steeper the drop, the worse you'll feel. That's why low-quality carbohydrates can lead to feeling irritable, depressed, sluggish, and foggy-headed. If you eat low-quality carbs regularly, your blood sugar won't have a chance to stabilize . . . and neither will your moods. That's why I recommend making sugary and refined foods an occasional treat, not a regular part of your diet. Try to limit the amount of these inferior carbs to no more than about 10 percent of your total daily calories. (See Weight Loss, page 19, for information on how to calculate and use calorie information.)

For an even keel all day, the majority of your daily diet should come from high-quality carbohydrates combined with protein. Protein is critical to moderating mood because it is the great stabilizer. It does not add to blood sugar. Instead, it helps slow the absorption of carbohydrates from the blood. That's why when it comes to a better mood, I recommend incorporating at least some protein into your meals whenever possible—breakfast, lunch, dinner, and snacks.

BEST FOODS FOR PROTEIN: *Turkey breast, chicken breast, seafood and fish, veal, pork tenderloin, lean ham, lean beef, egg whites, yogurt (fat-free, low-fat), milk (fat-free, 1% reduced-fat, skim plus), enriched/fortified soy milk, cheese (fat-free, reduced-fat), beans (lima, black, navy, pinto, garbanzo), lentils, split peas, tofu, tempeh, soybeans, nuts (soy nuts, peanuts, almonds), peanut butter*

FAQS

You say that protein is important for stabilizing blood sugar, but when I was on the Atkins diet, I felt terrible all the time. How come? Did I do something wrong?

Protein is important, but it is just one part of the mood-balancing equation. Protein must be combined with high-quality carbohydrates for the best possible mood-regulating results. Because carbs provide the blood sugar to give us energy and are needed for the conversion of tryptophan to serotonin in the brain, people who severely restrict their carbohydrates may end up feeling more irritable than usual, an effect I call low-carb crabbiness. Mix moderate amounts of high-quality carbohydrates with protein and you'll inevitably feel better.

OMEGA-3 FATTY ACIDS

In our diet-conscious society, *fat* has become a synonym for *bad*. But some fat in the body *and* in your diet is necessary for good health. For example, the type of polyunsaturated fat known as *omega-3 fatty acids* make up part of the structure of our brain membranes, and

FAQS

I've been taking an antidepressant for about a year, and I feel like my mood is back to normal. Can I stop taking the medication if I promise to eat right and take omega-3 supplements?

Please don't stop taking any medication without consulting your doctor. Clinical depression is a medical condition that should be taken seriously ... thank goodness your medicine is working! Good nutrition can help, but it may not be enough for everyone. At the very least, it can make anyone feel healthier and stronger. But if you're determined to get off the antidepressants, I recommend that you follow this plan (while continuing your medication) for a couple of months. Then, together with your doctor, make the decision about whether tapering off the medication is a good idea for you.

they seem to help brain cells use neurotransmitters more efficiently. So it makes sense that omega-3s seem to help regulate mood.

The relationship between depression and omega-3 fatty acids is complex and not completely understood. Studies have shown that people who are clinically depressed have low blood levels of omega-3s, but their mood did not improve when they took omega-3 supplements. *However* . . . when depressed people took omega-3s *along with* antidepressants, the supplements reduced depressive symptoms better than the medication alone. If you have been diagnosed with depression and would like to try a therapeutic dose of omega-3s, see the Supplements section, page 311.

For people with milder problems—let's call them *mood issues*—I recommend going the food route (although you can certainly consider supplements if you can't get enough omega-3s through food). I believe that foods rich in omega-3 fatty acids could help regulate brain function and level out everyday moods. Omega-3s are most abundant in fatty fish so I recommend eating one serving of fatty fish at least two or three times per week. My list includes only the fatty fish that have been shown to be low in mercury, PCBs, and dioxins.

BEST FOODS FOR OMEGA-3 FATTY ACIDS: *Wild salmon (fresh, canned), herring, mackerel (not king), sardines, anchovies, rainbow trout, Pacific oysters, omega-3–fortified eggs, flaxseed (ground and oil), walnuts, butternuts (white walnuts), seaweed, walnut oil, canola oil, soybeans*

VITAMIN D

In the past few years, research has suggested that vitamin D might help relieve mood disorders because it seems to increase levels of serotonin, one of the neurotransmitters responsible for mood. In particular, vitamin D seems to help the type of depression called *seasonal affective disorder* (SAD), or the winter blues. More than 10 million Americans are thought to suffer from SAD, leading to anxiety, fatigue, and feelings of sadness for three to six months of the year. Scientists believe this is due to the shortened days and limited sunlight of winter. You see, our bodies can make plenty of vitamin D on their own from sunlight. Just 10 to 15 minutes of sun on the bare skin of your arms three or four times a week is enough to keep most of us healthy. The problem is that sunlight isn't always safe—too much causes skin damage and premature aging, and may lead to skin cancer—and while using sunscreen protects your skin, it also prevents your body from making its own vitamin D. It becomes important, then, to get healthy amounts of vitamin D from the foods you eat and/or from supplements.

Scientists have discovered that people with SAD have normal blood levels of vitamin D in the summer, but that their levels drop by as much as one-third in winter. No wonder they feel moody and tired! Those who took vitamin D supplements for a year had stable blood levels, and most experienced a significant improvement in their depression. If you would like to try supplementation, see my guidelines for choosing a multivitamin on page 311. But everyone with minor depression and anxiety issues should strive to eat more foods rich in vitamin D to improve their mood profile.

BEST FOODS FOR VITAMIN D: *Wild salmon (with bones), mackerel (not king), sardines (with bones), herring, milk (fat-free, 1% reduced-fat), enriched/fortified soy milk, egg yolks, mushrooms (especially shiitake), fortified margarine (soft tub, trans fat–free), fortified whole grain cereals*

B VITAMINS: FOLATE AND B$_{12}$

Two B vitamins—folate and vitamin B$_{12}$—seem to be important for mood. Studies have shown that low blood levels of these vitamins are related to depression, although no one is exactly sure why. Some scientists believe that these vitamins are used by the body to create serotonin, which, as mentioned earlier, is one of the key neurotransmitters that help normalize mood. It would seem logical, then, that low intake of these vitamins would contribute to mood problems.

Research is coming close to showing exactly that. One study found that people who have low blood levels of folate have a higher risk of depression. Other studies tracked people who had been hospitalized for depression, and revealed that about 30 percent were deficient in vitamin B$_{12}$. When researchers tracked 700 women over age 65, they discovered that the women who had low blood levels of vitamin B$_{12}$ were twice as likely to be depressed as women who did not have a deficiency. In addition, researchers found that both vitamins seem to help depressed people respond better to antidepressant medications, which means that adding these B vitamin may help people suffering from depression feel better faster.

If you are clinically depressed, it is important to continue to follow your doctor's treatment recommendations, but you may want to consider taking a multivitamin with appropriate amounts of folate and B$_{12}$ (see Supplements section, page 311), in addition to your antidepressant medications. Of course, eating a diet rich in these nutrients is important for maintaining mood, even if you are not clinically depressed.

BEST FOODS FOR FOLATE: *Fortified whole grain cereal, lentils, black-eyed peas, soybeans, oatmeal, turnip greens, spinach, mustard greens, green peas, artichokes, okra, beets, parsnips, broccoli, broccoli raab, sunflower seeds, wheat germ, oranges and juice, Brussels sprouts, papaya, seaweed, berries (boysenberries, blackberries, strawberries), beans (black, pinto, kidney, garbanzo, navy), cauliflower, Chinese cabbage, corn, whole grain bread, pasta (preferably whole wheat)*

BEST FOODS FOR VITAMIN B₁₂: *Shellfish (clams, oysters, crab), wild salmon (fresh, canned), fortified whole grain cereal, enriched/fortified soy milk, trout (rainbow, wild), tuna (canned light), lean beef, veggie burgers, cottage cheese (fat-free, 1% reduced-fat), yogurt (fat-free, low-fat), milk (fat-free, 1% reduced-fat), eggs, cheese (fat-free, reduced-fat)*

BONUS POINTS

- **Eat consistently throughout the day.** If your blood sugar flags, your energy will fade and your mood can take a nasty turn, as well. You need to eat at least once every four to five hours in order to keep your brain well-fueled and happy. Some people who are extremely sensitive to frequent blood sugar dips may need to eat every three hours or so to keep from feeling that post-meal letdown. To keep from gaining weight, make absolutely sure the meals and snacks are calorie-controlled. And each meal and snack should contain a mix of high-quality carbohydrates and protein to best stabilize your blood sugar levels (see meal plans, page 317, for examples).

- **Exercise.** Too many people underestimate the benefits of exercise—it's not just for weight loss or fitness (although it is terrific for accomplishing those goals). Exercise can make you feel stronger, more confident, and more self-assured. That alone is enough to improve your overall mood. But exercise exerts other mood-enhancing effects: It raises blood levels of endorphins, those natural body chemicals that scientists believe might induce feelings of well-being. Plus, exercise improves blood flow, which means that the brain gets more oxygen, helping improve its function. Most studies that have looked at the effects of exercise on mood find that nearly any kind of exercise reduces anxiety, tension, stress, and feelings of depression. These amazing results are most powerful after several weeks of regular exercise, but research shows that mood can improve even on the first day of exercise.

  Researchers at the University of Texas Southwestern put people with mild to moderate depression on a exercise program—30 minutes three to five times per week for 12 weeks. The study participants who did a moderately intense workout on a treadmill or stationary bike reduced their depressive symptoms by nearly half, similar to what might be seen after starting antidepressant medications. Less intense exercisers reduced their symptoms by 30 percent—even those participants doing only stretching exercises reduced their symptoms by 29 percent.

  For mood improvement, then, my recommendation is to do some sort of exercise—any sort of exercise—at least three times per week, 30 minutes per session. The more your intense your workout, the more your mood will improve, so do what you can. Happiness really could be just around the corner . . . as long as you walk there!

- **Make time for your life.** Feeling frazzled, crazed, overextended, and overworked is a sure way to end up angry, anxious, or depressed . . . or all three. As impossible as it may seem, your family and friends may be your best "vaccine" against the daily stresses and strains that can wear us down. But it's not enough just to *have* family and friends, you have to make time to relax with them and enjoy the simple pleasures they can bring. On the same note, you need to find a way to enjoy your work. If you're like most people, you probably spend a minimum of eight hours a day at your job. That's one-third of your day, five days a week . . . and that's not counting your commute. If you hate what you do, it will eventually affect your emotions. I understand that not everyone can just quit a job or change careers, but everyone can learn to enjoy some aspect of their work (or at least meditate for relaxation). Alternatively, psychological counselors can help you develop a new set of responses to stressful circumstances, or to "reframe" how you think about them so that you can learn to enjoy something that you once found intolerable. If you're retired, then your challenge becomes finding ways to fill your days that are challenging and emotionally rewarding.

■ **An occasional cup of coffee may perk you up.** When many people feel low, they often turn to caffeine in cola, coffee, or tea. The problem is that it doesn't necessarily work. Researchers have studied and studied *and studied* caffeine, but there are no consistent results. Some researchers find that caffeine improves concentration and mood all the time. Others find that caffeine works only if you use it periodically, but stops working for mood improvement if you use it every day. Still other studies show that caffeine doesn't improve mood at all. This means that how you use caffeine is up to you. If you find that an occasional cup of coffee or tea helps you get through the day, there is no reason to deny yourself. But it doesn't work for everybody—if you find yourself becoming jittery or irritable after drinking caffeinated drink, try decaf instead.

SUPPLEMENTS

If you are concerned about mood and want to consider supplements *in addition to* the food fixes, here are some that might be beneficial:

1. **A multivitamin.** For mood concerns, I typically recommend a senior formula multivitamin. These formulations often provide higher amounts of folate and vitamin B_{12} compared to regular multivitamins. Simply look for a brand that contains at least 100% DV of vitamin D (400 IU) and folate (400 micrograms), and at least 6 micrograms of vitamin B_{12}.

2. **Fish oil.** If you find that you can't eat enough fatty fish or other foods to get your share of omega-3 fatty acids, you can always take fish oil capsules. I recommend taking 650 milligrams of omega-3s. (There are two sub-types of omega-3s called DHA [docosahexaenoic acid] and EPA [eicosapentaenoic acid]. When buying fish oil supplements, choose brands that contain at least 220 milligrams of DHA, and at least 220 milligrams of EPA. The remaining 200+ milligrams can come from either DHA or EPA. Check labels for these details).

   Doses of omega-3s greater than 3 grams (3,000 milligrams) per day are often used along with prescription antidepressants to treat clinical depression. I cannot recommend self-treatment at these doses, however. If you have been diagnosed with depression, talk with your doctor about whether you should add omega-3 fatty acid supplements to your treatment.

To prevent rancidity, always store bottles of fish oil supplements in the fridge. To lessen the chance of fishy burps or aftertaste, buy enteric-coated capsules, which are digested in your intestines instead of your stomach. Avoid getting omega-3 fats from cod liver oil because it may contain too much vitamin A.

3. **St. John's wort.** This herbal supplement, which seems to prolong the action of mood-stabilizing serotonin and other neurotransmitters in the brain, is a popular treatment for depression. Some scientific studies have demonstrated that St. John's wort works nearly as well as antidepressant medications for mild or moderate depression, although a few studies failed to find any benefits at all. (It is clear, however, that St. John's wort does not help people suffering from severe depression.)

    Just because St. John's wort is a natural herb doesn't necessarily mean it's safe. This is not a supplement to be taken casually—it is only recommended for people with documented depression because it has physiological effects that need to be monitored by a doctor. General side effects can include dry mouth, dizziness, fatigue, nausea, diarrhea, and sensitivity to sunlight. Like some prescription antidepressant medications, St. John's wort can have sexual side effects in some people, including an inability to become aroused or reach orgasm. It can also interact with many other medications, and can weaken oral contraceptives, which means that there may be an unintended pregnancy. So my advice is this: Please don't try this herb on your own—if you suffer from mild to moderate depression and want to try St. John's wort, talk with your doctor first.

4. **SAMe.** Another "natural" treatment for mild to moderate depression is SAMe (S-adenosylmethionine), an amino acid derivative. Because SAMe seems to increase the availability of dopamine and norepinephrine in the brain, it is thought to work similarly to some of the older antidepressant medications known as tricyclic antidepressants. Studies have shown that most people can take SAMe for up to two years with few side effects, and that it is pretty effective. Still, it is important to talk with your doctor before taking SAMe to make sure that your depression is being adequately treated. The usual recommended dose for depression is 400 to 800 milligrams twice a day. Be sure to look for the form of SAMe called *butanedisulfonate salt*—it is more stable and can be used more easily by the body. Here's the big drawback: the cost! SAMe can run $150 per month—much more expensive than a prescription for an antidepressant medication.

JOY'S 4-STEP PROGRAM
FOR MOOD

Follow this program if you find yourself feeling irritable, depressed, anxious, or angry more often than you would like.

STEP 1 ... START WITH THE BASICS

These are the first things you should do to take control of your moods.

- See your doctor if you have signs of depression that last longer than two weeks, including sadness, hopelessness, difficulty concentrating, a change in weight, or a change in sleep patterns.

- Limit the amount of sugary treats and refined foods you eat.

- Eat a small meal or snack at least once every four or five hours. Add a little protein to every meal and snack to avoid huge swings in blood sugar.

STEP2 ... YOUR ULTIMATE GROCERY LIST

A nutrition plan is only as good as the foods that you choose. This list contains high levels of nutrients that contribute to mood, plus some foods used as ingredients in the meal plans and recipes. You don't have to purchase every item . . . but these foods should make up the bulk of what you eat for the week. If you find yourself getting bored, try some unfamiliar foods from these groups—they may become favorites.

FRUIT

ALL fruits, but especially:	Berries (boysenberries, blackberries, raspberries, strawberries)	Dates	Papaya
Apples		Figs	Peaches
Apricots		Grapefruit	Pears
Bananas	Cantaloupe	Oranges (and orange juice)	Prunes
			Raisins

VEGETABLES

ALL vegetables, but especially:	Brussels sprouts	Mushrooms (especially shiitake)	Potatoes, sweet
Artichokes	Cabbage (including Chinese)	Mustard greens	Potatoes, white
Avocado	Carrots	Okra	Scallions
Beans (black, pinto, kidney, garbanzo, navy, lima)	Cauliflower	Onions (red, white, or yellow)	Seaweed
	Celery		Soybeans (edamame)
	Chickpeas (garbanzo beans)	Parsnips	Spinach
Beets	Corn	Peas (black-eyed, split)	Tomatoes
Broccoli	Cucumber	Peas (green)	Turnip greens
Broccoli raab	Lentils	Pepper, bell (red/green/yellow)	Yams
			Zucchini

SEAFOOD

ALL seafood and fish, but especially:	Salmon, wild (fresh, canned)	Shellfish (clams, oysters [especially Pacific], crab)
Anchovies	Sardines, canned (with bones)	Trout, rainbow
Herring		
Mackerel (not king)	Sea bass	Tuna (canned light)

LEAN MEATS/EGGS/SOY FOODS

Beef, lean	Ham, lean	Tofu	Turkey breast
Chicken breast	Ostrich burger	Turkey (lean ground)	Veal
Eggs (preferably omega-3–fortified)	Pork tenderloin	Turkey bacon, reduced-fat	Veggie burgers
	Tempeh		

NUTS AND SEEDS (PREFERABLY UNSALTED)

Almonds	Flaxseed, ground	Psyllium seeds, ground	Walnuts
Butternuts (white walnuts)	Peanut butter	Soy nuts	
	Peanuts	Sunflower seeds	

WHOLE GRAINS

Amaranth	Cereal, fortified whole grain	Pasta (preferably whole wheat)	Tortillas (whole grain)
Barley	Millet	Quinoa	Waffles, whole grain
Breads, whole grain (including crackers, pitas, English muffins)	Oat bran	Rice (brown, wild)	Wheat berries
	Oatmeal	Rice bran	Wheat germ

DAIRY

Cheese (fat-free, reduced-fat)	reduced-fat Cheddar, Parmesan	Cream cheese (fat-free)	Soy milk, fortified/ enriched
Cheese (for the meal plans): fat-free or	Cottage cheese (fat-free, 1% reduced-fat)	Milk, vitamin D– fortified (fat-free, 1% reduced-fat)	Yogurt (fat-free, low-fat)

MISCELLANEOUS

Artificial sweetener	Margarine spread, vitamin D–fortified, soft tub, trans fat–free	Oil, olive	Soup, lentil (low-fat)
Broth, chicken, low-sodium		Oil, walnut	Soup, vegetable or vegetable barley (low-fat)
Broth, vegetable, low-sodium		Parsley, fresh	
Cinnamon	Mayonnaise, reduced-fat	Salad dressing, raspberry vinaigrette, reduced-calorie	Sugar, brown
Garlic	Nonstick cooking spray	Salsa	Sugar substitute
Honey	Oil, canola	Salt substitute	Vinegar, balsamic or red wine
Hummus	Oil, flaxseed		

STEP3 ...GOING ABOVE AND BEYOND

If you want to do everything you can to improve your mood, here are some additional things you might try:

- Consider taking a multivitamin to make certain you get the recommended amounts of most nutrients necessary for a good mood, specifically a brand with 100% DV for vitamin D, folate, and B_{12}.

- Take 650 milligrams of fish oil supplements daily if you don't eat fatty fish and/or other omega-3–rich foods at least three times per week. Look for brands that contain at least 220 milligrams EPA, *and* at least 220 milligrams DHA.

- Add some sort of exercise to your weekly routine. Start with 30 minutes of any sort of exercise, at least three times a week. As you become comfortable with your routine, increase the intensity and length of your workout.

- If you have been diagnosed with depression, ask your doctor if St. John's wort or SAMe might be a good treatment option for you.

- Schedule downtime to spend with family and friends as actively as you schedule your work responsibilities.

- Take up a relaxing hobby, such as meditation or yoga.

GET MOVING FOR YOUR MOOD

We know exercise can help improve mood, but if you're feeling depressed, just getting up off the couch can be a major achievement. Here are some tips for turning exercise into a happy habit:

- Set up a pre-exercise routine, an unvarying sequence of events you do before starting. The prep helps signal your body that exercise is on the way.

- Do *something*. If the thought of a half hour of walking sucks your energy, then commit to walking for only five minutes. The first minutes are always the toughest. You'll usually find that if you can walk for five minutes, the next 25 minutes are no problem.

- Plan to exercise in the morning, so you have no chance to come up with excuses later.

- Invest in an MP3 player so you can listen to—and be energized by—your favorite music while exercising.

- Remember, the couch isn't going anywhere—let it be your reward for activity, instead of your excuse for avoidance.

STEP4 ...MEAL PLANS

These sample menus include some of the best mood foods—meals which incorporate both high quality carbohydrate and lean protein, and are rich in omega-3 fats, vitamin D, folate, B₁₂, and soluble fiber. Every day, choose *one* option for each of the three meals— breakfast, lunch, and dinner. When needed, choose from a variety of my suggested snacks. Be sure to eat consistently throughout the day—every four to five hours—to avoid potential blood sugar dips.

Approximate calories have been provided to help adjust for your personal weight management goals. If you find yourself hungry (and if weight is not an issue), feel free to increase the portion sizes for meals and snacks. Beverage calories are *not* included. Also, I strongly suggest a daily multivitamin-mineral to ensure you're getting adequate amounts of vitamin D.

BREAKFAST OPTIONS

(Approximately 300 to 400 calories)

Cereal with Nuts, Wheat Germ, and Fresh Fruit

1 cup whole grain fortified cereal mixed with 1 cup fat-free milk (or enriched/fortified soy milk) topped with 1 tablespoon chopped walnuts and 1 tablespoon wheat germ. Enjoy with 1 orange (or ½ grapefruit).

Breakfast Burrito

Scramble 1 omega-3–fortified egg with 2 egg whites on griddle coated with nonstick cooking spray; mix with ¼ cup black beans and 2 tablespoons shredded fat-free or reduced-fat cheese. Wrap in 1 whole grain or spinach tortilla (150 calories or less), adding optional onion, salsa, and/or hot sauce.

Banana-Berry Cottage Cheese with Almonds

1 cup fat-free or 1% reduced-fat cottage cheese (or fat-free flavored yogurt) mixed with ½ sliced banana, ½ cup chopped strawberries, and 1 tablespoon slivered almonds.

Apple-Cinnamon Oatmeal

½ cup dry oatmeal prepared with 1 cup fat-free milk (microwave for 1½ to 2 minutes); mix with 1 chopped apple and microwave for an additional 30 seconds. Sprinkle with optional cinnamon plus 1 teaspoon brown sugar, white sugar, or honey (or artificial sweetener).

Scrambled Eggs, Tomato, and Spinach with Toast

Beat 1 omega-3–fortified egg with 2 egg whites. Cook in a hot skillet coated with nonstick cooking spray, adding 2 tablespoons chopped tomato and unlimited spinach.

Serve with toasted whole grain English muffin (or 2 slices whole wheat toast), dry or with 1 to 2 teaspoons soft tub, trans fat–free margarine spread.

Waffles Topped with Yogurt and Berries

2 frozen whole grain waffles, toasted and topped with 1 cup fat-free flavored yogurt and ½ cup berries (or ½ sliced banana).

Hard-Boiled Eggs with Turkey Bacon and Fruit

2 hard-boiled omega-3–fortified eggs, 2 strips reduced-fat turkey bacon, and 3 prunes (or 1 orange or ½ grapefruit).

LUNCH OPTIONS

(Approximately 400 to 500 calories)

Wild Salmon Salad over Greens

1 serving Wild Salmon Salad (page 322), or drain and mash 6 ounces canned Alaskan salmon and mix with 2 teaspoons reduced-fat mayonnaise and minced onion. Serve over a bed of romaine lettuce or spinach leaves with 100 calories of whole grain crackers or a 70-calorie whole wheat pita.

Turkey Sandwich with Baby Carrots

4 ounces sliced turkey breast (or lean ham or grilled chicken breast) with unlimited romaine lettuce or spinach, sliced tomato, and onion on 2 slices whole grain bread or pita, plus optional 1 slice reduced-fat cheese, mustard, 2 teaspoons reduced-fat mayonnaise, or hummus). Serve with a large handful baby carrots.

Spinach-Cheese Omelet with Vegetable Salad

Beat 1 omega-3–fortified egg with 2 to 3 egg whites. Cook in heated skillet coated with nonstick cooking spray. When bottom is cooked, gently flip over. Top with unlimited raw or cooked spinach and 1 ounce reduced-fat or fat-free cheese. Fold omelet over and cook until egg mixture is firm and cheese melts. Enjoy with mixed salad greens topped with sliced beets and 1 tablespoon toasted walnuts (or sunflower seeds), 2 teaspoons olive oil and unlimited balsamic vinegar or fresh lemon juice (or 2 to 4 tablespoons reduced-calorie dressing).

Baked Potato with Broccoli and Cheese

1 baked potato topped with steamed or boiled chopped broccoli and 1 ounce melted reduced-fat or fat-free cheese. Serve with 1 cup Vegetable Oatmeal Bisque (page 323) or any prepared vegetable soup.

Grilled Chicken Vegetable Salad

4 ounces grilled skinless chicken breast on large bed of mixed greens (romaine, spinach, mustard greens, endive), topped with ½ cup cherry tomatoes, sliced beets, 1 chopped sweet pepper (red, yellow, or green), artichoke hearts, and ½ cup chickpeas (garbanzo beans), soybeans, or any other type of beans. Toss with 2 teaspoons olive oil and unlimited vinegar or fresh lemon juice (or 2 to 4 tablespoons reduced-calorie dressing).

Yogurt with Fruit, Wheat germ, Nuts, and Seeds

1 cup fat-free vanilla yogurt mixed with ½ chopped apple (or pear), ½ banana, and ½ cup berries (or orange, grapefruit, peach, raisins, papaya, dates, figs, or prunes), plus 2 tablespoons wheat germ, 1 tablespoon sunflower seeds, and 1 tablespoon chopped walnuts.

Peanut Butter Toast with Lentil Soup

1 slice toasted whole grain bread topped with 1 level tablespoon peanut butter. Serve with 2 cups lentil soup (or any other non-creamy bean soup).

DINNER OPTIONS

(Approximately 500 to 600 calories)

Grilled Wild Salmon with Brussels Sprouts and Brown Rice

5 ounces grilled wild salmon (or flounder, sole, or shrimp). Serve with 1 to 2 cups Brussels sprouts and ½ cup cooked brown rice tossed with 1 tablespoon slivered almonds.

Pork Tenderloin with Black-Eyed Peas and Cauliflower

5 ounces baked, grilled, or broiled pork tenderloin. Serve with 1 cup cooked black-eyed peas and 1 to 2 cups cooked cauliflower or Brussels sprouts.

Whole Wheat Pasta with Sea Bass and Green Peas

1 serving Whole Wheat Penne with Sea Bass and Pea Sauce (page 324). Serve with a side salad of leafy greens, beets, carrots, and 1 tablespoon chopped walnuts tossed with 2 teaspoons olive oil and vinegar or fresh lemon juice (or 2 to 4 tablespoons reduced-calorie dressing).

Vegetable Bisque with Grilled Chicken and Sautéed Spinach

2 servings (2 cups) Vegetable Oatmeal Bisque (page 323) or any prepared brand plain vegetable or vegetable-barley soup. Enjoy with 5 ounces grilled chicken breast topped with unlimited spinach sautéed in 1 teaspoon olive oil and crushed garlic.

Cheddar Burger with Sliced Tomato and Onion over Greens

1 (5-ounce) turkey burger, ostrich burger, or veggie burger topped with 1 ounce melted reduced-fat cheese and sliced tomato and onion (no bun) on a bed of unlimited leafy greens (lettuce, spinach, mustard greens, turnip greens) tossed with 2 tablespoons reduced-calorie vinaigrette. Serve with 1 cup boiled edamame (soybeans in the pod) lightly sprinkled with optional salt or salt substitute.

Chopped Chicken Salad with Apples and Walnuts

1 serving Chopped Chicken Salad with Apples and Walnuts (page 325).

Turkey Chili with Brown Rice and Salad

2 cups Turkey Chili (page 367) topped with 1 ounce shredded fat-free Cheddar cheese. Serve with ½ cup cooked brown rice (or amaranth or quinoa) and salad of leafy greens (and optional peppers, carrots, beets, and artichokes) tossed with 1 teaspoon olive oil and unlimited balsamic vinegar or fresh lemon juice (or 2 tablespoons reduced-calorie dressing).

SNACK OPTIONS

100 calories or less

Choose any one of the protein foods, *and* couple with any one of the high-quality carbohydrate foods for an ideal mood combination snack:

- **Protein foods** (choose one): ½ cup fat-free milk, ¼ cup plain fat-free yogurt, 2 tablespoons Parmesan cheese, 1 slice fat-free cheese, 2 tablespoon fat-free cream cheese, ¼ cup fat-free or 1% reduced-fat cottage cheese, 1 ounce sliced turkey (or ham or chicken), 5 almonds, 1 teaspoon peanut butter, or 2 hard-boiled egg whites

- **High-quality carbohydrate foods** (choose one): 1 cup raw or cooked turnip greens, mustard greens, spinach, artichokes, broccoli, broccoli raab, Brussels sprouts, seaweed, cauliflower, cabbage, carrots, okra, beets, or parsnips; 1 orange; ½ apple; ½ pear; ½ cup blueberries, blackberries, raspberries, or boysenberries; 10 strawberries; 1 to 2 tablespoons raisins; 2 dates, 1 fig; 2 prunes; 2 apricots; ¼ melon; ½ banana; 1 peach; ½ papaya; ½ grapefruit

Other great combination snacks:

- 1 level tablespoon peanut butter with celery sticks

- 6 ounces fat-free, flavored or plain yogurt

- 10 almonds, unsalted

- Skim café latte or cappuccino (decaffeinated, if caffeine makes you jittery or if you have PMS or insomnia)

- Handful baby carrots and 2 level tablespoons hummus
- 1 cup Vegetable Oatmeal Bisque (page 323)

100 to 200 calories

- 10 almonds with 1 apple
- ¼ cup walnuts, lightly toasted
- ¼ cup sunflower seeds in the shell
- ½ cup fat-free or 1% reduced-fat cottage cheese mixed with 2 tablespoons wheat germ
- 1 slice whole grain toast with 1 level tablespoon peanut butter (or 2 ounces turkey, ham, or chicken)
- ½ cup dry fortified whole grain cereal with ½ cup fat-free milk
- 1 cup fat-free plain yogurt mixed with ½ cup berries and 1 tablespoon wheat germ
- ½ cup chickpeas (garbanzo beans)
- Handful baby carrots with ¼ cup hummus
- 1 sliced apple with 1 level tablespoon peanut butter
- 1 frozen banana with 1 cup fat-free milk. (For frozen banana, peel banana, slice into several ½" wheels, place in a small plastic bag, and freeze.)
- Fruit smoothie: in a blender, mix 1 cup fat-free milk, 1 cup frozen strawberries, ½ frozen banana.

WILD SALMON SALAD

Everybody seems to have a favorite tuna salad recipe, but it is just as easy to create fabulous salads using canned salmon, which has much more omega-3 fatty acids. This recipe can also be made using leftover fresh salmon. Serve over a bed of lettuce, or in a sandwich with whole wheat bread.

Makes 3 servings, about 1 cup each

1	can (6 ounces) wild Alaskan salmon, well drained (remove skin)
1	can (19 ounces) chickpeas (garbanzo beans), rinsed and drained
1/2	cup chopped red onion
1/2	red bell pepper, chopped
2	tablespoons extra-virgin olive oil
2	tablespoon red wine vinegar

In a medium bowl, mash the salmon. Mix in the chickpeas, onion, and red pepper. In a separate bowl, whisk together the oil and vinegar. Pour the dressing over the salmon mixture and stir thoroughly. Cover and refrigerate up to 2 days.

PER SERVING
339 calories, 19 g protein, 33 g carbohydrate, 14 g fat (2 g saturated), 26 mg cholesterol, 60 mg sodium, 9 g fiber; plus 203 mg folic acid (50+% DV), 2 mg vitamin B_{12} (35% DV), and lots of Omega 3s and Vitamin D from the salmon

VEGETABLE OATMEAL BISQUE

You're probably thinking that veggies and oatmeal are one strange combination! But I promise, this hearty soup is easy to make and one of my most favorite (and filling!) low-calorie recipes. For less than 100 calories, you'll get plenty of high-quality carbohydrate, fiber, and folate. Plus, you'll have lots of leftovers for the next few days.

Makes 10 servings, 1 cup each

1	bag (16 ounces) frozen broccoli florets
1	bag (16 ounces) frozen cauliflower florets
1	bag (16 ounces) fresh baby carrots
1	zucchini, peeled and chopped
½	chopped medium onion
6	cups low-fat, reduced-sodium chicken broth
	Salt or salt substitute
	Ground black pepper
1	cup traditional oatmeal (not quick-cooking)

1. In a large pot over medium-high heat, combine the broccoli, cauliflower, carrots, zucchini, onion, broth, and salt (or salt substitute) and pepper to taste. Cover and bring to a boil. Reduce the heat and simmer, stirring occasionally, 1 hour.

2. Add the oatmeal and mix thoroughly. Simmer, stirring occasionally, 40 minutes longer. With an immersion blender or in a food processor or blender, puree the soup. Serve hot.

PER SERVING
86 calories, 6 g protein, 16 g carbohydrate, 0 g fat, 0 mg cholesterol, 386 mg sodium, 4 g fiber

WHOLE WHEAT PENNE
WITH SEA BASS AND PEA SAUCE

This meal tastes as decadent as it sounds . . . but it is low in calories and simple to prepare. If you prefer, substitute shrimp or wild salmon for the sea bass.

Makes 8 servings (1½ to 2 cups per serving)

1	package (16 ounces) whole wheat penne (or other preferred shape)
4	tablespoons extra-virgin olive oil
½	medium onion, chopped
2	cups fresh or thawed frozen peas
2	cups low-sodium vegetable broth,
	Salt
	Ground black pepper
¾	pound sea bass, cut into ½" dice
4	plum tomatoes, peeled, seeded, and diced
1	teaspoon chopped fresh parsley

1. Cook the pasta in a large pot of boiling water 8 minutes, until al dente. Drain and keep warm.
2. Meanwhile, in a saucepan, heat 1 tablespoon oil over medium-low heat. Add the onion and cook about 3 minutes, until softened. Add the peas and broth, and bring the mixture to boil. Simmer for 5 minutes. Working in two batches, transfer the broth mixture to a blender or food processor, and puree. Return to the saucepan, and season with salt and pepper to taste, and keep warm.
3. Heat the remaining 3 tablespoons oil in a large skillet over moderate heat. Add the sea bass and cook, stirring, 2 minutes, until almost cooked through. With a slotted spoon, transfer sea bass to a bowl. Add the tomatoes to the skillet and cook for 5 minutes. Return the sea bass to the skillet, and season with salt and pepper to taste. Add the cooked pasta and toss to coat.
4. To serve, ladle some of the warm pea sauce into each serving dish and mound some of the sea bass and pasta on top. Garnish with parsley.

PER SERVING
359 calories, 18 g protein, 51 g carbohydrate, 9 g fat (1 g saturated), 17 mg cholesterol, 520 mg sodium, 8 g fiber

CHOPPED CHICKEN SALAD WITH APPLES AND WALNUTS

This salad is delicious, and provides generous amounts of protein, high-quality carbs, soluble fiber, and 80 percent of your daily requirement for folate.

Makes 1 serving

1	to 2 cups chopped romaine lettuce
4	to 5 ounces chicken breast, cooked, cooled, and chopped
½	cup canned chickpeas (garbanzo beans)
½	medium Fuji or McIntosh apple (with skin), chopped
¼	cup chopped cucumber (with peel)
¼	cup chopped tomato
¼	cup chopped avocado
¼	cup chopped celery
2	scallions, finely chopped
1	tablespoon chopped walnuts
2	to 4 tablespoons reduced-calorie raspberry vinaigrette

Place the lettuce in a large bowl. Add the chicken, chickpeas, apple, cucumber, tomato, avocado, celery, scallions, and walnuts. Drizzle with the vinaigrette and toss to coat.

PER SERVING
569 calories, 44 g protein, 53 g carbohydrate, 23 g fat (2.5 g saturated), 91 mg cholesterol, 700 mg sodium, 14 g fiber; plus 320 mcg folate (80% DV)

CHAPTER 14

MIGRAINE HEADACHES

One of my friends describes her migraines as a pain storm that splits her skull across her right temple, liquefying her brain until it feels like it's oozing out through her ears. The sound of a phone ringing is like a cartoon frying pan slamming the top of her head. Bright light is like a paintball gun filled with needles shot straight through her eyeballs. Once they strike, these intense, throbbing headaches last anywhere from a few hours to three days. For however long the migraine lasts, all she can do is take rescue medication, lie in a darkened room, and wait for the incapacitating pain to resolve.

About one of every ten Americans has had at least one migraine. Some experience an *aura* that presages the coming pain. An aura is typically some unusual visual experience, such as blind spots, distortion, jagged lines running through the visual field, sparkling or flashing lights, or enhanced color or depth perception. But some auras can cause a feeling of pins-and-needles in arms or legs, speech difficulties, excessive thirst, sleepiness, food cravings, or unexplained mood changes, particularly feelings of depression and irritability. More often, however, there is no warning before the pain sets in.

Migraine headaches usually start on one side, but often spread and encompass the other hemisphere too. During an episode, most migraine sufferers become extremely

I've figured out how to avoid my trigger foods at home, but eating out seems like a chore. Do you have any guidelines for foods to avoid, or foods that are safe to eat in restaurants?

It's safest to avoid the following: cheap buffets that leave food sitting and use suspect ingredients; Chinese food due to added MSG and soy sauce; Japanese food due to soy sauce, tofu, and miso; Mexican food due to the assortment of dishes with beans, cheese, and sour cream (and guacamole!). Your safest bets are high-quality American, seafood, or Italian restaurants. My suggestions for relatively safe ordering include:

- Grilled chicken or fish (request no MSG or vinegar, and ensure the dish does not contain citrus juice)
- Steamed or sautéed vegetables in olive oil and garlic with a plain baked potato (or sweet potato or rice, preferably brown)
- Pasta with broccoli and grilled chicken tossed in an olive oil–based sauce
- For dessert, a non-chocolate treat like strawberries with whipped cream, rice pudding, or herbal tea with plain biscotti

sensitive to light and sound, and some may vomit or feel nauseated. Migraines can come just once or twice a year, or several times each month. My friend used to get migraines three times a week. Working with her doctor she was able to find the right preventive medication, and cut the frequency by half. A real improvement, but that still meant six migraines a month. Then, after identifying and eliminating food triggers from her diet, the number fell to about one or two.

You're probably thinking, "That's great for her, but how much pain relief can *I* expect?" Unfortunately, no one can say with any certainty. Everyone has different triggers, so what worked for my friend may have no effect on you. However, everything mentioned in this chapter helps some people. I recommend that you try everything, keep what works . . . and never lose hope that you'll someday be able to avoid or control your headaches.

WHAT AFFECTS MIGRAINE HEADACHES?

Migraines are a mystery. Scientists don't know precisely what causes them or what exactly happens in the body once a migraine is triggered. They believe that there is a genetic component, and that the headaches are a result of abnormal functions in certain brain structures. Early research suggested that migraine headaches were caused solely by changes in the way blood vessels in the head dilated and constricted. Now, scientists understand that while blood vessels are part of the migraine process, they are just one event in a cascade of events. For example, we know from brain scans that during migraine headaches there is increased blood flow in the brain stem and the cerebral cortex. Inflammatory chemicals, such as substance P, and other substances are released; nerve centers are stimulated; and there are changes in levels of brain chemicals called neurotransmitters. The main lessons are that migraines are physiologically complex, and that they absolutely, positively are not "all in the mind" of the sufferer.

But for our purposes, the more important questions are: What sets off the headache in the first place? And, Can it be stopped? Migraines are triggered by specific factors, many of which are understood . . . but what triggers one person's headache may not affect you in the least. The most common triggers are:

Foods. Many everyday foods are big, *big* triggers. I provide a specific list in the next section.

Stress. When we are stressed, our bodies react physically—muscles tense, hormones become elevated, and migraines can be triggered.

Hormonal changes. Because estrogen and progesterone are such potent migraine triggers, women are nearly three times more likely than men to experience migraines. In fact, there is a subset of headache known as the *menstrual migraine,* which can occur one or two days before the start of a woman's period, or during the first day or two of her period. Women with hormone triggers can take comfort in knowing that many women whose migraines are primarily menstrual find that they get complete relief after menopause.

Intense sensory stimuli. Bright light, loud noises, and strong smells—such as cleaning chemicals, cigarette smoke, raw onions, and perfume—can trigger migraines.

Physical exertion or abrupt lifestyle changes. Jumping into an extreme exercise program can cause migraines, as can sexual activity, changing sleep patterns, alternating work shifts, or anything else that breaks your body out of its normal rhythms. If you push yourself in a demanding job all week long, you'll be more likely to get a migraine when you finally slow down over the weekend. On the flip side, if you enjoy a weekend with a little too much fun, you may develop a Monday migraine.

Environmental factors. Some people get migraines when there are changes in the air . . . literally. Their headaches coincide with the arrival of thunderstorms, sudden changes in altitude or barometric pressure, wind storms, seasonal changes, pollen levels. Others are sensitive to the switch to daylight savings time or travel across time zones.

Medications. Medications can have a wide range of side effects, so it is no surprise that some can cause migraines. You need to be especially wary of antihistamines, decongestants, blood pressure medications, oral contraceptives, hormone replacement therapy, and prescription pain medications. Interestingly, migraines can also be triggered if you stop taking prescription or over-the-counter pain medications (such as aspirin, acetaminophen, or ibuprofen), a phenomenon called rebound.

Some neurologists believe that all those trigger factors can be additive. They theorize that everybody has a tolerance limit for triggers, and once that limit is exceeded, a migraine is in the near future. If you have extreme sensitivity, then a single mild trigger may be enough to cause a headache. But if you have a greater tolerance, it may take two or three triggers occurring in close succession to push you past that limit. So you may be just fine if you have to use strong-smelling cleaning products. But if you clean, and then a thunderstorm hits, that combination of triggers may be enough to send you over the top. That's why it is critical to try to eliminate as many potential "controllable" triggers from your life as possible.

HOW FOOD AFFECTS MIGRAINE HEADACHES

The most important role food plays in migraines is as a trigger. Not all the foods on my list will cause migraines in all sufferers, and some people have no food sensitivities. In order to determine what your particular triggers are, I recommend keeping a migraine diary for at least three months (see page 333). If you discover that one of the foods listed here is a trigger for you, then you know that you should avoid that particular food if you want to remain pain free.

It's important to remember, however, that you and your migraines are unique; what causes headaches for someone else might be perfectly safe for you. Don't eliminate foods permanently without confirming that they are triggers . . . many of the foods on this list contain healthful nutrients.

NUTRIENTS AND FOODS TO AVOID . . .

■ *Chocolate, cheese, and other foods containing* **tyramine** *or* **phenylethylamine.** Although many other foods contain these 2 amino acids, the following specific foods can often be powerful migraine triggers: chocolate (and anything made with cocoa), aged or fermented cheeses (including Cheddar, bleu, brie, and all hard cheeses and "moldy" cheese), yogurt, sour cream, buttermilk, soy products (including tofu, tempeh, miso, and foods made with soy protein/isolate), soy sauce, red wine vinegar and balsamic vinegar (including salad dressings, and condiments made with vine-

POSSIBLE TRIGGER FOODS: THE ANTI-GROCERY LIST

I tell my new migraine clients to eliminate every potential food trigger from their diets for at least one month. Note whether your migraines improve. Then, add back one food at a time . . . no more than one new food every two days. If you get a migraine within 24 hours of eating the add-back food, stop eating it again. (When you get through the whole list, you can always test it again if it is a particular favorite.)

FRUIT
Apple juice and cider
Apples (red-skinned only)
Bananas
Citrus fruits (oranges, grapefruit, lemons, limes, tangerines, clementines, pineapple)
Citrus juice (orange, grapefruit, lemonade, pineapple, and other citrus blends)
Dried fruits (including apricots, figs, prunes, dates)
Grapes (and grape juice)
Papaya
Passion fruit
Pears (red-skinned only)
Plums, red
Raisins
Raspberries

VEGETABLES
Avocado
Beans (fava, lima, navy, broad beans, lentils)
Canned tomato sauce
Canned vegetables
Eggplant
Onions (can be used for flavoring, but not to eat)
Peas
Pickles
Relish

Sauerkraut
Snow peas
Tomatoes (not often)

FISH
ALL cured, smoked, canned, pickled, or aged fish
Anchovies
Caviar
Lox
Pickled herring
Sardines

MEATS
ALL cured, smoked, canned, pickled, or aged meats
Bacon (including beef, pork, and turkey)
Beef (all cured, smoked, canned, pickled, or aged)
Beef jerky
Bologna (including beef, turkey, and low-fat)
Chicken (all cured, smoked, canned, pickled, or aged)
Corned beef
Deli meats (cured or smoked)
Ham (canned, cured, smoked, pickled, or aged)
Hot dogs (including chicken, turkey, and soy)
Liver and liverwurst
Organ meats (such as kidneys or liver)
Pastrami

gar), sauerkraut, relish, pickles, breads made with yeast extracts (including fresh baked bread, bagels, doughnuts, sourdough, pizza dough, soft pretzels, and coffee cake), organ meats (including liver, kidney, and pates), processed meats and fish (any smoked, pickled, cured, aged, or canned), beans (specifically lima, fava, navy, Italian or broad, and lentils), all nuts (including peanuts, cashews, almonds, and nut butters), seeds (specifically pumpkin, sunflower, and sesame), eggplant, avocado, onions, citrus fruits (pineapple, oranges, grapefruit, lemons, limes, tangerines, and clementines—and all of their juices), bananas, grapes, raisins, plums, papaya, passion fruit, and raspberries.

- **Alcohol.** Beer, red wine, sherry, and vermouth contain large amounts of tyramine, which can cause migraines. In addition, all alcohol can cause dehydration, which also can trigger headaches.

MEATS *(cont.)*
Pâté
Pepperoni
Pork (all cured, smoked, canned, pickled, or aged)
Salami
Sausages (including beef, chicken, turkey, and soy)
Turkey (all cured, smoked, canned, pickled, or aged)
Turkey jerky

SOY
Miso
Products made with soy protein isolate (check labels!)
Soy sauce (including reduced-sodium)
Tempeh
Tofu

NUTS AND SEEDS
All nuts
All nut butters
Seeds (pumpkin, sesame, sunflower)

DAIRY
Aged cheese (including Cheddar, bleu, Brie, Camembert, Parmesan, Gouda, Gruyère, mozzarella, provolone, Romano, Roquefort, Swiss, Stilton, and all other aged or "moldy" cheeses)
Buttermilk
Chocolate ice cream
Chocolate milk

Chocolate pudding
Foods prepared with cheese (check labels)
Sour cream
Yogurt

GRAINS
Bagels
Baked goods with yeast extracts (doughnuts, coffee cake)
Yeast bread, freshly baked

MISCELLANEOUS
Additives (check labels and avoid if products have MSG, HVP, HPP, kombu extract, or natural flavorings)
Alcohol (especially beer, red wine, sherry, and vermouth)
Chocolate
Cocoa
Coffee
Diet beverages/products that use the artificial sweetener aspartame (also known as NutraSweet and Equal)
Soft drinks (Red Bull, Mountain Dew, Coke, and others; check label for caffeine)
Tea (green and black)
Vinegar (especially balsamic and red wine vinegar, including salad dressings and condiments made with these vinegars)
Yeast extract

- **Avoid eating leftovers:** Because tyramine content increases over time, *especially* if food is improperly stored, avoid eating leftovers containing any of the "off limit" foods.
- *Tea, red skinned apples and pears, apple juice and cider, coffee, and red wine, which contain* **tannins**.
- *Deli meats and other food containing* **nitrites**. These include pepperoni, bacon, hot dogs, sausages (including chicken, turkey and soy sausages/bacon/hotdogs that list nitrites in their ingredients), bologna, pastrami, jerky (beef and turkey), corned beef, and all other beef/poultry/pork/wild game/fish that have been cured, smoked, pickled, canned, or preserved with nitrites.
- *Wine and other foods containing* **sulfites**. This preservative is commonly found in wine (more so in red), most dried fruits are typically preserved with sulfites (including prunes, figs, apricots, etc.), canned vegetables, and many processed foods.
- **Additives.** Check labels carefully and avoid foods that contain monosodium glutamate (MSG), hydrolyzed vegetable protein (HVP), hydrolyzed plant protein (HPP), kombu extract, any products claiming to have "natural flavor" or "natural flavorings."
- **Aspartame.** Can trigger migraines in some people. Avoid all foods made with this artificial sweetener (also known as Nutrasweet and Equal).
- **Caffeine.** People with sensitivity to caffeine can develop migraines after drinking black tea, green tea, coffee, cola soft drinks, or other caffeinated soft drinks. But caffeine can also be used to stop a migraine that is just beginning—that's why many over-the-counter migraine medications contain caffeine. Test your personal response to caffeine. If it gives you headaches, avoid it. Otherwise, try drinking one cup of coffee or two cups of strong black tea at the start of your next migraine to see if it helps. In 2005, German researchers reported that when people took a combination of 250 milligrams of aspirin, 200 milligrams of acetaminophen, and 50 milligrams of caffeine (an average 8-ounce mug of coffee has 100 milligrams caffeine) at the start of their migraines, they had better and faster pain relief than people who did not take the caffeine.

NUTRIENTS AND FOODS THAT MAY REDUCE MIGRAINE FREQUENCY

The list of potential trigger foods seems long, I know, but remember it's just a list of possibilities—most likely, when you're done systemically eliminating and then reintroducing these foods, you will find there are just a few things you need avoid. Now for the good news—some nutrients you should try to eat more often:

LIQUIDS

Dehydration is a common migraine trigger. When everyone seems to be rushing from house to work to meeting to the gym and back home again without much thought to food or drink, migraine sufferers need to stay hyper-vigilant about how much liquid they drink. While the latest government guidelines say that most people can allow thirst to guide how much they drink, migraine sufferers should aim to pre-empt thirst. Try to drink about nine

8-ounce cups of liquid a day if you're a woman, or about thirteen 8-ounce cups a day if you're a man. Eight ounces is a lot less than you think! I ask my clients to fill their favorite drinking glass with water, then transfer to a liquid-measuring cup to see exactly how many ounces they drink each time they fill the glass. Please remember that water is the single best way to stay hydrated—it is inexpensive, calorie-free, and efficient. The worst hydrating liquids are sodas, sugary fruit drinks, sweetened tea or coffee, and juices because they add too many calories to your daily diet (and in some instances are often migraine triggers).

BEST HYDRATING LIQUIDS: *Water, herbal tea, decaffeinated coffee, decaffeinated tea, milk (fat-free, 1% reduced fat)*

OMEGA-3 FATTY ACIDS AND OLIVE OIL

Adding some healthy fats into your diet may help reduce inflammation, which is part of what is thought to cause the pain of migraines. Omega-3 fatty acids, found in large quantities in fatty fish and fortified foods, and monounsaturated fats found in olive oil have both been shown to reduce the frequency, duration, and severity of headaches. I recommend eating fresh wild salmon high in omega-3s two to three times per week, and adding other omega-3 foods as a regular part of your diet. Try to use olive oil or canola oil instead of butter in your cooking whenever possible.

BEST FOODS FOR OMEGA-3 FATTY ACIDS: *Fresh wild salmon, Rainbow trout, Pacific oysters, omega-3–fortified eggs, flaxseed (ground and oil), seaweed, walnut oil, canola oil*

MIGRAINE DIARY

Some neurologists believe that becoming too obsessive about tracking migraine triggers can be stressful, and we all know that stress can trigger a migraine. But unless you keep a basic diary, it will be difficult to spot patterns. If you see a doctor, you'll be required to complete a diary, so starting now will put you one step ahead.

For each migraine episode, note on a regular calendar or in a journal:

- Date and day of the week
- The location and type of pain. For example, would you describe the pain as stabbing, throbbing, steady, dull, sharp? Use whatever adjectives come to mind—there is no wrong answer.
- Intensity level, on a scale of 1 to 10, where 1 = mild pain, and 10 = the worst pain you've ever felt
- Duration, in number of hours
- Any warning signs that the migraine was on its way
- Weather, at the time the migraine started and any changes during the subsequent 12 hours
- Activities or stress level in the 24 hours prior to the migraine
- Foods eaten in the 24 hours prior to the migraine
- What you did to try to stop the migraine, and whether those treatments were effective
- If you are a woman, where you are in your menstrual cycle

RIBOFLAVIN

Riboflavin—also called vitamin B_2—is involved with the body's production of energy at the level of the cell. Some research suggests that people with migraines may have a genetic defect that makes it difficult for their cells to maintain energy reserves, and this lack of basic energy could trigger migraines. Many neurologists recommend that their migraine patients take riboflavin supplements along with their prescription medications. Although it is difficult to get enough riboflavin to prevent migraines from food sources alone, I recommend adding some additional riboflavin-rich foods to your diet. If you would like to try riboflavin supplements, I recommend a 400 milligram dose or a combination product called *MigreLief.* See the Supplements section, next page, for more information.

BEST FOODS FOR RIBOFLAVIN: *Fresh lean beef, whole grain fortified cereal, milk (fat-free, 1% reduced-fat), eggs, mushrooms (portobello, white), asparagus, kale, broccoli, spinach*

MAGNESIUM

Magnesium deficiency has been linked to migraines. Getting enough magnesium through diet or supplements may help to prevent all kinds of migraines, but seems to be particularly valuable for women who get menstrual migraines. Eating a diet high in magnesium is safe, and will contribute to headache prevention. However, studies of the effects of magnesium on migraine have used supplements, not food sources. If you would like to try magnesium supplements, I recommend a combination product called *MigreLief.* See the Supplements section, next page, for more information.

BEST FOODS FOR MAGNESIUM: *Spinach, Swiss chard, fresh amaranth, quinoa, sweet potatoes, white potatoes, millet, artichoke hearts (fresh or frozen only, not canned), chickpeas (garbanzo beans), brown rice, whole wheat pasta, whole grains (see best varieties on grocery list), flaxseed, wheat germ*

BONUS POINTS

- **Eat regularly.** Anyone who skips a meal risks developing a headache, but migraine sufferers are particularly sensitive to the effects of low blood sugar. Don't let a crazy schedule stop you from eating regularly—at least every five hours, but it's possible you need to eat more often than that. Look at it this way . . . if you don't take the time to eat lunch and then get a migraine, you'll lose a lot more than your lunch hour nursing the headache. My friend who suffers migraines claims to eat like a cow—she grazes all day long, rarely going more than two hours without eating something—*and* like a bird, with just the tiniest portions at each sitting. She carries a small snack and a small bottle of water in her purse at all times so she can keep well-fueled and well-hydrated. Although it took a little experimentation, she has made frequent eating work for her, keeping migraines at bay without weight gain.

- **Lose weight, if you are overweight.** A study published in a 2006 issue of the journal *Neurology* looked at the relationship between weight and migraines. After interviewing more than 30,000 people, the researchers discovered that weight had no relation to whether a person suffered migraines. However, people who were overweight had more frequent and severe migraines . . . and the more overweight, the worse the migraines. This study relied on telephone interviews, so we don't know whether these results would hold up in a clinical setting, where the participants could be examined and evaluated by a doctor. But the relationship makes sense. Fat creates inflammation, and inflammation contributes to migraines, so it's not a big leap to think that fat could make migraines worse.

- **Quit smoking.** Smoking increases inflammation and can trigger migraines, so quitting could be a quick way to get rid of pain. If you need a more potent reason, how about stroke? Smoking increases the risk of stroke, and some types of migraine—migraine with aura—can also increase the risk of stroke, even in people under age 50. Adding the two together can be disastrous.

- **Exercise gently, but regularly.** Intense or unusual exercise can cause migraines . . . but regular exercise can reduce the frequency or severity of headaches by reducing tension. The trick is to warm up before exercising, and, if you are new to physical activity, to start slowly. Try walking, gentle cycling, or swimming to start.

- **Practice relaxation.** Because stress can trigger migraines, relaxation can help prevent them. Relaxation can be as simple as taking a bubble bath, listening to music, or spending an afternoon fishing. But more structured relaxation programs are custom-designed to put body and mind at ease. I recommend practicing yoga, progressive relaxation, or meditation for at least 30 minutes each day. Look for classes at your local community college or hospital wellness center.

- **Get enough sleep, without oversleeping.** In these over-busy, over-scheduled times, it is so easy to sleep too little or develop an erratic sleep pattern. But if you suffer with migraines, you need to pay attention to this detail. Both lack of sleep and too much sleep can trigger migraines, so it is important that you make your sleep pattern as regular as possible . . . no matter how busy you are.

- **Consider physical therapy along with acupuncture, biofeedback, or massage.** There are lots of different physical treatments that can help control or even prevent migraines. Research shows that physical therapy, when performed by a licensed physical therapist, is effective at treating migraines when paired with acupuncture, biofeedback, or massage. Acupuncture is an ancient Asian therapy that involves the placement of hair-thin needles into the skin along energy pathways called *meridians*. The precise placement of needles will reopen blocked energy meridians, thereby reducing pain. Biofeedback uses sensitive electronic measuring devices to teach the body how to control muscle tension, heart rate, and other "automatic" body processes that we usually think are not controllable. It is a way to help disrupt that chain of action and reaction that starts with stress, and ends with a migraine. Massage is . . . well, absolutely relaxing and wonderful. Although more research is needed before a definitive case can be made for any of these treatments, they all look promising.

SUPPLEMENTS

If you suffer from migraine headaches and want to consider supplements, research suggests that these might be helpful:

1. **MigreLief.** This supplement is a patented formulation designed specifically for people with migraines. Just two capsules a day—one in the morning and one at night—contain 300 milligrams of magnesium, 400 milligrams of riboflavin, and 100 milligrams of a specific form of the herb *feverfew,* which has been used for centuries to treat headaches. More recent research has found that taking feverfew, particularly in the standardized form found in MigreLief, can reduce the frequency and severity of migraines. People who take it notice improvements after one to three months. This product may cause diarrhea in some people. MigreLief should not be taken by anyone taking potassium-sparing diuretics, or with renal failure, or by women who are pregnant or nursing. To find stores near you that sell MigreLief, check the store locator at www.migrelief.com, or call 1-877-MIGRELIEF. One additional note of warning, just to prevent an unexpected shock: At these dosages, riboflavin will turn urine a bright fluorescent yellow. It isn't dangerous, just colorful.

2. **Omega-3 fish oil.** If you can't get enough omega-3 fats through diet alone, try fish oil supplements. I recommend the same amount used by researchers who studied its effects: 1,500 milligrams (1.5 grams). Check the label to ensure the majority of fish oil content is coming from a combination of DHA and EPA. Store in the fridge to prevent rancidity. To prevent fishy burps, take with food, and choose enteric-coated varieties, which are designed to dissolve in the intestines instead of the stomach. Because fish oil acts as a blood thinner, it should not be taken by people who have hemophilia, or who are already taking blood thinning medications or aspirin. People with diabetes should talk with their doctors before trying fish oil supplements because they may affect blood sugar.

3. **Coenzyme Q_{10} (CoQ_{10}).** CoQ_{10} is a vitamin-like substance that helps enzymes create energy at the cellular level. Without it, cells can't work properly. The first major scientific study of CoQ_{10} showed that about 60 percent of the participants who took 150 milligrams per day (at breakfast) were able to cut the frequency of their migraines by more than half. Although there are very few side effects from CoQ_{10}, some people may experience flu-like symptoms, itching, rashes, heartburn, lack of appetite, or gastrointestinal distress. If you have liver disease, diabetes, or thyroid disease, see your doctor before trying CoQ_{10}.

JOY'S 4-STEP PROGRAM
FOR MIGRAINE HEADACHES

Follow this program if you suffer from migraine headaches.

STEP 1 ... START WITH THE BASICS

These are the first things you should do to try to reduce the frequency and intensity of your headaches:

- If you haven't been diagnosed, see your doctor. Many disorders can cause severe headaches—everything from a simple sinus infection to a brain tumor. Get a professional evaluation. If you are diagnosed with migraines, your doctor will become your new best friend. Ask if there are medications that might be helpful for preventing or stopping a migraine.

- Begin keeping a migraine diary.

- Eliminate all potential migraine trigger foods from your diet.

- Carry sunglasses at all times to shield your eyes from bright lights. Also, wear ear protection (or block your ears with cotton) if you know you will be around loud noises, such as in a movie theater or at a children's party.

- Delegate chores that require chemical cleaners to someone else, or look for products that have less of a noxious odor, such as the natural orange cleaners available in most supermarkets.

- Make your routine as regular as possible. Stick to regular eating and sleeping schedules, work habits, exercise routines, and everything else. Migraine sufferers are sensitive to schedule changes of every sort.

- If you smoke, quit.

STEP 2 ... YOUR ULTIMATE GROCERY LIST

Many foods on this list have high levels of nutrients that can help give you some relief from migraine headaches (foods rich in magnesium, riboflavin, and omega-3 fats). I have also included additional foods used as ingredients in the meal plans and recipes. All foods on this list are generally considered "safe" for migraine sufferers. Conduct your month-long elimination diet by eating ample foods from this list only. After one month, begin to introduce potential trigger foods (one at a time at two-day intervals). This will help you determine a personal (shortened!) list of foods to avoid.

FRUIT

Apples (yellow and green only, no red-skinned)	Berries (blackberries, blueberries, strawberries) Cantaloupe	Cherries Cranberries Mangos Nectarines	Peaches Pears (brown and green only; no red-skinned) Watermelon

VEGETABLES

Artichoke (fresh or frozen only, not canned) Asparagus Beets Broccoli Brussels sprouts Carrots	Cauliflower Celery Chickpeas (garbanzo beans) Cucumbers Kale Lettuce (all varieties)	Mushrooms (portobello, white) Olives Peppers (red/green) Potatoes, sweet Potatoes, white Pumpkin Rhubarb	Seaweed Spinach Squash Swiss chard Turnips Yams Zucchini

SEAFOOD

Black cod (sablefish) Flounder Oysters, Pacific	Salmon, wild (fresh) Scallops Scrod	Snapper Tilapia Trout, rainbow

LEAN MEATS/EGGS

Beef (lean cuts; made to order or prepared yourself at home)	Chicken (skinless; made to order or prepared yourself at home)	Eggs (preferably omega-3–fortified) Turkey, ground (lean, extra-lean)	Turkey breast (made to order or prepared at home)

NUTS AND SEEDS

Flaxseed, ground

YEAST-FREE GRAINS (CHECK LABELS)

Amaranth

Cereal, fortified whole grain

Couscous, whole wheat

Crackers, whole grain

Matzo (preferably whole wheat)

Millet

Oatmeal

Pancake and waffle mix (preferably whole wheat—check labels to ensure no buttermilk)

Pasta (preferably whole wheat or spinach)

Quinoa

Rice (preferably brown or wild)

Rice cakes, plain and flavored

Taco shells

Tortilla wraps (preferably whole grain; tomato or spinach)

Wheat germ

DAIRY

Cheese, ricotta (fat-free, reduced-fat)

Cottage cheese (fat-free, 1% reduced-fat)

Cream cheese (fat-free, reduced-fat)

Milk (fat-free, 1% reduced-fat)

MISCELLANEOUS

Basil, fresh

Cardamom pods (green, crushed)

Chili powder, sweet

Cinnamon stick

Coffee, decaffeinated

Coriander seed, crushed

Cranberry juice

Garlic

Ginger, fresh

Jelly and Jam (strawberry, blackberry, blueberry, or other acceptable fruits)

Margarine spread, soft tub, trans fat–free

Oil, canola

Oil, flaxseed

Oil, olive

Oil, walnut

Paprika, sweet

Pepper, black

Rosemary, fresh

Salt (Kosher, sea, regular)

Sugar, brown

Tea, decaf or herbal (without citrus or caffeine)

Vinegar, distilled white only

STEP3 ...GOING ABOVE AND BEYOND

If you want to do everything you can to reduce the number and intensity of your migraines, here are some additional things you might try:

- Generally speaking, medical doctors are not big fans of supplements, but migraine supplements seem to be an exception. Discuss supplements with your doctor for help in choosing the right one for you. Ask about riboflavin, magnesium, CoQ_{10}, feverfew, and fish oil supplements

- Start a low-intensity exercise program.

- If you are overweight, try to lose weight.

- Get enough sleep, but not too much.

- Practice relaxation, in whatever form works best for you.

- Talk with your doctor about physical therapy.

BOTOX FOR MIGRAINES

One of the newer migraine treatments may help you look younger, too. Researchers have discovered that some migraine sufferers get almost total relief from their headaches after receiving injections of Botox. That's the same substance used by dermatologists and cosmetic surgeons to reduce facial wrinkles by paralyzing the muscles that, when tense, create frown lines and crow's feet. Researchers from Harvard found that people who describe their migraines as a "crushing" pain went from an average of 16 migraine days per month to about 1 migraine day after Botox therapy. They believe that these types of headaches are caused—at least partly—by muscle spasms of the face and head. On the other hand, people who described their pain as "exploding" didn't experience the same benefits. If the usual treatments haven't helped your pain, ask your doctor about whether Botox therapy might work for you.

STEP 4 ...MEAL PLANS

These sample menus contain no foods that are known to trigger migraines. You'll also be eating foods rich in omega-3 fats, riboflavin, and magnesium—nutrients which may be protective against migraine headaches. It is very important that you eat regularly.

Every day, choose *one* option for each of the three meals—breakfast, lunch, and dinner. Then, one or two times per day, choose from a variety of my suggested snacks. Approximate calories have been provided to help adjust for your personal weight-management goals. If you find yourself hungry (and if weight is not an issue), feel free to increase the portion sizes for meals and snacks. Beverage calories are *not* included.

BREAKFAST OPTIONS

(Approximately 300 to 400 calories)

Egg Tortilla Wrap with Spinach, Mushrooms, and Peppers

Sauté ½ cup each spinach, sliced mushrooms, and red or green peppers in 1 teaspoon olive oil or canola oil until soft. In small mixing bowl, beat 1 whole egg with 2 egg whites and scramble in heated pan. Warm whole wheat or spinach tortilla (150 calories or less) in microwave for 15 seconds (or wrap in foil and place in oven for a few minutes). Place scrambled eggs, spinach, mushrooms, and peppers in center of tortilla. Roll up!

Cantaloupe Stuffed with Cottage Cheese and Wheat Germ

Fill ½ cantaloupe with 1 cup fat-free or 1% reduced-fat cottage cheese and top with 1 to 2 tablespoons wheat germ or ground flaxseed.

Whole Grain Cereal with Milk and Berries

1 cup whole grain breakfast cereal with 1 cup milk (skim or 1% reduced-fat milk) topped with 1 cup of blueberries or strawberries.

Rice Cakes with Peach Ricotta Cheese

Combine ½ cup reduced-fat ricotta cheese (or 1 cup fat-free or 1% reduced-fat cottage cheese) with 1 chopped fresh peach or nectarine. Spread over 3 rice cakes (or 1 sheet whole wheat matzo or 100 calories of whole grain crackers).

Oatmeal with Berries and Flaxseed

½ cup dry oatmeal (or 1 instant packet) prepared with ½ cup water and ½ cup fat-free milk. Top with ½ cup blueberries (or cranberries or chopped strawberries), and 1 to 2 tablespoons ground flaxseed or wheat germ. (If you like, add 1 or 2 teaspoons of sugar, honey, or jam to taste).

LUNCH OPTIONS

(Approximately 400 to 500 calories)

Grilled Chicken Salad with Cranberry Basil Vinaigrette

Large portion of a mix of romaine lettuce and baby spinach leaves topped with 4 ounces cooked skinless chicken breast. Feel free to add: chopped pepper (red, yellow, or green), broccoli, sliced mushrooms, cucumbers, beets, carrots, and/or celery. Toss with 2 tablespoons Cranberry Basil Vinaigrette (page 346).

Turkey Burger over Greens with Baked Potato

5 ounces turkey burger (or extra-lean hamburger) on bed of leafy green vegetables (lettuce, endive, spinach leaves, etc.). Enjoy with a 1 baked potato topped with optional 1 teaspoon soft tub, trans fat–free margarine spread.

Spinach Omelet with Rice Cakes and Fresh Fruit

Beat 1 whole egg with 2 to 3 egg whites. Cook in heated skillet coated with 1 teaspoon olive or canola oil. When bottom is cooked, gently flip over. Top with unlimited fresh or cooked spinach. Fold omelet over and cook until egg mixture is firm. Enjoy with 150 calories of whole grain crackers or 3 rice cakes and ½ cantaloupe, 1 green apple, or 1 cup cherries.

Chicken and Tri-Colored Pepper Wrap

5 ounces grilled chicken mixed with unlimited red, yellow, and green peppers sautéed in 1 teaspoon olive or canola oil. Wrap in a whole wheat, spinach, or tomato tortilla (150 calories or less).

Turkey Roll-Up with Baby Carrots and Fruit

1 Fresh Turkey Tortilla Roll-Up (page 346). Serve with 1 cup baby carrots and ½ mango (or 1 peach or 1 cup blueberries, sliced strawberries, or blackberries).

DINNER OPTIONS

(Approximately 500 to 600 calories)

Sirloin Steak with Sautéed Spinach and Baked Potato

5 ounces grilled sirloin steak (or other lean beef). Serve with unlimited spinach sautéed in 1 teaspoon olive oil and garlic. Enjoy with ½ baked potato with optional 1 teaspoon soft tub, trans fat–free margarine spread.

Grilled Salmon with Brown Rice and Broccoli

1 serving Easy! 3-Step Microwave Salmon (page 345), or 5 ounces grilled salmon with 1 teaspoon olive oil and seasonings. Enjoy with ½ cup cooked brown rice (or amaranth or quinoa), sliced cucumbers, and 1 to 2 cups steamed broccoli or cauliflower.

Rosemary Chicken with Sautéed Swiss Chard and Potato

5 ounces grilled Rosemary Chicken (page 347) with 1 serving (1 cup) Sautéed Swiss Chard (page 348). Serve with 1 medium, plain baked white or sweet potato.

Whole Wheat Linguini with Vegetables

In a large pan, sauté minced garlic in 1 teaspoon olive oil. Add 1 cup broccoli florets, 1 cup sliced zucchini, and 1 cup cut asparagus spears and sauté until slightly soft. Add 1½ cups cooked whole wheat linguini or penne with 1 additional teaspoon olive oil. Thoroughly mix until pasta is coated with vegetables and oil. Season with salt and freshly ground black pepper.

Baked Fish with Brown Rice and Asparagus

6 ounces grilled or baked fillet of sole, flounder, trout, black cod, or tilapia. Season with preferred herbs, salt, pepper, and 1 teaspoon olive oil (or 1 tablespoon soft tub, trans fat–free margarine spread). Serve with 1 cup cooked brown rice, quinoa, amaranth (or 1 plain baked potato) and 1 cup steamed asparagus, cauliflower, or kale.

SNACK OPTIONS

100 calories or less

- *Best Vegetables:* 1 cup raw or cooked spinach, kale, red/green peppers, broccoli, cauliflower, asparagus, carrots, artichokes, Brussels sprouts, celery, cucumbers, or zucchini
- *Best Fruits:* 1 apple or pear (yellow and green only), peach, or nectarine; 1 cup blueberries, blackberries, cherries, or watermelon; 20 strawberries; ½ mango; ½ cantaloupe
- 8 to 10 olives
- 1 hard-boiled, omega-3–fortified egg
- ½ whole wheat matzo with 1 tablespoon fat-free or reduced-fat cream cheese
- Celery with 2 to 3 tablespoons fat-free or reduced-fat cream cheese
- 2 rice cakes, lightly salted
- Hot Spiced Tea (page 349)

100 to 200 calories

- 1 whole wheat matzo sheet with 1 tablespoon strawberry jam (or ½ cup fat-free or 1% reduced-fat cottage cheese)

- 2 hard-boiled, omega-3–fortified eggs

- ½ cup fat-free or 1% reduced-fat cottage cheese mixed with 1 cup berries

- 1 cup whole grain cereal with ½ cup fat-free milk

- 2 rice cakes, each topped with 1 tablespoon fat-free or reduced-fat cream cheese and 1 teaspoon strawberry jelly

EASY! 3-STEP MICROWAVE SALMON

If you're looking for the easiest way to prepare salmon, you've found the perfect recipe—dinner will be ready in less than 10 minutes. Plus you'll receive a healthy dose of omega-3 fats, olive oil, and magnesium—three ingredients that have been shown to help fight migraines. If you serve with green vegetables (such as asparagus, broccoli, or spinach) then you'll also add riboflavin to the mix.

Makes 2 servings

2	wild salmon fillets (6 ounces each), $\frac{1}{2}$" thick
1	tablespoon olive oil
2	cloves garlic, minced
$\frac{1}{4}$	teaspoon kosher salt
	Ground black pepper

Arrange the salmon fillets in microwaveable dish, skin down. Brush the oil evenly over the salmon and sprinkle with the garlic. Season with the salt and pepper to taste. Cover and microwave on high 1 to 2 minutes, until the edges are flaky and the fish is cooked through. Let stand 1 to 2 minutes before serving.

PER SERVING
306 calories, 34 g protein, 1 g carbohydrate, 17 g fat (2.5 g saturated), 93 mg cholesterol, 219 mg sodium, 0 g fiber; plus 50 mg magnesium (13% DV)

FRESH TURKEY TORTILLA ROLL-UP

This safe-food wrap also provides a good amount of riboflavin and magnesium. For some extra flavor, try adding 1 to 2 tablespoons of my Cranberry Basil Vinaigrette (below).

Makes 1

- 4   large romaine lettuce leaves
- 1   whole wheat tortilla wrap (150 calories or less; check label to make sure it is yeast-free)
- ¼   pound fresh sliced turkey breast
- 4   medium-thick slices red tomato (omit if tomatoes are one of your migraine triggers)

Layer the lettuce on the wrap. On one side of the wrap, arrange the turkey. (This makes the roll a little neater.) Top with the tomato. Now roll!

PER SERVING
275 calories, 38 g protein, 20 g carbohydrate, 4 g fat (1 g saturated), 94 mg cholesterol, 380 mg sodium, 6 g fiber; plus 50 mg magnesium (13% DV), 0.17 mg riboflavin (16% DV)

CRANBERRY BASIL VINAIGRETTE

Salad dressings are often filled with ingredients that could trigger a migraine—the wrong vinegars, MSG, citrus fruits, artificial coloring, and more. The next time you're craving a salad at home, try this one. It's a tasty combination of safe ingredients . . . and easy to make. Be sure to whisk thoroughly before each use (oil will separate) and store in the fridge.

Makes 13 servings, 2 tablespoons each

- 1   cup olive oil
- ¾   cup cranberry juice
- ¼   cup plus 1 tablespoon white distilled vinegar
- ¼   cup fresh basil, finely chopped
- ½   teaspoon sea salt
- ½   teaspoon black pepper

In medium mixing bowl, combine the oil, cranberry juice, vinegar, basil, salt, and pepper. Whisk thoroughly for a few minutes. Store leftovers in the fridge.

PER SERVING
150 calories, 0 g protein, 1 g carbohydrate, 16 g fat (2 g saturated), 0 mg cholesterol, 90 mg sodium, 0 g fiber

ROSEMARY CHICKEN

While you conduct an elimination diet, it's important to have a scrumptious, staple chicken recipe that uses only trigger-free ingredients. By the way, this chicken is a huge hit with kids—my own and the neighbors'! Serve with Sautéed Swiss Chard (page 348) for a blast of magnesium.

Makes 4 servings

1	tablespoon olive oil
2	teaspoons fresh rosemary, minced
1	teaspoon sweet paprika
1	teaspoon sweet chili powder
1	teaspoon crushed coriander seed (optional)
½	teaspoon freshly ground black pepper
4	skinless chicken cutlets, pounded to ⅛"-thickness (6 ounces each)
	Salt

1. Preheat a grill pan over medium-high? heat or an outdoor grill.
2. Mix the oil, rosemary, paprika, chili powder, coriander (if using), and pepper in a small bowl. Rub the spice mixture over the chicken and season with salt.
3. Grill the chicken, turning once, about 8 minutes, until no longer pink and the juices run clear.

   To bake the chicken in the oven, preheat the oven to 450°F. Line a baking sheet with foil and coat with nonstick olive oil spray. Place the chicken on the baking sheet and coat with olive oil spray. Bake, turning once half way through cooking, until no longer pink and the juices run clear, 6 to 7 minutes.

PER SERVING
227 calories, 40 g protein, 2 g carbohydrate, 6 g fat (1 g saturated), 98 mg cholesterol, 263 mg sodium, 1 g fiber

Tip: Once your grill is preheated, rub it lightly with canola oil to season the surface. If it's not grilling season, a wide variety of easy-to-care-for grill pans, some nonstick, are available for healthy, tasty grilling indoors. In a well-ventilated kitchen, simply preheat the grill pan on a gas or electric stovetop over high heat. Seasoning with canola oil is not necessary with a nonstick grill. If you would like to use nonstick spray, apply a thin layer to a clean grill before you heat it.

SAUTÉED SWISS CHARD

This vegetable is naturally loaded with magnesium. Sauté in olive oil, and you'll get the added benefits of monounsaturated fat. If you'd like to save some calories, skip the oil. When steamed or microwaved, 1 cup of Swiss chard contains only 35 calories!

Makes 4 servings, 1 cup each

- 2   tablespoons olive oil
- 2   cloves garlic, thinly sliced
- 2   pounds red or green Swiss chard, thinly sliced
       Salt
       Ground black pepper

In a large nonstick skillet over high heat, warm the oil. Add the garlic and cook, stirring constantly 1 to 2 minutes. Add the Swiss chard and sprinkle with salt and pepper. Cook 4 to 5 minutes, until the Swiss chard is soft and reduced by half in volume. Serve immediately.

PER SERVING
106 calories, 4 g protein, 9 g carbohydrate, 7 g fat (1 g saturated), 0 mg cholesterol, 483 mg sodium, 4 g fiber; plus 185 mg magnesium (46% DV), 0.21 mg riboflavin (19% DV)

HOT SPICED TEA

Delicious and low-calorie, this hot beverage treat delivers a shot of riboflavin, thanks to the fat-free milk!

Makes 2 servings

2	cups water
1	1" piece of fresh ginger, sliced
1	small cinnamon stick
4	green cardamom pods, crushed
1	cup fat-free milk
2	decaffeinated Earl Grey or English Breakfast tea bags
1	tablespoon brown sugar

In a small saucepan, combine the water, ginger, cinnamon, and cardamom pods. Bring to a boil. Add the milk, reduce the heat, and simmer 5 minutes. Remove from the heat and add the tea bags. Steep for 3 to 4 minutes. Strain through a sieve or coffee filter. Add the brown sugar. Serve immediately, or chill and serve over ice.

PER SERVING
62 calories, 4 g protein, 11 g carbohydrate, 0 g fat, 0 mg cholesterol, 60 mg sodium, 0 g fiber; plus .257 mg riboflavin (23% DV)

CHAPTER 15

PREMENSTRUAL SYNDROME

Many years ago, I had a client come to see me specifically to address her little problem with premenstrual syndrome (PMS). For about one week of the month, just before she got her period, Michelle would descend into a nightmare when she turned into what she called her "serial-killer self." During that time, she was prone to wildly changing and unpredictable moods, mostly rage with occasional bouts of weeping. She would cry at the soft look a father and his son exchanged on a fast food commercial . . . scream at the cabbie who dared to stop at a yellow light when she was in a hurry . . . fume or cry at the office over things that normally rolled off her back . . . and, just once, she took her car, stomped on the accelerator and rammed into the back of a car belonging to an ex-boyfriend's current lover. She hadn't dated the guy in over a year. It ended up costing her a small fortune in car repair bills, not to mention the increase in her premiums.

For Michelle, every month followed a predictable pattern: one week of being totally out of control, followed by two weeks spent begging forgiveness and writing letters of apology to all the people she hurt or offended the previous week. By the time she came to see me, she was desperate.

FAQS

There are lots of herbal "cures" for PMS ... do they help?

There's no doubt about it: herbal remedies come in and out of fashion just like hemlines. You may have heard that black cohosh, wild yam root, dong quai, and evening primrose oil can help relieve your symptoms. The only problem is there's no scientific evidence that shows any of them relieve PMS symptoms. Not only are they ineffective, some of them can be downright dangerous for some women so I cannot recommend any of them. St. John's wort and SAMe (S-adenosylmethionine) may be beneficial, but they are too potent to take without a doctor's guidance. If you want to try them, talk with your physician. (More information about St. John's wort and SAMe can be found on page 312.)

PMS is estimated to affect about 40 percent of American women of childbearing age. Between 3 and 9 percent of women have a more extreme form of PMS called *premenstrual dysphoric disorder* (PMDD). PMS and PMDD cause physical and emotional symptoms—including irritability, sadness, mood swings, low self-esteem, difficulty concentrating, bloating, water retention, lack of energy, and breast tenderness—for some portion of each month, triggered by the normal hormonal changes associated with the menstrual cycle. PMDD, the form of the disorder Michelle probably had (although she hadn't had a formal diagnosis when I knew her) is casually defined as PMS that is so severe that it negatively affects a woman's life. PMS feels uncomfortable and unpleasant, but PMDD can turn social lives, work lives, families, and marriages upside-down. In fact, I can remember a married couple—close friends—having a drag-out fight after the woman's husband asked a pharmacist working at a local drugstore for "Motrin with extra bitch control."

Regardless of whether you experience a little extra moodiness near your period, or car-crashing emotional breakdowns, nutrition can help alleviate many premenstrual symptoms. I worked with Michelle to level out her moods, and we had great results. Once she felt that she was able to make it through a month without potentially litigious behavior, we decided that she might benefit from talking with a therapist. I haven't heard from Michelle in a long while, but the last time I saw her, she was calm, happy, and—in a testament to her self-control—still in possession of her driver's license. My fighting friends . . . well, they are a whole other story.

WHAT AFFECTS PMS?

No one knows exactly why some women experience symptoms while others do not. The main theory is that some women have a greater sensitivity to the effects of the female hormones estrogen and progesterone, and to the effects of these hormones on serotonin. Research and clinical results seem to confirm that serotonin plays an important role—when women with the most severe premenstrual symptoms are treated with a serotonin-enhancing antidepressant (similar to Prozac), about 70 percent get substantial relief.

What we do know is that for many women, PMS is an uncomfortable fact of life. The exact severity and cluster of symptoms will differ from woman to woman. Some will have fatigue, bloating, and depression . . . others will have breast tenderness and irritability, or any combination of any of the symptoms. Most typically, symptoms begin the week before a woman is due to get her period, peak the day before the start of her period, and then disappear within a day after her period starts. The vast majority of women with PMS have symptoms for five to seven days each month. But some women can have symptoms that last two, or even three, weeks each month.

If you are a woman of childbearing age experiencing mood issues, I recommend keeping a PMS diary. On a regular calendar, write down your primary moods, emotions, and unusual physical symptoms each day. On the same calendar, keep track of your menstrual cycle. If your troubling moods or other symptoms occur primarily within the two weeks prior to the start of your period, you may have PMS (in addition to all the regular aggravations of life). However, if the days you experience irritability or depression are evenly spaced throughout the month, you may not have PMS, but a simple mood problem.

It is important to note all your physical symptoms in your PMS diary. For reasons that aren't exactly clear, many the symptoms of many diseases or disorders get worse premenstrually, a phenomenon known as *premenstrual exacerbation*. Depression and anxiety are prone to this exacerbation, as are migraines, epilepsy, asthma, allergies, diabetes, irritable bowel syndrome, and many autoimmune disorders. Just because your symptoms aren't generally included in a list of the symptoms of PMS doesn't mean that they aren't related to your menstrual cycle. If your worst symptoms seem to occur the week before your period, talk with your doctor about whether there are things you can do to better control your particular disorder.

HOW FOOD AFFECTS PMS

Many women with PMS define their monthly nutrition needs in terms of their cravings for anything salty or chocolate. Although indulging in chocolate-dipped pretzels might seem like a fantasy-come-true, they won't improve your mood or reduce the bloat. There are many better options:

CALCIUM

Calcium deficiency and PMS share many symptoms, which led researchers to test to see if they might be related. The results suggest that they very well might be. Compared with women who don't have premenstrual symptoms, women with PMS have lower blood levels of calcium around their time of ovulation. And when PMS sufferers take 1,000 to 1,200 milligrams of calcium supplements daily, their mood and bloating improve after just a few months. I consider calcium-rich foods an absolute must for women with PMS.

BEST FOODS FOR CALCIUM: *Yogurt (fat-free, low-fat), milk (fat-free, 1% reduced-fat), enriched/fortified soy milk, calcium-fortified fruit juice, cheese (fat-free, low-fat), tofu with calcium, canned sardines (with bones), wild salmon (with bones, fresh), soybeans, frozen yogurt (fat-free, low-fat), low-fat ice cream, calcium-fortified whole grain waffles, bok choy, kale, white beans, broccoli, almonds*

VITAMIN D

Our bodies can't absorb or use calcium without vitamin D. That's why the two are so often mentioned together, and why some high-calcium foods (such as milk) are often fortified with vitamin D. In addition, research suggests that vitamin D may act on its own to prevent PMS. In a study that followed more than 3,000 women for more than 10 years, women who ate a diet high in vitamin D reduced their risk of PMS by about 40 percent.

> **BEST FOODS FOR VITAMIN D:** *Wild salmon (with bones), mackerel (not king), sardines (with bones), herring, fortified milk (fat-free, 1% reduced-fat), enriched/fortified soy milk, egg yolks, mushrooms (especially shiitake), vitamin D–fortified soft tub trans fat–free margarine spread, fortified whole grain breakfast cereal*

MAGNESIUM

Just as was found with calcium, women with PMS seem to have lower blood levels of magnesium compared with women who did not have PMS symptoms. Women with PMS who took magnesium supplements had better mood and less water retention than women who did not get enough magnesium. (And really, doesn't less water retention sound good for everybody?) It is thought that magnesium might help regulate the activity of serotonin, the so-called feel-good neurotransmitter. Magnesium-rich foods are second only to calcium foods for improving your chances for symptom reduction.

> **BEST FOODS FOR MAGNESIUM:** *Pumpkin seeds, spinach, Swiss chard, amaranth, sunflower seeds, cashews, almonds, quinoa, tempeh, sweet potatoes, white potatoes, soybeans, millet, beans (black, white, navy, lima, pinto, kidney), artichoke hearts, peanuts, peanut butter, chickpeas (garbanzo beans), brown rice, whole grain bread, sesame seeds, wheat germ, flaxseed*

VITAMIN B$_6$

Your body can't make dopamine—one of the mood neurotransmitters—without vitamin B$_6$. Research studies into the effects of vitamin B$_6$ on PMS have been mixed—some show that taking supplements reduces irritability, depression, and breast tenderness, while others don't find any effect at all. Still, I highly recommend eating vitamin B$_6$–rich foods because they seem to have helped many of my clients with PMS.

> **BEST FOODS FOR VITAMIN B$_6$:** *Fortified whole grain breakfast cereal, chickpeas (garbanzo beans), wild salmon (fresh, canned), lean beef, pork tenderloin, chicken breast, white potatoes (with skin), oatmeal, banana, pistachio nuts, lentils, tomato paste, barley, rice (brown, wild), peppers, sweet potatoes, squash (winter, acorn), broccoli, broccoli raab, carrots, Brussels sprouts, peanut butter, eggs, shrimp, tofu, apricots, watermelon, avocado, strawberries, whole grain bread*

MANGANESE

Manganese is found in minute quantities in foods, but that's OK because we don't need a lot to stay healthy. If you eat a relatively balanced diet, you're probably getting enough manganese. But blood levels of manganese vary throughout the menstrual cycle, so it is not surprising that this mineral might be involved in PMS. A handful of studies have suggested that manganese, in combination with calcium, may reduce the irritability, depression, and tension associated with PMS. One study found that women who did not get enough manganese in their diets had more pain and worse moods premenstrually. Therefore, I encourage you to go out of your way to incorporate manganese-rich foods, specifically around the time of PMS.

> **BEST FOODS FOR MANGANESE:** *Pineapple, wheat germ, spinach, collard greens, pecans, amaranth, lima beans, pumpkin seeds, walnuts, oats, tempeh, quinoa, brown rice, flaxseed, raspberries, chickpeas (garbanzo beans), sunflower seeds, peanuts, tofu, soybeans, soy nuts, lentils*

OTHER FOOD FIXES

- **Avoid salt and salty foods.** PMS causes bloating and water retention. Salt can cause bloating and water retention. Ergo, salt can make those problems of PMS worse.
- **Avoid alcohol.** Premenstrually, alcohol can cause increased breast tenderness. Also, alcohol can lower blood sugar, which may make typical PMS mood symptoms worse. If you cannot totally avoid alcohol premenstrually, at least try not to drink to excess.
- **Avoid caffeine.** Some research suggests that the effects of caffeine are magnified premenstrually, leading to greater breast tenderness, more nervousness, and potentially more irritability. Instead of coffee, tea, or caffeinated soft drinks, try herbal teas and other decaffeinated beverages.

MAGNESIUM-RICH AMARANTH

Although amaranth (pronounced *AM-uh-ranth*) is touted as a "super grain," it is actually not a grain at all. It is a plant related to the common garden weed called pigweed. Its leaves cook and taste much like spinach, but amaranth is mostly prized for its abundance of tiny, high-protein seeds, or *grains*. The whole seeds, when simmered, produce a thick, oatmeal-like porridge that has a gelatinous texture (translation: it's not for everyone!). To make amaranth more appetizing, mix it with a grain such as brown rice or buckwheat (amaranth should make up no more than 15 percent of the total mixture), then follow the cooking instructions for the predominant grain. Amaranth can be found in many natural food stores and some supermarkets alongside rice, barley, and other grains. Sticker shock alert! Because harvesting amaranth is labor intensive, it is relatively expensive.

Cooking amaranth: Simmer 1½ cups liquid (such as broth, apple juice, or water) and ½ cup amaranth seeds for about 30 minutes, or until the seeds are tender. Add fresh herbs or gingerroot to the cooking liquid to make it tastier, or mix with beans for a main dish. For a breakfast cereal, increase the amount of cooking liquid and sweeten with a bit of honey or brown rice syrup, and add 1 to 2 tablespoons raisins, dried cranberries, allspice, and/or nuts.

■ **Drink chamomile tea.** Premenstrually, chamomile tea may be particularly helpful because it contains properties that relieve muscle spasms, and may therefore help reduce the severity of menstrual cramps. In addition, chamomile seems to reduce tension that may lead to anxiety and irritability.

BONUS POINTS

■ **Read the chapter about mood (page 303).** All the good-mood advice about getting appropriate amount of exercise, eating regularly throughout the day, getting the right mix of proteins and high-quality carbohydrates, and decreasing stress apply to PMS as well.

■ **Get enough sleep.** Hormonal shifts can make some women lose sleep, which in turn may make them irritable. It is generally important to get enough sleep to level out moods. Premenstrually, sleep becomes crucial. Many women even feel the need to nap during the premenstrual week—if you can manage a quick few minutes of sleep in the middle of the day, indulge. It may make the difference between a good day, and a day of snapping and tears.

SUPPLEMENTS

If you experience PMS and want to consider supplements *in addition to* the food fixes, I recommend:

1. **Multivitamin.** In order to assure that you get all the nutrients important for mood and physical symptoms of PMS, look for a multivitamin that contains 100% DV of vitamin D (400 IU), 100% DV manganese (2 milligrams), at least 20% DV of magnesium (80 milligrams or more), and 100% DV of B$_6$, all of which may help improve mood and reduce bloating. (The vitamin D is necessary to help the body absorb calcium.)

2. **Calcium plus vitamin D$_3$ and magnesium.** Most women need calcium supplements, regardless of whether or not they have PMS. That's why I recommend taking calcium supplements—500 to 600 milligrams two times a day (with food if it's in the form of calcium carbonate), for a total of 1,000 to 1,200 milligrams. The calcium supplements should also provide vitamin D$_3$ (cholecalciferol, the most potent form of vitamin D) and magnesium. This should be taken *in addition to* a multivitamin that includes vitamin D and magnesium.

3. **Vitamin B$_6$.** The studies of this vitamin have been mixed, with about half showing no benefit at all. Although I can't give it my unadulterated endorsement, women with *severe* PMS symptoms may want to consider taking a separate supplement of 50 to 100 milligrams of vitamin B$_6$ daily. *Important note:* Taking amounts in excess of 100 milligrams per day may cause permanent nerve damage in hands, arms, feet, and legs. Take no more than 100 milligrams daily.

4. **Chasteberry extract.** If the food and nutritional supplements aren't enough to calm your premenstrual symptoms, scientists have found that chasteberry extract may also help. Typical dosage is a 20 milligram tablet, one to two times a day. This extract has been shown to relieve mood swings, irritability, anger, headache, and breast tenderness in about half the women who took it for three months. Scientists believe that the actions of chasteberry are due to flavonoids and other phytochemicals that seem to relieve anxiety and reduce inflammation. *Important note:* If you experience headache, gastrointestinal distress, or rash while taking chasteberry extract, discontinue using it. Chasteberry lowers prolactin levels, so it should not be used by women who are pregnant or nursing. Because of possible interactions, do not use chasteberry if you are also taking drugs or hormones that affect the pituitary, such as bromocriptine.

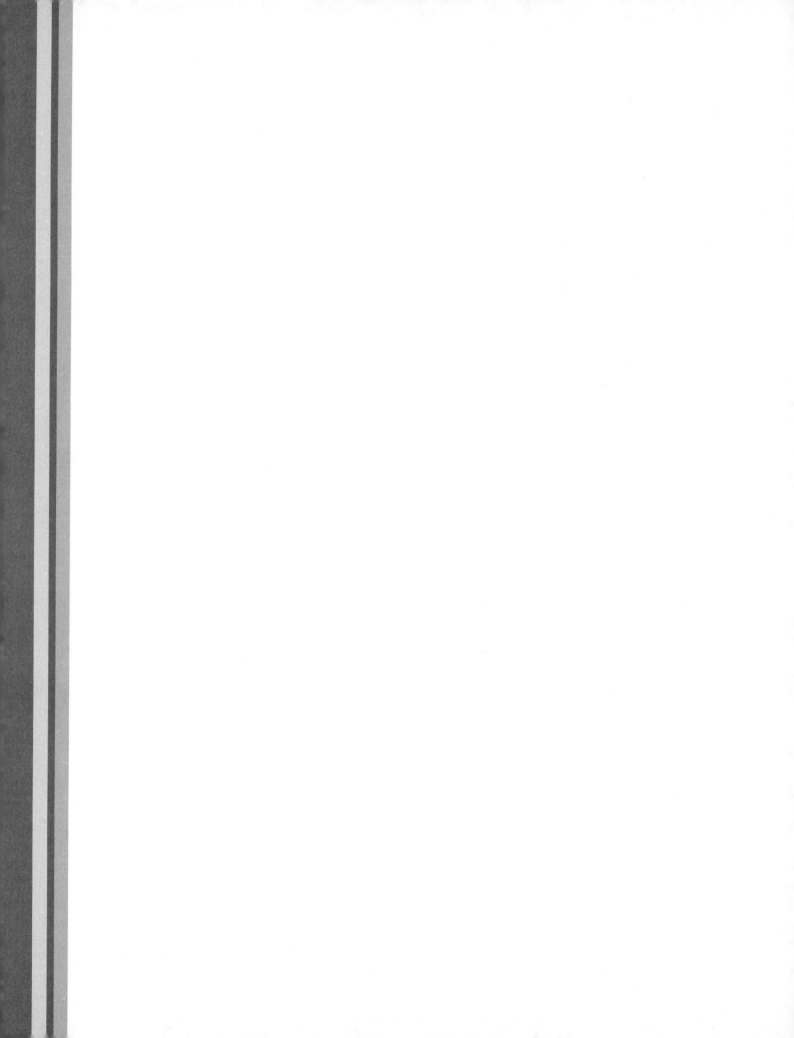

JOY'S 4-STEP PROGRAM
FOR PREMENSTRUAL SYNDROME

Follow this program if you are a woman who feels moody, emotional, irritable, or bloated—or have other symptoms of PMS—at predictable times corresponding to your menstrual cycle.

STEP 1 ... START WITH THE BASICS

These are the first things you should do to take control of your PMS.

- Keep a mood diary to see whether your mood and physical symptoms are related to your menstrual cycle. If not, you probably don't have PMS.

- If your moods or physical symptoms are overly distressing, or if they have caused problems in your life, see a doctor. There are prescription medications that you can take for only part of the month, whenever you feel symptoms.

- Avoid alcohol, salty foods, and foods with caffeine, all of which can aggravate premenstrual symptoms.

- You may also want to read the chapter on mood (page 303). Many of the recommendations there may also help PMS, particularly the information about leveling out blood sugars, and about exercise.

STEP 2 ... YOUR ULTIMATE GROCERY LIST

A nutrition plan is only as good as the foods that you choose. This list contains foods with high levels of nutrients that can help relieve PMS symptoms, plus some additional foods used as ingredients in the meal plans and recipes. These foods are high in vitamin B$_6$, calcium, vitamin D, magnesium, and/or manganese.

FRUIT

Apples	Berries	Juice, calcium-fortified	Watermelon
Apricots	(raspberries,	Lemons	
Bananas	strawberries)	Pineapple	

VEGETABLES

Artichoke hearts	Carrots	Onions	Tomato paste
Avocado	Celery	Peppers (red/yellow/	Tomatoes (fresh;
Beans (black, white,	Chickpeas	green)	canned, crushed
navy, lima, pinto,	Collard greens	Potatoes, sweet	without paste)
kidney, garbanzo)	Corn	Potatoes, white	
Bok choy	Kale	Soybeans (edamame)	
Broccoli	Lentils	Spinach	
Broccoli raab	Mushrooms (especially	Squash (winter, acorn)	
Brussels sprouts	shiitake)	Swiss chard	

SEAFOOD

Herring	Salmon, wild (with	Shrimp
Mackerel	bones)	
(not king)	Sardines (with bones)	

LEAN MEATS/EGGS/SOY FOODS

Beef, lean	Pork tenderloin	Turkey breast (fresh	Turkey breast (lean
Chicken breast	Tempeh	sliced)	ground)
Eggs	Tofu (with calcium)		

NUTS AND SEEDS (UNSALTED)

Almonds	Peanut butter	Pistachio nuts	Soy nuts
Cashews	Peanuts	Pumpkin seeds	Sunflower seeds
Flaxseed, ground	Pecans	Sesame seeds	Walnuts

WHOLE GRAINS

Amaranth	Cereal, fortified whole	Pasta, whole wheat	Tortilla, whole wheat
Barley	grain	Pita, whole wheat	Waffles, calcium-
Bread, whole grain	Millet	Quinoa	fortified whole grain
Bread, whole grain	Oatmeal	Rice (brown, wild,	Wheat germ
reduced-calorie	Oats	long-grain)	

DAIRY

Cheese (fat-free,	Cheese, string, reduced-	Soy milk, enriched/	
reduced-fat)	fat	fortified	
Cheese (for meal plan):	Ice cream, low-fat	Yogurt (fat-free, low-fat)	
fat-free or shredded	Milk (fat-free, 1%	Yogurt, frozen (fat-free,	
Cheddar, Swiss,	reduced-fat)	low-fat)	
Parmesan, and	Sour cream (fat-free,		
Romano	reduced-fat)		

MISCELLANEOUS

Chili powder	vitamin D–fortified	Pepper, black	Vinegar, balsamic or
Cumin	trans fat–free	Pepper, ground red	red wine
Garlic	Mayonnaise, reduced-fat	Salad dressing,	
Garlic powder	Mustard, spicy brown	low-calorie	
Guacamole	or Dijon	Salsa	
Hot cocoa, diet	Nonstick cooking spray	Salt, kosher	
Hummus	Oil, olive	Salt substitute	
Margarine spread,	Oregano, dried	Tea, chamomile	
reduced-fat soft tub	Paprika	Vinegar	

STEP3 ... GOING ABOVE AND BEYOND

If you want to do everything you can to reduce PMS symptoms, here are some additional things you might try:

- I strongly recommend taking a calcium supplement with added vitamin D_3 and magnesium. Calcium should equal 500 to 600 milligrams. Take twice daily (with food if it is calcium carbonate) for a total dose of 1,000 to 1,200 milligrams.

- A multivitamin with 100% DV vitamin D, vitamin B_6, manganese, and at least 20% DV magnesium.

- Women with severe PMS symptoms may also want to try an additional vitamin B_6 supplement, or chasteberry extract. See the Supplements section, page 356, for more information.

- Get enough sleep.

MAKE IT TO MENOPAUSE

I have good news and bad news when it comes to PMS. The good news is that it eventually ends. The bad news is that you'll have to go through menopause first, and women who are most bothered by emotional symptoms of PMS also have the roughest time with menopause. In your 40s, you may notice your PMS symptoms becoming erratic as your ovulation and periods become less predictable. If you experience more physical or emotional pain than usual as you head into your hot flash years, talk with your doctor—there are many treatments that can help ease this transition.

STEP 4 ...MEAL PLANS

The following meals are rich in nutrients that may ease PMS symptoms—calcium, vitamin D, magnesium, manganese, and vitamin B$_6$—and low in those foods that aggravate symptoms. Be sure to drink lots of water with (and between) your meals . . . and if you'd like, enjoy chamomile tea and calcium-rich drinks, such as fat-free milk, enriched/fortified soy milk, and fortified fruit juice. (The calories for beverages are not included in the following sample days.)

Every day, choose *one* option for each of the three meals—breakfast, lunch, and dinner. Then, one or two times per day, choose from a variety of my suggested snacks. Approximate calories have been provided to help adjust for your personal weight management goals. If you find yourself hungry (and if weight is not an issue), feel free to increase the portion sizes for meals and snacks.

BREAKFAST OPTIONS

(Approximately 300 to 400 calories)

Whole Grain Cereal with Milk and Fruit

1 cup whole grain cereal (120 calories or less) with 1 cup milk (fat-free, or 1% reduced-fat) and 1 cup sliced pineapple (or 1 cup raspberries). Serve with chamomile tea.

Oatmeal with Wheat Germ and Berries

½ cup dry oatmeal prepared with 1 cup milk (fat-free, 1% reduced-fat or enriched/fortified soy) and topped with 2 tablespoons wheat germ (or ground flaxseed) and ½ cup berries (sliced strawberries and/or raspberries). Enjoy with chamomile tea.

Broccoli-Cheese Egg-White Omelet with Toast

Sauté 1 cup broccoli florets in a heated pan coated with nonstick cooking spray until soft. Beat 1 whole egg with 3 egg whites and pour around the broccoli. When bottom is cooked, gently flip. Top with 2 tablespoons shredded fat-free cheese. Fold omelet over and cook until cheese is melted and egg mixture is firm. Season with salt substitute and ground black pepper. Enjoy with 1 slice whole grain bread (or 2 slices reduced-calorie bread—45 calories or less per slice), toasted and topped with 1 to 2 teaspoons reduced-fat, soft tub, trans fat–free margarine spread and enjoy with chamomile tea.

Strawberry-Banana Cottage Cheese with Sunflower Seeds

1 cup fat-free or 1% reduced-fat cottage cheese (or 8 ounces fat-free, plain or flavored yogurt) mixed with ½ sliced banana, ½ cup chopped strawberries, and 1 tablespoon sunflower seeds. Enjoy with chamomile tea.

Peanut Butter Pita with Yogurt

1 whole wheat pita (150 calories or less), lightly toasted and topped with 1 level table-spoon peanut butter. Enjoy with 1 cup fat-free plain or flavored yogurt (120 calories or less). Serve with chamomile tea.

LUNCH OPTIONS

(Approximately 400 to 500 calories)

Chicken-Spinach Sandwich with Broccoli

4 ounces grilled chicken breast with spinach leaves, tomato, and onion (and 1 optional tablespoon hummus, ketchup, barbecue sauce, or Dijon mustard) on 2 slices whole wheat bread (or pita). Serve with 1 cup steamed broccoli or Swiss chard topped with 2 tablespoons grated Parmesan cheese.

Veggie-Bean Burrito with Guacamole

1 whole wheat tortilla (150 calories or less) filled with ½ cup black beans, unlimited steamed vegetables (preferably collard greens, Swiss chard, chopped broccoli), 1 ounce shredded fat-free Cheddar cheese, and 2 tablespoons guacamole.

Yogurt Fruit Fiesta

1 cup fat-free, plain or vanilla yogurt (or 1 cup fat-free or 1% reduced-fat cottage cheese) mixed with ½ cup pineapple, ½ chopped apple (or pear), and ½ sliced banana; top with 2 tablespoons ground flaxseed, 1 tablespoon sunflower seeds, and 1 tablespoon chopped walnuts.

Turkey, Swiss Cheese, and Avocado Sandwich

4 ounces sliced turkey breast (or grilled chicken or lean ham), 1 ounce reduced-fat Swiss cheese, 2 to 3 thin slices avocado, and lettuce, tomato, and onion on 2 slices reduced-calorie, whole wheat bread (45 calories or less per slice). You may choose to add mustard (or 2 teaspoons reduced-fat mayonnaise or 2 teaspoons hummus). Enjoy with 1 cup green/yellow/red bell pepper sticks.

Baked Potato with Broccoli and Cheese

1 medium baked potato topped with 1 cup steamed or boiled chopped broccoli and 1 ounce fat-free or reduced-fat cheese (or ½ cup fat-free or 1% reduced-fat cottage cheese). Serve with 2 tablespoons fat-free or reduced-fat sour cream and optional salsa. Enjoy with 1 cup crunchy baby carrots.

DINNER OPTIONS

(Approximately 500 to 600 calories)

Turkey Chili with Brown Rice and Salad

1 serving (2 cups) Turkey Chili (page 367) topped with 1 ounce shredded fat-free Cheddar cheese. Serve with ½ cup cooked brown rice (or amaranth or quinoa) and a tossed salad of leafy greens and optional peppers, carrots, and artichokes tossed with 1 teaspoon olive oil and 2 tablespoons balsamic vinegar or fresh lemon juice (or 2 tablespoons low-calorie dressing).

Grilled Salmon with Edamame and Swiss Chard

1 cup boiled edamame (soybeans in the pod) seasoned with salt substitute and 5 ounces grilled wild salmon seasoned with 1 teaspoon olive oil, preferred herbs, and fresh lemon. Serve with 1 cup steamed Swiss chard (or spinach).

Whole Wheat Penne with Chicken and Broccoli

1 serving Whole Wheat Penne with Chicken and Broccoli (page 368). Enjoy with side salad of leafy greens, tomatoes, peppers, and 1 tablespoon chopped walnuts tossed with 1 teaspoon olive oil and 2 tablespoons balsamic vinegar or fresh lemon juice (or 2 tablespoons low-calorie dressing).

Pork Tenderloin with Brussels Sprouts and Sweet Potato

5 ounces grilled, baked, or broiled lean pork tenderloin (or grilled chicken breast). Enjoy with 1 cup steamed Brussels sprouts (or collard greens, spinach, broccoli, or kale), topped with 1 tablespoon reduced-fat, soft tub, trans fat–free margarine. Serve with 1 medium plain baked sweet potato.

Sweet and Sour Tofu-Veggie Stir-Fry with Brown Rice

1 serving Sweet and Sour Tofu-Veggie Stir-Fry (page 251), with 1 cup cooked brown rice (or 1 medium baked white or sweet potato topped with 1 teaspoon reduced-fat, soft tub trans fat–free margarine or 1 tablespoon fat-free or reduced-fat sour cream.)

SNACK OPTIONS

100 calories or less

- *Best Vegetables:* 1 cup raw or cooked kale, broccoli, broccoli raab, bok choy, mushrooms, spinach, Swiss chard, peppers, carrots, Brussels sprouts, collard greens, or artichokes

- *Best Fruits:* 1 cup watermelon (or 1 wedge), sliced strawberries, pineapple, or raspberries; ½ banana; 4 apricots; 20 whole strawberries

- 1 reduced-fat string cheese (or 1 ounce any variety reduced-fat cheese)
- 1 cup fat-free milk
- Celery sticks with 1 level tablespoon peanut butter
- 1 hard-boiled egg (or 4 hard-boiled egg whites)
- ½ cup fat-free or 1% reduced-fat cottage cheese

100 to 200 calories

- 1 cup fat-free flavored yogurt topped with 1 tablespoon chopped pecans or sunflower seeds (or 2 tablespoons wheat germ)
- 10 raw almonds plus 1 serving fruit (see Best Fruits list)
- ¼ cup sunflower seeds or pistachio nuts in the shell
- Unsalted nuts: 1 ounce (about ¼ cup) plain or toasted walnuts, pecans, cashews, almonds, peanuts, or soy nuts
- 1 level tablespoon peanut butter on 70-calorie whole wheat pita bread
- 1 frozen banana
- ½ cup low-fat ice cream (200 calories or less)
- 1 cup diet hot cocoa with 1 serving fruit (see Best Fruit list)
- 1 cup edamame (soybeans boiled in the pod), seasoned with salt substitute
- Red/yellow/green pepper sticks with 2 heaping tablespoons guacamole or hummus
- ½ cup fat-free or 1% reduced-fat cottage cheese mixed with ½ cup raspberries (or sliced strawberries) and 2 tablespoons wheat germ
- 1 serving (2 cups) Tropical Mango-Citrus Smoothie (page 123)

TURKEY CHILI

You won't miss the high-fat beef in this hearty, well-seasoned dish, which relies on extra-lean ground turkey and black beans for its thick, crowd-pleasing consistency. Plus, you'll receive a healthy dose of magnesium, folic acid, manganese, and fiber. Freeze leftovers in a tightly covered container, or store in the fridge for up to 3 days.

Makes 8 servings, 2 cups each

2	pounds extra-lean ground turkey breast
1	can (28 ounces) crushed tomato (without paste)
2	cups water
2	large onions, coarsely chopped
2	tablespoons chili powder
2	teaspoons garlic powder
1	teaspoon paprika
1	teaspoon black pepper
1	teaspoon cumin
1	teaspoon dried oregano
½	teaspoon ground red pepper (or more for hotter chili)
2	teaspoons all-purpose flour
2	cans (15 ounces each) black beans, well drained and rinsed
1	can (15 ounces) corn, well drained and rinsed

1. In a large skillet over medium-high heat, brown the turkey, stirring to break up the meat. Drain the fat. Add the tomatoes, water, onions, chili powder, garlic powder, paprika, black pepper, cumin, oregano, and red pepper. Mix thoroughly. Cover and simmer, stirring occasionally, 25 to 30 minutes.

2. Stir in the flour, and cook, stirring, 2 minutes. Stir in the beans and corn and cook, uncovered and stirring occasionally, for 20 minutes.

PER SERVING
269 calories, 34 g protein, 29 g carbohydrate, 2.5 g fat (1 g saturated), 45 mg cholesterol, 220 mg sodium, 8 g fiber; plus 120 mg folic acid (30% DV), 59 mg magnesium (15% DV), 0.38 mg manganese (15% DV)

WHOLE WHEAT PENNE WITH CHICKEN AND BROCCOLI

This low-cal, nutrient-rich pasta dish is a favorite dinner among all three of my kids (believe me, that's a feat). Even better, one serving provides 30% DV for vitamin B$_6$, 43% DV for manganese, and 17% DV for magnesium. Plus, the cheese and broccoli supply a healthy hit of calcium. Enjoy it with a colorful tossed salad and you've got a nutritional powerhouse!

Makes 8 servings, 2 cups each

¼	cup extra virgin olive oil
½	large onion, chopped
4	cloves garlic, minced
1	pound skinless, boneless chicken breast, cut into 1" cubes
8	cups broccoli florets
1	package (18 ounces) whole wheat penne
½	teaspoon Kosher salt
2	tablespoons grated Romano cheese
	Black pepper

1. Bring a large pot of water to a rolling boil over high heat.
2. Meanwhile, heat the olive oil in a medium-size saucepan over medium heat. Add the onion and garlic and cook, stirring, until translucent, being careful not to let the onion brown. Add the chicken and cook, stirring, until no longer pink throughout. Remove from the heat and set aside.
3. Once the water boils, add the broccoli and cook until firm yet tender. Using a slotted spoon or skimmer, transfer the broccoli to the saucepan with the chicken. Cook until the broccoli is soft.
4. Return the large pot of salted water to a boil, and add the pasta. Cook until al dente, about 8 minutes. Drain the pasta, reserving 1 cup of pasta water. Add the pasta, water, and salt to the broccoli mixture, and toss to mix. Add the cheese and mix again. Serve immediately on individual dishes and top with fresh ground pepper to taste.

PER SERVING
378 calories, 23 g protein, 51 g carbohydrate, 9 g fat (1.5 g saturated), 34 mg cholesterol, 231 mg sodium, 8 g fiber; plus 6 mg Vitamin B$_6$ (30% DV), 1 mg manganese (43% DV), 65 mg magnesium (17% DV)

CHAPTER 16

INSOMNIA

Catherine is 47 and for most of her life has been what she calls "a champion sleeper." Once, when Catherine was 12 years old, her younger sister got sick and passed out in the middle of the night. An ambulance came to the house, accompanied by two police cars and a fire engine. As the ambulance whisked the girl away with sirens blaring, neighbors heard the ruckus and came out on their lawns to see what was happening. Catherine, as you may have already guessed, slept through the entire incident. Thirty-five years later, the family members still tell the story with genuine astonishment that anyone could sleep so soundly.

Catherine lost her super-sleeper status after complex shoulder surgery two years ago. For eight weeks after surgery, she had to spend her nights sitting bolt upright on the couch; and for another eight weeks after that, she could only lean back on a huge pile of pillows—no lying down. For those four months the pain was so bad that she barely slept—three solid hours of sleep was a good night. Months later, after she was done with physical therapy, she could lie down flat on the bed, but she still didn't sleep well. She said that it felt as though her body had forgotten how to sleep. No matter what time she turned in, no matter how many hours she had been awake, or how tired she was, she couldn't seem to sleep longer than four hours. Even the smallest sound would awaken her and then she was up for the rest of the night. She mourned the loss of her sleep as though she had lost a close friend.

Catherine's sister, Joanna, has a different problem. As a busy stay-at-home mom, Joanna had always managed to carve out time to relax in those precious hours between her daughters' bedtime and her own. Joanna stuck to her routine as the girls grew; the only problem was that their bedtime got later and later. Preserving those few hours of private time meant staying up until 2:00 a.m. In a way it's not a problem for her; she has no trouble staying awake, and no trouble falling asleep once she goes to bed. She gets up at 6:00 a.m. to get the girls off to school, and then settles in for a nap from 9:00 a.m. until 11:00 a.m. In the past two months, Joanna has decided to resume her career, but she can't seem to break her night owl ways. She doesn't want to apply for jobs until she knows that she can maintain a "normal" schedule, but she has been unsuccessful so far. Now she's wondering if she might have to take shiftwork.

Catherine and Joanna's father, Harry, is in his 80s. His insomnia has gotten steadily worse over the past decade, and he blames it on getting older. He has no trouble falling asleep . . . but *staying* asleep is a problem. No matter what time he goes to bed, he always wakes up between 3:00 a.m. and 4:00 a.m., and he can't get back to sleep. He stays wide awake until about noon, but then he feels exhausted. By evening, when friends and family can schedule time to get together, he's too tired to enjoy their company. He feels like he is missing half his life.

One family, three distinct sleep problems. Sadly, this family's problems are not unusual. Experts at the National Institutes of Health estimate that about 70 million Americans experience sleep problems, and about half of those can be considered chronic. Insomnia is more than frustrating; it can be downright dangerous. Excess sleepiness increases everyone's risk of injury from accidents. And lack of sleep can weaken the immune system, raising your chances of developing everything from a common cold to cardiovascular disease. Of course, long-term disease prospects are no help when you are lying in bed in the dark, wide awake with no hope of sleep. It is hard not to feel like you are the only person on earth staring at the ceiling. It's lonely, and depressing . . . and unnecessary. Nutrition has answers for many different cases and types of insomnia.

WHAT AFFECTS YOUR ABILITY TO SLEEP?

Insomnia has many different faces. It can mean difficulty falling asleep, frequent waking throughout the night, or waking up too early in the morning. (But just because you don't sleep much, that doesn't necessarily mean you have a problem—many people feel that three or four hours of sleep each night are sufficient. They are happy to have more time in their day, and do not have insomnia.)

It is not unusual for just about anyone to have difficulty sleeping once in a while, particularly in times of stress, or during travel, or if the room you're sleeping in is too hot, cold, noisy, or bright. These types of short-term insomnia are annoying, and can certainly affect the way you function the next day, but they are often easily remedied.

Temporary insomnia also can be caused by certain medications, including bronchodilators, pseudoephedrine (found in some over-the-counter cold medicines), antipsychotic medications, beta-blockers, calcium channel blockers, most antidepressants, and many, many others. If your insomnia started within two weeks of starting a new medication, talk with your doctor about whether there is a different medication or dose that might work better for you.

If insomnia occurs at least three nights a week for a month or longer, it is considered chronic. At this point, lack of sleep becomes more than just an annoyance, it can be life altering. Almost all cases of chronic insomnia can be traced to a medical condition, a lifestyle habit, or a psychological preoccupation. Let's take a closer look at all three.

MEDICAL CONDITIONS

Conventional wisdom had it that insomnia was age-related and you could reasonably expect your sleep habits to change after age 60. That's no longer considered true. Although people do seem to have more difficulty sleeping as they get older, the underlying reason is usually medical. In other words, insomnia is not an inescapable companion of aging. For example, we know that sleep can worsen in people who have depression, gastroesophageal reflux disease (GERD), sleep apnea, restless legs syndrome, arthritis, kidney or heart disease, osteoporosis, cancer, or Parkinson's disease—most of which occur more often in older people. Those disorders can affect neuron function, cause pain, interfere with breathing, or trigger major muscle movements—all of which can lead to sleeplessness. That's why it is important to have all new cases of insomnia checked out by a doctor, to rule out the possibility of a physical disorder.

Remember Harry, Catherine and Joanna's dad, who thought that his 10-year problem with insomnia was due to old age? It turned out that he had Parkinson's disease. Three months after starting medication for the disorder, he was surprised to find that his insomnia had disappeared. Now, he regularly sleeps until 7:00 a.m. (or later!), and he has more energy later in the day. But really, curing Harry's insomnia was just a side benefit—he was finally getting help for a disease that went untreated for years.

LIFESTYLE FACTORS

Everything that affects the rhythms of your life can affect your sleep pattern: the long work hours leading up to a deadline, a new exercise routine, a suddenly busy travel schedule.

FAQS

When I drink coffee, I only drink decaf, but on the nights I have a cup, I notice I have a hard time falling asleep. My friend told me that even decaffeinated coffees and teas contain small amounts of caffeine. Is that true? Do I need to stop drinking hot beverages at night?

The teeny-tiny amount of caffeine in decaffeinated drinks is so inconsequential that it really shouldn't affect your sleep (generally less than 5 milligrams per cup serving, compared to 100+ milligrams in regular coffee). There are a couple of reasons why your beverages might keep you awake. First, if you order decaf coffee at a restaurant, you may not be drinking real decaf. It is a sad fact that some restaurants accidentally serve full-caffeine coffee—instead of decaf. Even the color of the pot or the label on the tureen may be misleading. If caffeine is a real problem for you, I recommend you avoid coffee altogether when you eat out. Instead, order decaffeinated or herbal tea, and examine the tag to confirm that you received what you asked for. Another possibility is that there is a psychological reason...either you are worried about being kept awake, or you are too revved up from your evening's activities. If there is any lingering doubt, switch to herbal teas, which naturally contain no caffeine.

All that upheaval can be reflected in your sleep patterns. For example, when people retire, they may sleep later, or feel less stress than they did when they (or their spouses) were still working. These changes help some people sleep better, but others develop insomnia. It may take a while for the new lifestyle to become routine, and for new habits to assert themselves. Until then, sleeplessness can be a real problem.

Some lifestyle choices have an immediate effect on sleep. For example, caffeine and nicotine are common causes of insomnia because they can activate the brain. So if you need yet another good reason to quit smoking, do it to improve your sleep.

PSYCHOLOGICAL FACTORS

Mental preoccupation can have devastating effects on sleep. We all know how worrying over a plague-ridden work project can wreck a night's sleep. Imagine if those feelings lasted for *years*. A friend of a friend, a lovely man who had been the comedian of his suburban neighborhood, lost his 10-year-old daughter to a car accident. He started down a spiral of insomnia that continues to this day, eight years later. He is not clinically depressed, but he is chronically sad and he just doesn't sleep. He keeps himself in that personal hell as a way to assure that he doesn't ever live a normal day without his daughter.

I wish he would see a doctor. If you have experienced long-term insomnia, I encourage you to see one, no matter what you think the cause is, no matter whether it is based in physiology or psychology . . . because you don't have to live like that. Help is available.

HOW FOOD AFFECTS SLEEP

Combating insomnia through nutrition is about eating the right combination of foods in the evening, and—perhaps even more importantly—knowing what foods to avoid.

WHAT TO EAT FOR A GOOD NIGHT'S SLEEP

Among the best natural sedatives is tryptophan, an amino acid component of many plant and animal proteins. Tryptophan is one of the ingredients necessary for the body to make serotonin, the neurotransmitter best known for creating feelings of calm, and for making you sleepy. How sleepy? A 2005 study of people with chronic insomnia found that diet made a big difference. After three weeks, those who ate foods with high amounts of tryptophan with carbohydrates or who took pharmaceutical grade tryptophan supplements had improvements on all measures of sleep . . . and food sources worked just as well as the supplements.

The trick is to combine foods that have some tryptophan with ample carbohydrates. That's because in order for insomnia-busting tryptophan to work, it has to make its way to the brain. Unfortunately, amino acids compete with each other for transport to the brain. When you eat carbs, they trigger the release of insulin, which transports competing amino acids into muscle tissue . . . but leaves tryptophan alone, so it can make its way to the brain.

BEST LOW-PROTEIN/HIGH-CARB FOODS FOR SEROTONIN PRODUCTION: *whole grain breads, crackers, and cereal; whole wheat pasta; brown rice, wild rice; whole wheat couscous; buckwheat; oats; oatmeal; amaranth; fruits, especially mangos, bananas, grapes, papaya, oranges, grapefruit, and plums; vegetables, especially spinach, yams, sweet potatoes, white potatoes, corn, squash, green peas, broccoli, Brussels sprouts, kale, asparagus, cauliflower, sugar snap peas, pumpkin, celery, beets; milk (fat-free, 1% reduced-fat), yogurt (fat-free, low-fat), low-fat ice cream, low-fat frozen yogurt*

WHAT NOT TO EAT BEFORE BED

CAFFEINE

It seems obvious, but you'd be surprised how many caffeine junkies come into my practice complaining of sleep problems! You should avoid caffeinated drinks and foods—coffee, tea, many soft drinks, and chocolate—several hours before bed. Caffeine is a natural chemical that activates the central nervous system, which means that it revs up nerves and thought processes. For people who are sensitive to caffeine, that excitation is not pleasant. It leaves them feeling jittery and slightly ill. If you drink caffeinated drinks too close to bedtime, chances are it will keep you awake. Of course, what *too close* means varies from person to person. Sensitive people should stop drinking caffeine at least eight hours before bedtime (that means by 3:00 p.m., if you hit the sack at 11:00 p.m.). You can play with your particular timing . . . just don't experiment on a night when you're counting on getting a good night's sleep.

ALCOHOL

It's true that a drink (or two) can make you sleepy and may help you get to sleep. But after a few hours, alcohol can cause frequent awakenings and lighter, less restful sleep. I'm not saying you need to give up alcohol, but don't use it like a sleeping pill; and if you have insomnia, I strongly recommend omitting alcohol for a few weeks to see if your sleep problem resolves.

LARGE MEALS

Eating a huge dinner, or even a large before-bedtime snack, may make you feel drowsy, but the sleep won't necessarily take. When you lie down and try to sleep, there's a good

FAQS

I've been waking up with cookie crumbs in my pajamas and a mess in my kitchen. I think I'm getting up and eating at night, but I don't remember any of it. Is this possible?

Yes, it is possible, and more common than you might think. There are several different reasons why this happens. If you are on a very restrictive weight-loss diet, your body may be doing what comes naturally—seeking food it desperately wants. If this sounds like you, I recommend eating one of my bedtime snacks (page 383) to make sure you don't get hungry in the middle of the night.

Or, maybe you're eating enough during the day but "overly preoccupied" with food, even while you sleep. I've had some clients who were forced to put padlocks on the kitchen cabinets, and notes around the house reminding them to "Wake up" and "Do not eat!" In this case, I also recommend that you see a psychologist. Many times, sleep eating is a sign of an eating disorder of some sort. It's always better to have these kinds of extreme behaviors checked out by a professional.

chance you'll feel uncomfortably full, which can keep you awake. Even worse, you may develop heartburn or gas, which will only increase your discomfort. I recommend eating a dinner that has no more than 600 calories (and optimally at least three hours before bed). The good news: All the dinner meal plans in this book weigh in at 600 calories or less.

LIQUIDS

The single best piece of advice I can give to those of you who wake up in the middle of the night to visit the bathroom is to not drink water or fluids within 90 minutes of bedtime. It takes that long for your body to process liquid of any type. If you must have something to drink, for example to take a prescribed medication, take a small sip. If the medication requires a full glass of water, take it earlier in the evening if possible.

BONUS POINTS

- **Make the room you sleep in comfortable and peaceful.** If your bedroom is a place of distraction and chaos, it will be that much more difficult for you to fall asleep. Remove the alarm clock from sight—instead, put it under the bed or in a drawer. Adjust the room temperature for your comfort—for most people that's between 65°F and 70°F— and make sure you have comfortable pillows and enough blankets. Hang blackout curtains or wear an eye mask if you are easily awakened by light.

- **Add white noise.** For many people, noise that is steady and not easily identifiable is easier to tune out than the sound of snoring, the rumble of traffic, or the musical stylings of the amateur trumpet player who lives next door. For others, total silence is disturbing. White noise machines emit a steady whirring or purring sound, similar to the sound of wind rustling through leaves, which provides a welcome distraction for both these problems.

- **Practice good sleep habits.** Sleeping well is often as much about establishing the right habits as anything else. Our bodies can become programmed to respond to various cues in our environment—think of how the smell of your favorite dinner can make your mouth water, or how Sunday night can throw some people into a panic at the thought of returning to work on Monday morning. It's the same way with sleep. If your bed has become a place of tension from an extended bout of insomnia (or even just worrying about insomnia), then you have to work that much harder to associate *bed* with *sleep* again. First, get a different perspective and a fresh start on new habits by making the bedroom less familiar—move the furniture around . . . or buy a new set of bedding . . . or repaint the walls. Second, try to stick with a regular schedule of going to bed and waking up, even on the weekends. That way, your body will learn to associate certain times of day with a particular part of your sleep rhythm. Third, avoid using the bedroom for anything except sleeping and sex—no reading, no television, and definitely no eating. Finally, don't let insomnia back into the bedroom. If you are unable to fall asleep within about 20 minutes of when your head hits the pillow, get up, go to another room, and do something relaxing. Return to bed only when you feel sleepy again.

- **Eliminate naps.** People with insomnia often resort to afternoon naps to catch up on their missed sleep, but that's a mistake. Napping encourages insomnia because you'll be less likely to be tired at bedtime if you sleep during the day. It can also become a counterproductive habit. Fight the urge; but if you must nap, don't sleep for more than 20 minutes. After a day or two, your body will learn that the proper time for sleep is when you lie down in bed at the end of a day.

- **Make a to-do list.** People tend to lay awake in bed angst-ridden over the all the things they need to get done. Before you go to bed each night, draft a list of everything you need to do for the next day. Getting it down on paper helps get it out of your mind.

- **Relax.** You can't run a crazy life and expect to just unplug your mind when you slip into bed. Sleep requires relaxation of mind and body. Try to take 30 minutes out at the end of each day to unwind: meditate, read, do yoga, take a hot shower or candlelight bath . . . anything that helps you put worries away for the next eight hours.

- **Exercise regularly, early in the day.** Some scientists believe that regular exercise may be the single best and safest method for improving sleep. Exercise has many wonderful effects on the body, all of which may contribute to better sleep. Exercise forces the body to work harder than usual, which means that we generally need more sleep to recuperate from the physical exertion. Exercise also increases the body's production of endorphins and other hormones that lead to feelings of calm and well-being. However, time of day matters. In a 2003 study published in the journal *Sleep,* researchers looked at the effects of moderate-intensity exercise (such as brisk walking), low-intensity stretching, and time of day. They found that women who exercised *in the morning* for at least 225 minutes a week (three and three-quarter hours) had less trouble falling asleep than those who exercised less than 180 minutes per week (three hours). However, those who exercised *at night* had more trouble falling asleep. Women who stretched also had less trouble falling asleep, and they were less likely to need sleep medication, regardless of whether they stretched at night or in the morning. So for a good night's sleep, exercise in the morning and stretch at any point during the day that works for your personal schedule.

- **Don't rely on sleeping pills.** Only your doctor can determine if sleep medication is a good option for you. Sleep medication is designed to help with occasional bouts of insomnia—even if you have a prescription, it is never a good idea to take them for more than a week or two. Some medications are physically addictive, but all can cause psychological dependence, so that you may be unable to fall asleep without the pills simply because you believe you can't. For occasional use, medications can be helpful, but they are not magic . . . it is better to fix the underlying problem.

SUPPLEMENTS

If you are plagued by insomnia and want to consider supplements, two have been studied scientifically and shown to have beneficial effects:

1. **Valerian.** This herb has been used as a sedative for hundreds of years. Like sleep medications known as benzodiazepines (which include Xanax, Valium, Librium, and Ativan), valerian seems to enhance the action of the neurotransmitter GABA (gamma amino butyric acid), which acts to calm us down and make us sleepy. If you want to try valerian, look for an extract standardized to contain 0.4 to 0.6 percent of valerenic acid. Take 400 to 900 milligrams per day, two hours before bedtime. Although valerian has been well researched for safety, it shouldn't be taken for longer than 30 days. Common side effects include headache, itchiness, dizziness, and gastrointestinal distress. You should not take valerian if you are pregnant or nursing, or if you are also taking a prescription sedative. Although valerian has not been shown to have any significant interactions with medications, it is always best to talk with your doctor before beginning any herbal supplement.

2. **Melatonin.** This neurohormone has long been linked to sleep. Research shows that people with some forms of insomnia have lower-than-normal levels of melatonin. Reviews of the medical literature suggest that taking melatonin may help some people with insomnia—in particular, some older people and so-called night owls who naturally have a hard time falling asleep before 2:00 a.m. Other people may also benefit, but the research is less clear. Melatonin seems to be safe if taken for only a month or two, with no known cautions. The most common side effects are nausea, headache, and dizziness. If you want to try melatonin, the recommended dosage is 2 to 3 milligrams per day taken 30 to 60 minutes prior to bed time. (When buying supplements, remember that 1 mg = 1000 micrograms.) If you have trouble falling asleep, use immediate-release form; if you have trouble staying asleep, use sustained-release form. You may need to take it for several days before you see any results. If you don't see results after two weeks, chances are it won't work for you at all.

JOY'S 4-STEP PROGRAM
FOR INSOMNIA

Follow this program if you have trouble falling asleep or staying asleep for at least three nights a week for at least two weeks in a row.

STEP 1 ... START WITH THE BASICS

These are the first things you should do to improve your chance for a good night's sleep.

- If you have had insomnia for a month or longer, see your doctor to rule out a medical cause.

- Stop drinking caffeinated beverages after 3:00 p.m. (or at least eight hours before bedtime).

- If you're struggling with fragmented sleep, avoid drinking alcohol.

- To avoid having to get up in the middle of the night, don't drink any beverages within 90 minutes of going to bed.

- Avoid heavy dinners, especially within three hours of going to bed.

STEP 2 ...YOUR ULTIMATE GROCERY LIST

This list contains the types of foods that help promote sleep, including those with high-quality carbohydrate and tryptophan. Foods marked with an **asterisk** (*) are the best sleep-inducing foods. This list also contains other healthy foods that are part of the meal plans and recipes for this chapter.

FRUIT

ALL fruits, but especially:	Berries	Lemon	*Plums
Apples	Cantaloupe	*Mangos	Watermelon
*Bananas	*Grapefruit	*Oranges	
	*Grapes	*Papaya	

VEGETABLES

ALL vegetables, but especially:	*Celery	Onion	Scallions
*Asparagus	*Corn	*Peas, green	Shallots
*Beets	Cucumbers	*Peas, sugar snap	*Spinach
*Broccoli	Greens, leafy	Peppers (green/red/yellow)	*Squash
*Brussels sprouts	*Kale	*Potatoes, sweet	Tomatoes (regular, cherry)
Carrots	Lettuce	*Potatoes, white	*Yams
*Cauliflower	Olives (Kalamata, Niçoise)	*Pumpkin	

LEAN MEATS/EGGS/SOY FOODS

Beef, roast (lean)	Soy sausage	Turkey burger, lean
Chicken breast	Turkey bacon, reduced-fat	
Eggs	Turkey breast	
Ham		

NUTS AND SEEDS (PREFERABLY UNSALTED)

Almonds	Peanut butter	Walnuts

WHOLE GRAINS

*Amaranth	*Buckwheat	*Oatmeal	*Rice (brown, wild)
*Breads, whole grain (crackers, English muffins, pitas)	*Cereals, whole grain	*Oats	
	*Couscous, whole wheat	*Pasta, whole wheat (for meal plan)	

DAIRY

Cheese (fat-free, reduced-fat)	Cottage cheese (fat-free or 1% reduced-fat)	*Milk (fat-free, 1% reduced-fat)	low-fat; plain, flavored)
Cheese, Cheddar, fat-free (for the meal plans)	Cream cheese (fat-free or reduced-fat)	Pudding, vanilla, low-fat	*Yogurt, frozen (not coffee flavors)
Cheese, Parmesan	*Ice cream, low-fat (not coffee flavors)	Sour cream (fat-free)	
Cheese, ricotta, fat-free		*Yogurt (fat-free,	

MISCELLANEOUS

Basil, fresh	Granola bar, low-fat	Oil, olive	Soy crisps
Broth, chicken or turkey, fat-free, low-sodium	Honey	Oil, Walnut	Sugar, brown
	Hummus	Onion powder	Sugar substitute
Broth, vegetable, fat-free	Mayonnaise, reduced-fat	Paprika	Sugar, white
	Mint, fresh	Pepper, black	Vinegar
Cayenne pepper	Mustard	Sage, fresh	Vinegar, balsamic or red wine
Cinnamon, ground	Nonstick cooking spray	Salad dressing, low-calorie	
Cumin, ground	Nutmeg	Salsa	
Garlic	Oil, canola	Salt	

* Best sleep-inducing foods

STEP3 ...GOING ABOVE AND BEYOND

For a dreamy night's sleep, here are some additional things you might try:

- Talk with your doctor about whether you are a good candidate for taking valerian or melatonin supplements.

- Restructure your evening schedule and habits to be more conducive to sleep. Take some quiet time to relax, try to turn in at the same time each night, and make the bedroom a place for sleep (and sex) only.

- Try a white noise machine to block out distracting ambient sounds.

- Make a to-do list before going to bed each night.

- Exercise regularly, but early in the day.

LAVENDER POWER

Generations ago, people put lavender sprigs in the bedroom to encourage a good night's sleep. Now, it seems there is science behind the practice. Research suggests that aromatherapy with essence of lavender calms the nervous system, allowing us to relax and fall asleep more easily. There are many different ways to use lavender to treat insomnia. The most potent is to receive a massage with essential oil, or to use an aromatherapy diffuser. Alternatively, try aromatic bath oils, lotions, soaps, air sprays, and sachets that include lavender oil. You can find a wide variety of products at health food stores and bath and body shops.

STEP4 ...MEAL PLANS

These sample menus include foods that may help you sleep better. You'll notice that protein is generously spread out between breakfast and lunch, and then dramatically lowered with dinner. That's because in order to maximize serotonin production and induce sleepiness, your dinner and bedtime snacks should optimally be low in protein and high in carbohydrate (with foods that contain some tryptophan).

Every day, choose *one* option for each of the three meals—breakfast, lunch, and dinner. Between lunch and dinner, you may have one small healthy snack of your choosing (consider fresh fruit or vegetables, a handful of nuts, or a low-fat granola bar). Then, before bed each night, choose one option from my suggested bedtime snacks, listed below. Approximate calories have been provided to help adjust for your personal weight-management goals. If you find yourself hungry (and if weight is not an issue), feel free to increase the portion sizes for meals and snacks. Beverage calories are *not* included.

BREAKFAST OPTIONS

(Approximately 300 to 400 calories)

Hard-Boiled Eggs with Turkey Bacon and Fruit

2 hard-boiled whole eggs and 2 hard-boiled egg whites with 2 strips reduced-fat turkey bacon and 1 cup berries (or ½ grapefruit or ¼ cantaloupe).

Cottage Cheese with Cantaloupe and Almonds

½ cantaloupe filled with 1 cup 1% fat-free or reduced-fat cottage cheese (or fat-free flavored yogurt), topped with 1 tablespoon slivered almonds.

Scrambled Eggs with Vegetables and English Muffin

Beat 1 whole egg with 3 egg whites. Cook scrambled eggs in skillet coated with non-stick cooking spray or 1 teaspoon canola oil, adding preferred vegetables (onion, red and green peppers, tomato—pre-sautéed in non-stick cooking spray). Enjoy with 1 dry toasted whole grain English muffin.

Whole Grain Cereal with Milk and Breakfast Sausage

1 cup whole grain cereal with 1 cup fat-free milk. Enjoy with 1 lean turkey or soy sausage (120 calories or less).

Toast with Cream Cheese, Tomato, Onion, and Lox

2 toasted slices whole wheat bread, each topped with 1 tablespoon fat-free cream cheese, sliced tomato and onion, and 1 or 2 ounces smoked salmon.

LUNCH OPTIONS

(Approximately 400 to 500 calories)

Ham and Cheese Sandwich with Crunchy Carrots and Peppers

4 or 5 ounces sliced ham (or turkey breast, lean roast beef, or grilled chicken breast), lettuce, sliced tomato, and onion on 2 slices whole grain bread or pita. Add optional 1 slice reduced-fat cheese, mustard, 2 teaspoons reduced-fat mayonnaise, or hummus. Enjoy with large handful baby carrots and green/red pepper sticks.

Grilled Chicken–Vegetable Salad

5 ounces skinless grilled chicken breast on large bed of leafy greens mixed with ½ cup cherry tomatoes, unlimited sliced cucumbers, chopped carrots, chopped sweet pepper (red, yellow or green), and artichoke hearts. Toss with 2 teaspoons olive oil and unlimited vinegar or fresh lemon juice (or 2 to 4 tablespoons low-calorie dressing).

Turkey Burger with Veggies

1 (5-ounce) lean turkey burger on ½ whole grain bun (or in one 70-calorie pita pocket). Serve with 1 cup steamed vegetables (choose from broccoli, cauliflower, spinach) topped with optional 1 tablespoon grated Parmesan cheese.

Vegetable Tuna Salad with Whole Grain Pita

Veggie Tuna Salad (page 274). Enjoy with 150 calories of whole wheat pita bread or whole grain crackers plus ¼ cantaloupe (or 1 cup watermelon or mixed berries).

Turkey Chili with Mixed Green Salad

1 serving (2 cups) Turkey Chili (page 367) or 2 cups prepared turkey or vegetarian chili, topped with 1 ounce shredded fat-free Cheddar cheese. Enjoy with tossed salad (leafy greens and other preferred vegetables) with 1 teaspoon olive oil and unlimited vinegar or fresh lemon juice (or 2 to 3 tablespoons low-calorie dressing).

DINNER OPTIONS

(Approximately 500 to 600 calories)

Pasta with Roasted Pumpkin and Salad

1 serving Angel Hair Pasta with Roasted Pumpkin, Sage, and Walnuts (page 385). Enjoy with leafy green salad tossed with 2 teaspoons olive oil and unlimited vinegar or fresh lemon juice (or 2 to 4 tablespoons low-calorie dressing).

Parmesan Couscous and Ratatouille with Vegetables

1 serving Parmesan Couscous and Ratatouille with Olives, Tomatoes, and Basil (page 388).

Apple-Cinnamon Oatmeal for Dinner

1 cup dry instant oatmeal prepared with 1 cup fat-free milk and 1 cup water (microwave for 1½ to 2 minutes); mix with 1 chopped apple and microwave for an additional 30 to 60 seconds. Sprinkle with optional cinnamon and 1 teaspoon brown sugar, white sugar, or honey (or artificial sweetener).

Sweet Potato–Cauliflower Mash with Warm Turkey Bacon-Spinach Salad

1 serving Sweet Potato–Cauliflower Mash with Warm Bacon-Spinach Salad (page 386). Enjoy with 1 plain toasted whole wheat pita bread or 2 servings Tangy Pita Chips (page 389).

Baked Potato with Broccoli and Cheese

1 baked potato topped with cooked chopped broccoli and 1 ounce melted reduced-fat or fat-free cheese. Serve with 2 servings (2 cups) Vegetable Oatmeal Bisque (page 323), or 2 cups of any prepared vegetable soup.

BEDTIME SNACK OPTIONS

(Serotonin-producing)

100 calories or less

- *Best Vegetables for Sleep:* 1 cup raw or cooked spinach, broccoli, Brussels sprouts, kale, asparagus, cauliflower, sugar snap peas, celery, beets

- *Best Fruits for Sleep:* 1 cup grapes (plain or frozen), 1 orange, 1 plum, ½ grapefruit, ½ banana, ½ mango, ½ papaya

- Tangy Pita Chips (page 389) with salsa

- 1 cup fat-free milk

- 6 ounces fat-free flavored yogurt (100 calories or less)

100 to 200 calories

- Banana-Mango Parfait (page 390)

- Cinnamon Oatmeal: ½ cup dry instant oatmeal prepared with ½ cup fat-free milk and ½ cup water. Sprinkle with cinnamon and optional Splenda.

- Frozen banana

- 1 slice whole wheat toast topped with sliced tomato and 1 slice fat-free cheese

- 1 banana with 1 level teaspoon peanut butter

- 1 cup fat-free milk with 1 orange (or 1 cup grapes, 1 plum, ½ grapefruit, ½ banana, ½ mango, or ½ papaya)

- ½ cup frozen yogurt or low-fat ice cream (avoid coffee flavors)

- 1 low-fat ice cream pop (less than 200 calories, avoid coffee flavors)

- ½ cup low-fat vanilla pudding

- ¾ cup whole grain cereal (120 calories or less) with 1 cup fat-free milk

- 1 serving (1½ cups) Sweet Potato–Cauliflower Mash (page 386)

- ½ baked sweet or white potato with optional 1 tablespoon grated Parmesan cheese

ANGEL HAIR PASTA WITH ROASTED PUMPKIN, SAGE, AND WALNUTS

If you love pasta, but you're tired of eating the same old spaghetti with tomato sauce, definitely try this recipe. The unique combination of roasted pumpkin, walnuts, and sage create a colorful and delicious dish. Another bonus—two of three Bauer children like it!

Makes 3 servings (2 cups per serving)

	Nonstick cooking spray
1	pound fresh pumpkin, cut into $\frac{1}{2}$-inch cubes (about 2 cups)
	Salt
1	package (8 ounces) whole wheat angel hair pasta
1	tablespoon olive oil or walnut oil
$\frac{1}{4}$	cup fresh sage leaves, finely sliced
2	tablespoons walnuts, chopped
$\frac{1}{2}$	cup fat-free ricotta cheese, at room temperature
$\frac{1}{2}$	cup fat-free, low-sodium chicken or vegetable broth, heated
	Ground black pepper

1. Preheat the oven to 425°F. Cover a large baking sheet with parchment paper or aluminum foil, and coat with nonstick cooking spray.

2. Arrange the pumpkin cubes on the prepared baking sheet in a single layer so they are not touching. Coat the pumpkin with nonstick cooking spray, and sprinkle with salt. Roast 15 to 20 minutes, until the pumpkin has softened and begins to take on a gold color.

3. Cook the pasta according to the package instructions. Drain, reserving $1\frac{1}{2}$ cups of the cooking water.

4. Coat a large skillet with nonstick cooking spray Add the oil and heat over high heat. Add the sage and cook, stirring, 1 to 2 minutes, until the sage turns dark green (but not brown) and becomes crispy. Reduce the heat to low and add the pumpkin, pasta, walnuts, ricotta, broth, and 1 cup of the pasta cooking water. Stir to coat the pasta. Season with additional salt and black pepper. If the pasta is too dry, add more of the cooking water. Serve immediately.

PER SERVING
388 calories, 18 g protein, 60 g carbohydrate, 10 g fat (1 g saturated), 10 mg cholesterol, 200 mg sodium, 13 g fiber

SWEET POTATO–CAULIFLOWER MASH WITH WARM TURKEY BACON–SPINACH SALAD

My low-cal mashed potatoes were accidentally created one night when I didn't have enough sweet potatoes and used leftover cauliflower to beef up mashed sweet potatoes. Clearly, an accident meant to happen—only 122 calories in 1½ cups, yet still loaded with nutrition and fiber. Enjoy the sweet potatoes with any meal you prepare . . . or couple with the spinach salad.

Makes 2 servings

SWEET POTATO–CAULIFLOWER MASH

	1 large sweet potato (½ pound), peeled and cubed
¼	head cauliflower, cut into florets (about 1 cup)
½	cup fat-free, low-sodium chicken or turkey broth, heated
2	tablespoons fat-free sour cream
1	clove garlic, minced
¼	teaspoon freshly grated nutmeg
	Salt
	Ground black pepper
1	scallion, minced

Steam the sweet potato and cauliflower over 1" of water until fork tender, 9 to 10 minutes. In a large bowl, mash the potato and cauliflower with the broth. Stir in the sour cream, garlic, and nutmeg. Season to taste with salt and black pepper. Garnish each serving with scallion. *Makes 3 cups.*

PER SERVING
122 calories, 4 g protein, 27 g carbohydrate, 6 g total sugar, 0 g fat, 0 mg cholesterol, 236 mg sodium, 5 g fiber

WARM TURKEY BACON-SPINACH SALAD

	1 pound baby spinach (about 4 cups)
4	slices turkey bacon
1	tablespoon olive oil
1	small shallot, thinly sliced
¼	cup fat-free, low-sodium chicken or turkey broth, heated
2	tablespoons sherry vinegar or balsamic vinegar
½	teaspoon mustard
2	tablespoons toasted walnuts
	Salt
	Ground black pepper

Place the spinach in a large bowl, or divide evenly between two large plates. In a medium skillet over medium-high heat, cook the turkey bacon 3 to 4 minutes, until crisp and browned. Crumble, and sprinkle over the spinach. In the same skillet, heat the olive oil over medium-low heat. Add the shallot and cook, stirring, 1 to 2 minutes, until softened. Add the broth, vinegar, and mustard, and cook, stirring, until the mixture forms a dressing. Immediately pour over the salad. Top with the walnuts. Season to taste with salt and pepper.

PER SERVING
200 calories, 7 g protein, 4 g carbohydrate, 17 g fat (3 g saturated), 30 mg cholesterol, 450 mg sodium, 6 g fiber

PARMESAN COUSCOUS AND RATATOUILLE WITH OLIVES, TOMATOES, AND FRESH BASIL

Although this flavorful Mediterranean dish may appear complicated, it's not. I prefer it without the olives, but my husband (and son) insist on them. Of course, in your kitchen, you're the boss!

Makes 3 servings (1½ cups ratatouille; 1½ cups couscous per serving)

RATATOUILLE

½	pound kale, stems trimmed, thinly sliced
	Salt
¾	cup water
1	tablespoon olive oil
1	large yellow squash, cut into small dice (about 2 cups)
½	pound (about 2 medium) tomatoes, diced
¼	cup Kalamata or Niçoise olives (7 or 8 olives), pitted and chopped
	Pinch of cayenne pepper
¼	cup whole basil leaves, torn

COUSCOUS

1	cup whole wheat couscous
1	cup sugar snap peas, diced
1¼	cups fat-free, low-sodium chicken broth, heated
½	cup grated reduced-fat Parmesan cheese
	Salt
	Ground black pepper

To make the ratatouille: Heat a deep sauté pan over high heat. Add the kale, a sprinkle of salt, and the water. Cook, stirring occasionally, until softened, 13 to 15 minutes. If the kale becomes too dry, add more water. Stir in the oil, squash, tomatoes, olives, and cayenne. Cook 5 to 6 minutes, until the squash is tender and the tomatoes lose their shape. Remove from the heat, and stir in the fresh basil. Set aside.

To make the couscous: In a medium bowl, mix the couscous and sugar snap peas. Pour the hot broth on top, stir once, and cover with plastic wrap or aluminum foil. Allow the couscous to rest 5 to 6 minutes, until all the water is absorbed and the couscous is soft and fluffy. Fold the Parmesan cheese into the couscous, and season with salt and black pepper if necessary.

To serve: Mold the couscous into a coffee mug or ramekin, then turn it over onto a plate for a nice presentation. Or place couscous in a warm soup plate. Either way, serve the ratatouille over top.

PER SERVING
514 calories, 22 g protein, 88 g carbohydrate, 12 g fat (3 g saturated), 0 mg cholesterol, 561 mg sodium, 15 g fiber

TANGY PITA CHIPS

If you're looking for crunch, my tangy pita chips will hit the spot. In fact, if you're any-thing like me, make sure you ONLY prepare one portion at a time—it's too easy to gobble down several servings. Enjoy with your favorite prepared or jarred salsa!

Makes 1 serving

1	small whole wheat pita pocket
1	clove garlic, cut in half lengthwise
¼	teaspoon onion powder
⅛	teaspoon ground cumin
⅛	teaspoon paprika
⅛	teaspoon fine sea salt
	Pinch of cayenne pepper
	Pinch of freshly ground black pepper
	Nonstick cooking spray

1. Preheat the oven or toaster oven to 350°F. Split the pita pocket, and rub the top of each half with the cut side of the garlic clove.
2. In a small bowl, combine the onion powder, cumin, paprika, sea salt, cayenne, and black pepper. Sprinkle the spice mixture over the 2 pita halves. Coat the pita with nonstick cooking spray.
3. Toast directly on a wire rack for 8 to 9 minutes, until the spices give off fragrance and the pita is crispy. Eat whole, or cut into wedges.

PER SERVING
70 calories, 3.5 g protein, 16 g carbohydrate, 0 g fat, 0 mg cholesterol, 500 mg sodium, 3 g fiber

BANANA-MANGO PARFAIT

You'll love the rich, decadent flavor in this sleepy-time snack. And because it's comprised of three fabulous ingredients—banana, mango, and fat-free ricotta cheese—your body gets a blast of nutrition before bed. I like it super cold, chilled for at least an hour.

Makes 3 servings

1	ripe medium mango, peeled and cubed
2	tablespoons sugar
1	cup fat-free ricotta cheese
¼	cup mint leaves, finely sliced, plus 3 whole sprigs for garnish
1	large banana, thinly sliced

1. Puree the mango and sugar in a blender until smooth. Transfer to a large bowl and stir in the ricotta and sliced mint.
2. Spoon 2 tablespoons of the ricotta mixture into each of 3 parfait glasses. Top with half of the banana slices, and another layer of ricotta. Top with the remaining banana, and then the remaining ricotta mixture.
3. Garnish each glass with a sprig of fresh mint. Serve immediately, or chill up to 4 hours.

PER SERVING
164 calories, 8 g protein, 33 g carbohydrate, 0 g fat, 20 mg cholesterol, 201 mg sodium, 2 g fiber

CHAPTER 17

IRRITABLE BOWEL SYNDROME

Irritable bowel syndrome (IBS) is common, affecting about 20 percent of Americans, and yet it is a mystery. No one knows exactly what causes it and there is no way for a doctor to make a definitive diagnosis. There is no single trigger, and no single set of identifying symptoms, which can come and go in a day, or plague sufferers for months or years. So much uncertainty attached to very real physical discomfort makes coping with IBS frustrating in the extreme.

IBS is called a *functional bowel disorder,* and not a disease, because it doesn't cause permanent damage, it doesn't progress to serious illness, and it can usually be controlled with diet and lifestyle changes. There's another reason to be hopeful if your case is a persistent one—people with chronic symptoms like yours have been successfully treated with new medications, making the condition less disabling than ever before.

WHAT AFFECTS IBS?

The agony of IBS comes from the pain, discomfort, and embarrassing inconvenience of symptoms, which include diarrhea or constipation, cramping, bloating, excess gas, and mucus in the stool. To understand what happens in IBS, imagine a football stadium full of spectators doing "the wave." If everyone cooperates, you can see the forward progress of the wave as each section stands and then sits again—it's amazing to see so many bodies working in concert. Now imagine that you have some very nervous spectators . . . they see the wave coming at them, and they stand up too early, starting a secondary wave, so now there are two competing waves. The rhythm is disrupted. Or, imagine that one group stands up for the wave but doesn't sit back down again. The wave is "stuck," unable to move forward until the disrupting group decides to sit back down again.

Our intestines are lined with muscles that contract and relax in waves (ah-ha!) called *peristalsis,* which push the food you eat through the system. Along the way, nutrients are absorbed, and the residual is eventually eliminated in feces. In people with IBS, normally rhythmic waves are disrupted. Sometimes, the nervous bowel contracts too much or too forcefully, so food moves through the intestines too quickly, resulting in diarrhea.

Other times, the intestinal muscles contract but don't relax again, or they contract very slowly, resulting in constipation. These crazy, out-of-sync muscle movements are behind the pain of IBS, much like muscle spasms in your leg cause the pain of a charley horse. We all have intestinal gas, but for people with IBS, it can become trapped inside, resulting in bloating and distention. Some of my clients with IBS have admitted to buying two wardrobes—an everyday wardrobe and another specifically for their bloated, symptomatic days. Makes perfect sense—who wants to wear a snug pair of jeans or a fitted dress when they feel like the Pillsbury Dough Boy? In addition, the intestinal nerves of people with IBS are highly sensitive, so that even minor bloating can have them doubled over in pain.

An individual with IBS might experience just a few of these symptoms, or all of them. Although most sufferers have either diarrhea-predominant IBS or constipation-predominant IBS, some people alternate between diarrhea and constipation. No matter what type of IBS you have, the underlying problem is that the rhythm of intestinal muscle contractions periodically get messed up. There is no test for messed-up intestinal waves, however, and the symptoms of IBS are common to many other diseases, so arriving at a diagnosis of IBS is lengthy and full of guesswork. Your doctor will want to rule out all other possible disorders through a physical examination, blood tests, ultrasound, x-ray of your bowels, and sigmoidoscopy or colonoscopy, in which a lighted flexible tube is inserted into your lower intestines to get an up close and personal look at your intestinal lining. If there are no other problems, it's IBS by default. Once you have a diagnosis, you and your doctor can get to work to find a treatment that works for you—IBS *can* be controlled. It's important to remember that although IBS can be uncomfortable, and strictly speaking there is no "cure," it also won't turn into anything more serious.

We don't know what disrupts the workings of the intestines in the first place, but we do know what can trigger flares of the disorder. Food is a biggie, and I'll address that in the next section. Aside from food and eating issues, the only other significant IBS trigger is stress.

Stress can trigger a flare of IBS, and it can make food-triggered IBS symptoms worse. That's why many health experts recommend that people suffering from IBS actively explore a variety of ways to de-stress—there might be a terrific way to relax that you just haven't tried yet. Some doctors even talk about an *IBS personality,* one that is noticeably tense and anxious. I've seen this is my own practice. The client that comes to mind is Amy, a kindergarten teacher. The first time I saw Amy, I was struck by her rigid body language—every move she made told me she was a very controlled person—sitting or standing her posture was perfect, and she held her arms close to her body using minimal gestures. She spoke in a clipped, drill-sergeant sort of way. Everything Amy did, she did quickly. She was always on the run doing things for the kids in her class, running errands for her family, setting up the classroom, and gobbling down her food. Amy didn't sit down to eat. If she couldn't wolf down a meal in five minutes it wasn't worth eating. The challenge with Amy was getting her to recognize her food triggers, and also—perhaps more importantly—helping her to understand that her stressful, on-the-go lifestyle was only making her IBS worse.

FAQS

I've read that I should take fiber supplements for my IBS. Are they helpful?

Many experts recommend fiber supplements, but they are not always the best medicine. I say this because many of my clients have complained they've become *more* bloated and gassy after taking them. And this goes for both types—soluble and insoluble fiber supplements. That's because people with IBS are very sensitive to fiber. When I treat clients, I start by asking about their symptoms. If it's predominantly diarrhea, I'll have them take a rest from most fiber-rich foods. Then, ever so slowly, we start adding it back—focusing first on the soluble type. If a client complains of persistent constipation, I immediately incorporate soluble fiber–rich foods (along with some insoluble fiber) evenly sprinkled throughout the day. When my clients feel well enough, we add more. I can't explain why, but when it comes to fiber, I've had much more success with food than supplements. Skip the pills and instead, add fiber-rich foods (slowly!) along with lots of flat water to your diet.

On a very basic level, eating quickly is risky because you are more likely to swallow air, which can directly lead to bloating and distention. But stress can also stimulate spasms in the gastrointestinal tract—like feeling butterflies in your stomach when rumors about impending layoffs start flying around the water cooler. In people with IBS, those butterflies are on a rampage. Amy's IBS was certainly made worse by her tense, never-stop, full-of-stress lifestyle. Fortunately, we were able to get her symptoms under control in pretty short order. We identified her food triggers (soy-based foods, raw vegetables, gum, and coffee), which eliminated most of her problems, but stress education was the biggest eye-opener for her. Amy had no idea how much her driven personality affected her bowels. Although she still has a way to go, it's easier for her to relax now that she doesn't have to worry about whether her diarrhea will strike unexpectedly and she's made a determined effort to be more relaxed. Ironically, she's as driven about finding time to de-stress as she is about everything else, but she's on her way to achieving the type of balanced life that can keep her IBS symptoms to a minimum.

HOW FOOD AFFECTS IBS

A sensitive gut needs to be treated like a fussy baby—you have to put it on a regular feeding schedule, keep it calm, and protect it from potential irritants.

IDENTIFYING TRIGGER FOODS

Identifying your particular trigger foods can be difficult. Even people without IBS will have a gastrointestinal reaction to certain foods once in a while. It just happens, and it's perfectly normal. But people with IBS have a heightened sensitivity to foods; they know the awful consequences of a trigger food so they might eat a spicy bowl of chili, for example, have a reaction, and condemn chili to a list of foods to be avoided forever. But what if the reaction was really due to unusual stress, or a mild case of food poisoning, or just one of those normal gut reactions? You might avoid a food forever for no good reason. By the time some clients come to see me, they're downright food phobic. They are so afraid of an attack of diarrhea, constipation, or horrific gas that they err on the side of caution . . . but too much caution can result in low blood sugar, weight loss, malnutrition, and another kind of socially awkward situation—they can become afraid of eating with friends and going out for fear of an attack.

For people with *extreme* IBS, the simplest way to identify the right trigger foods is to first follow an elimination diet for five to seven days—a meal plan which avoids *all* potential offending foods, then slowly reintroduce those same foods one by one. Along the way you keep track of reactions to foods you are reintroducing in a food diary. Depending upon your symptoms, my guidelines for an elimination diet vary slightly. Please note: Following an elimination diet can be very difficult. It's just a week, but you still need to be pretty committed to put up with such a limited selection of food. Then again, if you're currently suffering, better to put up with a week of discomfort than a lifetime of untreated abdominal pain.

If you have severe diarrhea-predominant IBS, your five- to seven-day elimination diet will avoid all trigger foods *plus* all fiber, including soluble fiber (instructions are provided in my 4-Step Program under Extreme Elimination Diet—No Fiber, page 408).

If you have *severe* constipation-predominant IBS, your elimination diet will avoid all trigger foods, but *incorporate* foods rich in soluble fiber and small amounts of insoluble fiber (those instructions are provided in my 4-Step Program under Elimination Diet with Added Fiber, page 411). The addition of soluble fiber can help encourage your intestines to "wave" more effectively.

Whichever plan you follow, after about a week you'll be ready to test some of the potential trigger foods. I recommend trying one new food every two to three days, and carefully documenting what you eat and how you feel during the 24 hours afterward. Although this chapter provides all the instruction you need to do this on your own, it's a big job. If you try on your own and find it unmanageable, I encourage you to work with a registered dietitian who specializes in gastrointestinal issues.

As I said, these elimination plans are only for very severe cases of IBS. For less debilitating IBS, feel free to skip the elimination meal plan altogether and go straight to keeping an IBS journal. Your journal should list exactly what you eat, when you eat, what symptoms you experience, as well as your emotional state for the day. Make a special note if you feel particularly tense, anxious, or stressed.

When you have an IBS attack, consult your diary to see which foods you ate in the

COMMON IBS TRIGGER FOODS

The most common IBS trigger foods are:

- **Milk and dairy products,** including milk, yogurt, cheese, butter, cream, cream cheese, sour cream, ice cream, frozen yogurt, sherbet, pudding, custard, prepared foods that contain dairy (i.e., cream soups, creamy salad dressings, mashed potatoes, pancakes), and baked goods that contain dairy (i.e., cake, cookies, muffins, and donuts)

- **Soy foods,** including soy milk, edamame, tempeh, tofu, soy crisps, and soy nuts and snack bars that list soy protein as an ingredient. For some people, soy sauce is a trigger.

- **Citrus fruits,** including oranges, grapefruits, tangerines, mandarin oranges, tangelos, clementines, lemons, limes, and pomelo

- **Raw vegetables,** all, including lettuce

- **Cruciferous vegetables,** including broccoli, cauliflower, kale, cabbage, Brussels sprouts, bok choy, turnip greens, mustard greens, and collard greens; also, the nightshade vegetables—eggplant and peppers.

- **Wheat,** including all products made with wheat flour such as bread, crackers, pasta, and cereals

- **Foods high in insoluble fiber:** Some people are *only* sensitive to wheat products that are very high in insoluble fiber, such as wheat bran and high-fiber breakfast cereals.

- **Concentrated sources of fructose,** such as sugar, honey, fruit juice and beverages, dried fruit, and candies and syrup that contain high fructose corn syrup

- **Beans and lentils**

- **Whole nuts and seeds:** Nut butters are typically tolerated, but still test to be certain they are safe for you.

- **Corn and popcorn**

- **Garlic and onions**

- **Spicy foods**

- **Carbonated beverages:** any drinks that fizz with little bubbles

- **Caffeinated drinks,** such as coffee, tea, and colas

- **Alcohol**

- **Fatty foods,** especially fried foods such as French fries, onion rings, fried fish and chicken, or deep-fried anything

- **Red meat,** particularly steaks, hamburgers, hot dogs, cold cuts, and sausages

- **Sugar alcohol sweeteners:** all foods, gums, and candy containing sorbitol, malitol, and mannitol

- **Olestra** (fat substitute)

- **Chewing gum** (sugared and sugar-free)

- **Chocolate** (sorry!)

- **Condiments,** including ketchup, mustard, pickle relish, soy sauce, chutney, mayonnaise, and barbecue sauce previous 24 hours and start a list of your potential triggers. Keep eating normally, always noting which foods you ate in the 24 hours prior to an attack and adding new items to your potential trigger list. When a food already on your list precedes an attack, make a hatch mark next to it each time it comes up. After a few weeks, those marks should tell you which foods are most likely to trigger an episode. Narrow down your list to the three most likely triggers, and avoid those foods entirely for two weeks. Continue to keep your IBS journal, and repeat the process. Every once in a while, test your trigger foods again (one at a time) to make sure you're not avoiding them for no reason. Over time, you'll have a good handle on which foods you need to avoid to feel well, and which you can eat safely. NOTE: If you find yourself with more than five main trigger foods, see a dietitian to make sure that the rest of your diet is making up for whatever nutrients you're missing by eliminating those foods.

For everyone fighting IBS, there are a few mealtime guidelines that can make your life easier:

1. Try to eat meals at the same time each day to get your body used to a schedule.
2. Eat smaller, more frequent meals so you don't overload your gut at any one time.
3. Slow down—sit, relax, and take time to chew your food. Think of it as time invested in training your digestive system to behave.

GOOD FOODS TO CHOOSE

The best foods for IBS health are those that are gentle on the digestive system, and which encourage "smooth passage" through the intestines. Thus, vegetables, fruit, and whole grains—*it pains me to say*—should be limited until your symptoms subside and you identify foods that are problematic for you. It's hard to imagine I just said that! Truth be told, these healthful foods are a bit hard for the body to break down, but remember I'm only recommending you watch your intake *until* you've got a handle on your triggers—even with diarrhea-predominant IBS, you should eventually be able to tolerate moderate amounts of all three groups, although you'll probably need to cook vegetables.

SOLUBLE FIBER

Fiber comes in two main varieties: soluble and insoluble. Soluble fiber dissolves in water and turns into a kind of gooey, gummy consistency—think what happens to oatmeal after it sits in a pot of water for a time. Insoluble fiber is tougher. It doesn't dissolve, and pretty much keeps its form.

Although insoluble fiber is generally healthy, it can be hard on the intestines of people with IBS. Insoluble fiber speeds food through the colon, something that many diarrhea-predominant IBS sufferers want to avoid. People with constipation-predominant IBS may want to experiment with how much insoluble fiber they can eat without experiencing too much gas and bloating.

Soluble fiber, on the other hand, promotes gentle regularity, regardless of the type of IBS you have. That's why you'll find plenty of soluble fiber integrated into my Elimination

Diet with Added Fiber (it doesn't, however, include soluble fiber–rich foods that also act as potential triggers, such as beans, lentils, broccoli, and cabbage).

Most foods high in soluble fiber are considered safe for people with IBS. The trick is to eat a variety of foods in moderation, without eating too much of one particular food, or too much food in general at one time. If you have diarrhea-predominant IBS, I recommend slowly adding more foods high in soluble fiber to your diet. If you experience too much bloating or pain, back off a little, wait a few days, then add fiber again. The key is to eat just a little bit of extra fiber, building up to about six servings a day over a course of weeks, not days. However, for constipation-predominant IBS, you can be more aggressive, fiber-wise. The Elimination Diet with Added Fiber (for constipation-predominant IBS) works in three to six (or more) daily portions of soluble fiber, depending upon the meals and snacks you chose. Of course, even then you'll want to moderate the portions and spread them throughout the day—as opposed to eating them all at one sitting—to avoid the risk of excess gas. And . . . remember to drink plenty of water to help move it along.

In my Elimination Diet with Added Fiber, I incorporate at least one serving of soluble fiber–rich food at each meal. If you have diarrhea-predominant IBS, and you're

LACTOSE INTOLERANCE VERSUS IBS

Milk can trigger IBS, that's why you'll find dairy on the list of foods to initially avoid. But sensitivity to dairy foods may also be a sign of lactose intolerance. Lactose intolerance is not IBS. In fact, it's a completely different problem and one that's easily remedied. If you suspect you're lactose intolerant, make dairy the first thing you test.

Milk products contain a form of natural sugar called lactose. In order to digest lactose, our bodies produce a specific enzyme called lactase. For a variety of reasons, including genetic abnormalities, digestive disorders (i.e., celiac disease, Crohn's disease, IBS), intestinal injury, and/or the natural aging process, some people end up with very low levels of lactase. Depending on how much of the offending food you eat, and how much lactase enzyme your body can produce, symptoms can be mild or severe, and include nausea, cramping, gas, bloating, and diarrhea. Sound familiar? The symptoms can be remarkably like IBS symptoms. So, how do you tell the difference? Simple. Avoid milk and anything containing milk for three to five days (see full dairy list under Common IBS Trigger Foods, page 395). If your symptoms disappear, you're probably lactose intolerant. If you're willing to avoid those trigger foods indefinitely, it really doesn't matter whether you have lactose intolerance or IBS—as long as you don't eat them you'll feel fine.

On the other hand, you may want to know definitively which it is—IBS or lactose intolerance, if only to understand your options. Many people with lactose intolerance can enjoy lactose-reduced milk products without any symptoms. Others take lactase enzyme (such as Lactaid) in a tablet or liquid form with their first bite or sip of a milk product and voila—no digestive trouble. It's unlikely people with dairy-triggered IBS can tolerate these reduced-lactose products. But those aren't diagnostic tests. If you really want an answer ask your doctor about these: the Lactose Tolerance Test, which is a series of blood tests taken over a two-hour period after drinking a lactose-rich test drink; and the Hydrogen Breath Test, which looks for a higher-than-normal amount of hydrogen in the breath, caused by the extra gases produced by the bacteria fermenting the undigested lactose in the intestines.

If you test positive for lactose intolerance and avoid all milk products but still have gastrointestinal symptoms, talk with your doctor about whether you need additional testing. In the end, you may have both, lactose intolerance and IBS (I know—oy!).

ready to follow the less extreme Elimination Diet with Added Fiber, you may want to move more slowly . . . starting with a single serving for the entire day. All foods rich in soluble fiber included in Your Ultimate Grocery List have an asterisk (*), so you'll know what to include and what to avoid. Everything is explained in the 4-Step Program, page 403.

In addition, raw vegetables—*whether rich in soluble OR insoluble fiber*—tend to be difficult for IBS sufferers to digest and can often trigger diarrhea, gas, and bloating. When you're ready to introduce vegetables into your diet, I strongly recommend you stick to cooked vegetables.

> **BEST FOODS FOR SOLUBLE FIBER:** *Psyllium Seeds (ground), oat and rice bran, oatmeal, barley, peas, apple, blackberries, pears, apricots, cantaloupe, strawberries, bananas, peaches, cooked carrots, cooked spinach, sweet potatoes, yams, white potatoes, avocado, raspberries, flaxseed (ground)*

LIQUIDS

All people with IBS should strive to drink at least eight 8-ounce glasses of flat water every day. If constipation is your problem, water will help keep your stools moist so they pass more easily; the soluble fiber in your diet will help too. If diarrhea is your problem, you'll need to replenish the water you lose through loose stools. Plain water and naturally decaffeinated herbal teas should be your first choices. Carbonated beverages are the worst choices because the gas from the carbonation gets trapped in your intestines, causing discomfort. If you have diarrhea-predominant IBS, you'll also want to avoid drinking caffeinated beverages and alcohol, which can stimulate the intestines and make symptoms worse.

BONUS POINTS

- **Rule out other disorders.** Please don't assume that your symptoms are due to IBS unless your doctor has told you so. You need to get a thorough medical workup to rule out other, more serious diseases, including Crohn's disease, ulcerative colitis, celiac disease, and colorectal cancer. Even if you've had a diagnosis of IBS, be sure to go back to your doctor if your symptoms change or worsen.
- **Talk with your doctor about medications.** The standard of care is to treat IBS with diet and lifestyle changes. But if you can't get your symptoms under control, and if the pain and other symptoms are affecting your life, ask your doctor about medications that have been approved for IBS. There are a variety of possible medications, including antispasmodics, antidiarrheals, and antidepressants. Yes, antidepressants—for your intestines, not your brain—because they seem to modulate intestinal pain and regulate gut regularity. Many antidepressants regulate the neurotransmitter serotonin and (who knew?) 95 percent of serotonin is found in your gut, where it helps maintain smooth,

regular contractions of the intestines. Some scientists believe that the intestines of people with IBS require more serotonin than they're getting for normal function. The theory is that antidepressants that make more serotonin available (the serotonin reuptake inhibitors—SSRIs—such as Prozac, Zoloft, or Paxil), will fix the problem. More research needs to be done before antidepressants are a first-line treatment, but if you've tried everything else, you may want to discuss this possibility with your physician.

- **Don't self-medicate without guidance.** You may be tempted to take control of IBS by stocking up on over-the-counter laxatives or anti-diarrhea medication. Don't do it unless you get the go-ahead from your doctor. IBS is a chronic disorder, and over-the-counter medications are short-term solutions. Laxatives in particular can be hard on the intestines if used inappropriately. If you find yourself relying on over-the-counter meds, talk with your doctor to find a better solution.

- **Maintain healthy eating patterns.** Eat small meals regularly throughout the day. Try to eat at about the same time each day. Slow down during meal time—try to avoid on-the-run (or over-the-kitchen-sink) eating.

- **Put a lid on stress.** Stress is a complex problem. Although circumstances outside our control can *feel* stressful, psychologists remind us that events don't *create* stress. Stress is of our own making. It's how we interpret events or think about future outcomes that leads to stress. Those perceptions trigger a variety of physiologic responses, including changes in the way our gastrointestinal systems function. That's how the mind-body connection works—the things we think have very real effects on our bodies. But just as we create stress, we can also learn to respond in different ways to life events. People with IBS can have extreme physical reactions to stress, so relaxation is especially important. Stress can be controlled. Your IBS symptoms may depend on it.

The first thing to try is deep breathing, which is breathing from the diaphragm instead of the chest. To get started: Lie down on the floor on your back. Bend your knees, and put your feet on the floor. Put one hand over your diaphragm, just under your ribs. Keeping your shoulders as flat as possible against the floor, take a deep breath. As you breathe in, focus on letting your diaphragm push your hand up, expanding your abdomen. Exhale naturally, and notice how your hand gently falls as the air leaves your lungs. (After you get the hang of this type of breathing, try it while standing or sitting up straight.) This type of deep breathing triggers a relaxation response in the body.

Along with deep breathing, you can bring in an arsenal of relaxation techniques, including massage, yoga, and meditation. Even taking quiet time for yourself—a half-hour to read, take a bubble bath, garden, or just enjoy nature—may be enough to give your mind and body a much-needed break.

If stress has gotten out of control, you might want to consider a short course of counseling with a psychologist to help you learn how to change the way you respond to the stressful events in your life. There are specific techniques that can help you experience life without tension, anxiety, or that feeling of being overwhelmed. In fact, researchers from Mount Sinai School of Medicine in New York found that people with IBS who were treated by both a gastroenterologist and a psychologist got better faster than those treated by just one type of specialist.

■ **Make exercise a daily prescription.** Exercise is important for two main reasons. First, exercise is a great stress reliever. Dozens of studies have shown that no matter what the cause of the stress, no matter what symptoms the stress causes, regular moderate exercise can help make you feel better. Second, exercise is critically important for the proper functioning of the gastrointestinal system. If your body is sluggish, your gut can follow suit. If your body is fit and active, your gut will be healthier. Although there have been just a few studies that focus on the effects of exercise on IBS symptoms, at least one study found that regular physical activity was protective. If you don't already exercise, you may want to consider walking for 30 minutes a day, every day at a moderate pace. But really, any activity will be helpful, so choose something fun to do every day.

SUPPLEMENTS

If you suffer from IBS and want to consider supplements *in addition to* the food fixes, I recommend:

1. **Multivitamin.** I recommend a multivitamin to ensure that you always get the basic nutrition you might otherwise miss if you're tip-toeing around a sensitive stomach. Unfortunately, many people with IBS find that vitamins upset the delicate balance of their digestive systems. Look for liquid or chewable multivitamins—any brand, even children's chewables, are great for people with IBS. Read the label, and take the amount recommended for adults.

2. **Calcium and vitamin D$_3$.** If you have IBS triggered by milk products, you may not get enough calcium in your diet to stay healthy. Women may want to consider taking a calcium supplement with added vitamin D$_3$ (cholecalciferol, the most potent form). The vitamin D is necessary, otherwise your body can't absorb and use the calcium. I recommend taking 500 to 600 milligrams of calcium (plus 100 to 400 IU of vitamin D) twice a day. (If you are a man, talk with your doctor before taking a calcium supplement. There is some evidence that too much calcium may be related to an increased risk of developing prostate cancer.) I recommend brands that contain calcium citrate (instead of the more common calcium carbonate), because it is easier on the stomach. One of my favorite brands is Citracal Plus, which also contains vitamin D and magnesium (take two tablets twice a day). If you can't swallow a pill, look for chewy supplements. *Important note*: Some chews contain lactose, so if milk bothers your stomach, avoid the chews. Instead, buy the pill form, crush them with a pill crusher, and mix with natural applesauce to help them go down more easily.

3. **Probiotics.** Our intestines are full of microorganisms, but that's not necessarily bad. Some of the bacteria and yeast microorganisms are good for us, and can help keep us healthy. Some experts believe that people with IBS don't have enough of the good microorganisms, which is why their intestines seem to be out of balance. Probiotics are supplements that provide more of the good stuff, which can prevent the bad stuff

from causing diarrhea or constipation. There are many varieties of probiotics, but the brand I recommend most often for IBS is Florastor (which contains *Saccharomyces boulardii*), a non-harmful yeast. You should take one capsule twice a day, morning and evening. Although most probiotics require refrigeration, the Florastor brand should *not* be stored in the fridge—always read labels. Research shows that other probiotics, including *Lactobacillus plantarum* (Lp299v) and *Bifidobacterium infantis*, also help reduce pain, bloating, and abnormal bowel movements. Another respected brand to consider is VSL#3—take ½ to 1 packet per day for IBS. When taking probiotics, keep in mind that for the first two to seven days, your symptoms may worsen. Don't panic, the supplements are just doing their job. Your body will soon adjust and you'll most likely feel better than baseline. Florastor and other probiotics are often sold behind the pharmacy counters at mainstream drug stores. Speak with your local pharmacist if you have trouble finding them.

4. **Enteric-coated peppermint oil.** Peppermint naturally reduces gastrointestinal muscle spasms. It also acts as an antimicrobial agent, capable of stopping the growth of some strains of bacteria—particularly some harmful bacteria. For both those reasons, researchers have studied peppermint oil as a way to control IBS symptoms. The results have been mixed, but there is some strong evidence that peppermint oil may work as well as some smooth muscle relaxant medications (called *anticholinergics*). Treatment with peppermint oil capsules seem to help reduce abdominal pain, distention, flatulence, and diarrhea. Studies have found that participants get some relief if they take a total of 0.2 to 0.4 mL, three times a day 15 to 30 minutes before meals for one or two weeks. Choose a brand that is enteric-coated, which means that the supplements are specially designed to bypass the stomach and dissolve only in the intestines, reducing the possibility of heartburn and stomach distress.

5. **Beano**. When we eat beans, we get gas. It's a fact of life. That's because we don't have enough of an enzyme called *alpha-galactosidase*, which breaks down certain components of complex carbohydrates. The bacteria naturally found in our intestines break down the undigested complex carbs, creating gas in the process. The product Beano contains alpha-galactosidase, so it helps break down more of the gas-producing foods. It works with beans, of course, but also with vegetables (including cruciferous vegetables) and whole grains. Follow the directions on the label for best results. I suggest you keep a bottle on hand at all times—you'll thank me when you're unexpectedly dining out at a restaurant of someone else's choosing!

6. **Artichoke leaf extract.** Studies by researchers in the United Kingdom have shown that artichoke leaf extract (*Cynara scolymus*) can reduce IBS symptoms of pain and flatulence by more than 25 percent with just two months of use. About half of the IBS patients who claimed to have alternating constipation and diarrhea reported having "normal" bowel habits after treatment with the extract. The recommended dosage is 320 to 640 milligrams, two to three times per day.

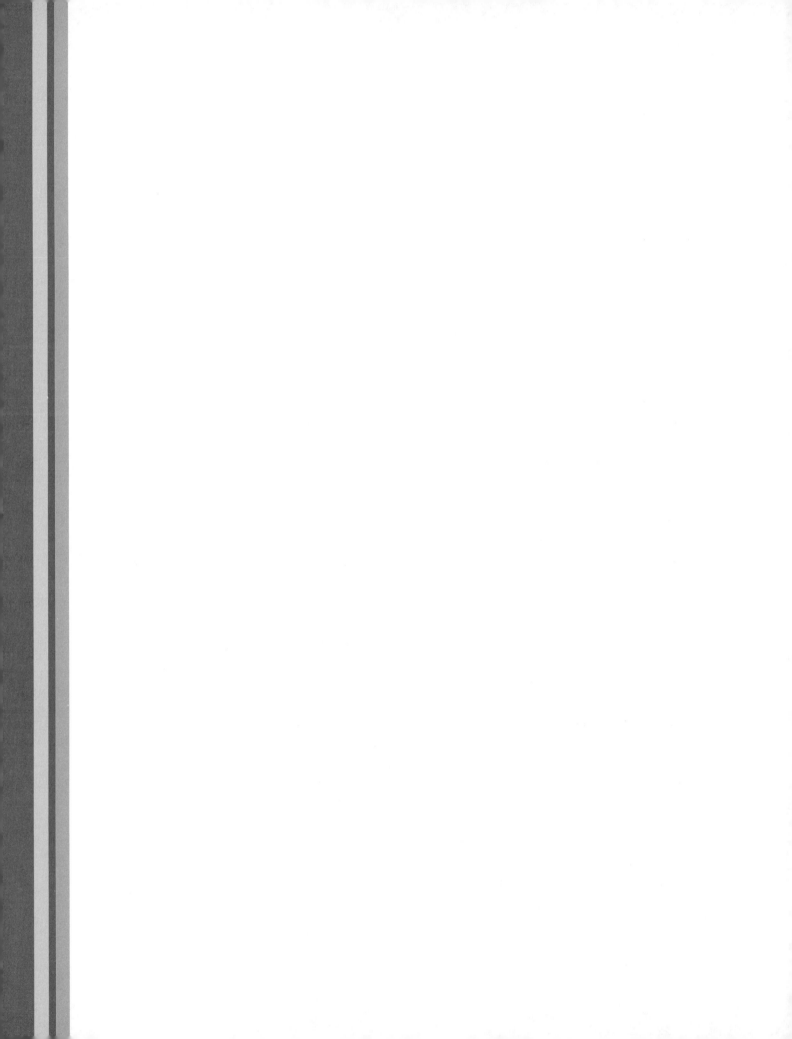

JOY'S 4-STEP PROGRAM
FOR IRRITABLE BOWEL SYNDROME

Follow this program if you have been diagnosed with Irritable Bowel Syndrome.

STEP 1 ... START WITH THE BASICS

These are the first things you should do try to take control of your IBS symptoms:

- If you haven't been officially diagnosed with IBS, see a doctor to rule out other possible causes of your discomfort.

- For severe diarrhea-predominant IBS, start the Extreme Elimination Diet—No Fiber on page 408.

- For severe constipation-predominant IBS (along with other persistent types that cause gas, cramping, or pain) start the regular Elimination Diet with Added Fiber on page 411.

- For less debilitating IBS, begin keeping an IBS Diary to keep track of your symptoms, your diet, and your stress levels. Learn to identify which factors trigger your IBS attacks.

- Eat all your meals sitting down. Chew your food thoroughly. Make meals a time of relaxation, not a race.

- Remember, stress hurts. Make relaxation a priority.

- Exercise daily.

- Take Beano at meals to reduce the potential for gas.

STEP 2 ... YOUR ULTIMATE GROCERY LIST

A food plan for IBS is more about avoiding your personal trigger foods than about specific nutrients that will help alleviate your symptoms. The foods on this list are considered generally "safe," avoiding *all* known triggers, common allergens, and then some! If you have severe diarrhea-predominant IBS, go easy on foods marked with an **asterisk (*).** These foods are rich in fiber, and although they can often help control diarrhea in the long run, they need to be slowly and cautiously introduced into your diet. (See Extreme Elimination Diet—No Fiber, page 408.)

There are *so* many potential trigger foods that affect different people in different ways, which is why my grocery list is, unfortunately, both short and limited. This is where *you* come in. Take a few minutes to add healthful foods you know you can personally tolerate without a problem. For example, if you regularly eat whole wheat bread, peanut butter, fat-free yogurt, and pasta without symptoms, add them to your personal grocery list. As you keep an IBS journal or perform an elimination diet, you'll identify many more safe and healthy foods. Use the allotted spaces below each food category for your personal notes.

FRUIT

*Apples	*Bananas	*Cantaloupe	*Pears
Applesauce, natural unsweetened	*Berries (strawberries, blackberries, raspberries)	*Mango	*watermelon
*Apricots (fresh)		*Nectarines	
		*Peaches	

Personal Safe Items

_____

_____

_____

_____

VEGETABLES

*Avocado	*Green beans, cooked	*Peas, green	*Spinach, cooked
*Carrots, cooked	*Peas, black-eyed	*Potatoes, white and sweet	*Yellow squash, cooked
			*Zucchini, cooked

Personal Safe Items

_____

_____

_____

_____

SEAFOOD

ALL fresh or frozen seafood with no breading, no	sauce (avoid shellfish) Flounder	Salmon, wild (fresh and canned) Tilapia	Sole Trout

Personal Safe Items

LEAN MEATS/EGGS/SOY FOODS

Chicken breast, skinless	Turkey breast, skinless	Turkey burgers, lean

Personal Safe Items

NUTS AND SEEDS (PREFERABLY UNSALTED)

*Flaxseed, ground	*Psyllium seeds, ground

Personal Safe Items

GRAINS

*Amaranth	Cereal, hot cream of rice	peas, potato, quinoa, or rice	Rice cakes, plain and brown
*Barley			
*Buckwheat	*Oatmeal	Rice (white, yellow, brown, wild)	Tortillas (made only from rice flour)
Cereal, puffed rice	*Pasta made only from		

Personal Safe Items

DAIRY

Personal Safe Items

_____

_____

_____

MISCELLANEOUS (INCLUDING CONDIMENTS)

Almond extract	Margarine, soft tub	Potato chips, plain	Salt
Baking powder	reduced-fat, trans	baked (no olestra)	Sugar
Baking soda	fat–free (no dairy)	Preserves, strawberry	Vanilla
Cinnamon, ground	Nonstick cooking spray	(low-sugar)	
Flour, barley	Oil, olive	Rice milk, low-fat plain	
Flour, oat	Pepper, black	and vanilla	

Personal Safe Items

_____

_____

_____

*Foods rich in soluble fiber that should be slowly introduced if you have severe diarrhea-predominant IBS

STEP 3 ...GOING ABOVE AND BEYOND

If you want to do everything you can to try to alleviate your IBS symptoms while still staying healthy, here are some additional things you might try:

- Consider taking a chewable or liquid multivitamin to assure that you get the basic level of nutrition, even if your food choices are limited.

- If your IBS symptoms are triggered by dairy products, take a calcium citrate supplement that also includes vitamin D_3 to make up for any shortfall in dietary calcium.

- Consider taking supplements to reduce your symptoms, such as a probiotic, peppermint oil, or artichoke leaf extract.

- If you can't get relief from dietary and lifestyle changes, talk with your doctor. There are new medications that can help you get control over your worst symptoms.

HYPNOTHERAPY FOR IBS

If nothing else helps relieve your IBS symptoms, you might want to try hypnotherapy. Researchers from Sweden tested 135 people who had IBS that did not respond to any other treatment. After 12 weekly one-hour hypnotherapy sessions, they found significant improvements in abdominal pain, distension, and bloating. People felt better, even though their bowel habits did not change. These improvements held for at least one year. To find a qualified hypnotherapist, check with the National Board for Certified Clinical Hypnotherapists, www.natboard.com or 1-800-449-8144.

STEP4 ...MEAL PLANS

For severe diarrhea-predominant IBS, follow the Extreme Elimination Diet—No Fiber, which follows.

For severe constipation-predominant IBS, follow the Elimination Diet with Added Fiber, page 411.

EXTREME ELIMINATION DIET—NO FIBER
For severe diarrhea-predominant IBS (follow for five to seven days)

This elimination diet is extreme and should not be followed for longer than one week. It's designed to help people who suffer from severe persistent diarrhea-predominant IBS determine which foods may be aggravating their condition. It avoids ALL IBS potential trigger foods *plus* additional common allergens (including shellfish and eggs). This plan is very low in dietary fiber and is based on the few foods I've found that clients with this type of IBS can tolerate. Fiber *and nutrition* will be slowly increased as you introduce new foods. Rice cereal (hot and cold varieties) and rice milk can be purchased at a local health food store or online. Make sure you buy a soft tub reduced-fat, trans fat–free margarine spread that does not contain dairy.

If you're a candidate for this extreme plan, follow it for one week. Every day, choose *one* option for each of the three meals—breakfast, lunch, and dinner. Then, one or two times per day, choose from the variety of my suggested snacks. Eat slowly and thoroughly chew your food. Approximate calories have been provided to help adjust for your personal weight-management goals. If you find yourself hungry (and if weight is not an issue), feel free to increase the portion sizes for meals and snacks. Stick with flat water as your beverage, and drink at least 8 cups throughout each day.

After following this plan for one week, you can start experimenting by adding new foods. You should add one new food every two to three days (it's best to stick with one portion of a new food per day). Keep an IBS diary and write down everything you eat . . . and everything you feel. Pay close attention to how you feel after eating each new food, which will help you determine if it can be permanently reintroduced into your diet. If any food bothers your stomach, stop eating it and add it to your list of problem foods. Move on to the next food category. You can always retest a problem food at a later date.

At the end of this tough assignment, you will (we hope) have identified most of the foods that aggravate your IBS. Let's hope it's a short list. For the sake of good nutrition and food variety, here's my suggested order for reintroducing new foods:

1. Dairy (fat-free and reduced-fat milk, yogurt, cheese, etc.)
2. Sweet potatoes and/or yams
3. Eggs
4. Wheat products: Stick with white versions of bread, crackers, and pasta. In the future when symptoms subside, you can slowly test small amounts of whole wheat varieties.

5. Oats, oatmeal, and barley
6. Brown and wild rice
7. Nut butters
8. Cooked vegetables (noncruciferous, no corn, no peppers, no eggplant)
9. Fruit (peel fruits with tough outer skins at first; avoid citrus)
10. Shellfish
11. Soy foods
12. Whole nuts and seeds
13. Garlic and onion
14. Citrus fruits
15. Cooked cruciferous vegetables (plus cooked peppers and eggplant)
16. Beans and lentils
17. Raw vegetables
18. Corn
19. Ketchup, mustard, soy sauce, and other condiments (test one at a time)
20. Dried fruit
21. Chocolate
22. Fruit juice, sugar, and honey
23. Alcohol
24. Coffee or tea

BREAKFAST OPTIONS

(Approximately 300 to 400 calories)

Hot Cereal with Banana Slices

1½ cups cooked cream of rice cereal prepared with water and 1 tablespoon soft tub reduced-fat trans fat–free margarine spread. Enjoy with 1 sliced banana.

Cold Cereal with Rice Milk

2 cups puffed rice cereal with 1½ cups plain or vanilla low-fat rice milk.

Breakfast Potato with Cinnamon Applesauce

1 medium baked potato; serve with 1 cup natural unsweetened applesauce mixed with optional cinnamon. Do not eat the potato skin.

LUNCH OPTIONS

(Approximately 400 to 500 calories)

Grilled Chicken with Rice

5 ounces grilled chicken breast. Enjoy with 1 cup cooked white or yellow rice.

Turkey Burger with Baked Potato

5 ounces plain turkey burger. Serve with 1 medium baked potato topped with 2 teaspoons soft tub reduced-fat trans fat–free margarine spread. Do not eat the potato skin.

Turkey and Avocado on Rice Cakes

5 ounces sliced turkey breast (or grilled chicken) divided over 3 plain rice cakes, each topped with 1 thin slice avocado. Enjoy with ½ cup natural unsweetened applesauce.

DINNER OPTIONS

(500 to 600 calories)

Grilled Fish with Rice

Easy! 3-Step Microwave Salmon (page 345, omit the garlic) or 5 ounces grilled salmon (or sole, trout, or tilapia) seasoned with 1 teaspoon olive oil and pinch of salt. Serve with 1 cup cooked white or yellow rice.

Rosemary Chicken with Baked Potato

5 ounces Rosemary Chicken (page 347) with 1 medium baked potato topped with 1 tablespoon soft tub reduced-fat, trans fat–free margarine spread. Do not eat the potato skin.

Roast Turkey with Mashed Potatoes

6 ounces roast turkey breast. Serve with 1 medium baked potato scooped and mashed with 1 tablespoon soft tub reduced-fat, trans fat–free margarine spread (or 1 cup cooked white or yellow rice). Do not eat the potato skin.

SNACK OPTIONS

100 calories or less

- 2 plain rice cakes
- ½ cup natural unsweetened applesauce
- 1 small banana

100 to 200 calories

- 3 to 5 plain rice crackers
- 1 ounce baked potato chips (no olestra, check labels)
- 1 cup natural unsweetened applesauce

- ½ baked potato with 1 teaspoon soft tub reduced-fat, trans fat–free margarine spread; do not eat the potato skin.

ELIMINATION DIET WITH ADDED FIBER
For severe constipation-predominant IBS, and follow-up for the extreme elimination diet

This elimination diet is extreme and should not be followed long term. It's designed to help people who suffer with persistent constipation-predominant IBS (and other debilitating types that cause gas, cramping, and pain) finally figure out which foods may be aggravating their condition. It avoids *all* IBS potential trigger foods *plus* additional common allergens (including shellfish and eggs). It provides a moderate amount of dietary fiber—with a good amount specifically coming from soluble fiber sources. All foods rich in soluble fiber are marked with an **asterisk** (*)—if you're feeling gassy or uncomfortably distended, go easy on these foods. Your total fiber intake *(and nutrition!)* will slowly increase when you start introducing new foods. Puffed rice cereal and low-fat rice milk can be purchased at your local health food store (or online). Make sure your soft tub reduced-fat, trans fat–free margarine spread does not contain dairy.

If you're a candidate for this plan, follow it for one week. Every day, choose *one* option for each of the three meals—breakfast, lunch, and dinner. Then, one or two times per day, choose from a variety of my suggested snacks. Eat slowly and thoroughly chew your food. Approximate calories have been provided to help adjust for your personal weight-management goals. If you find yourself hungry (and if weight is not an issue), feel free to increase the portion sizes for meals and snacks. Stick with flat water as your beverage and drink at least 10 cups throughout each day.

After following this plan for one week, you're ready to experiment by adding new foods. You should add one new food every two to three days (it's best to stick with one portion of a new food per day). Keep an IBS diary and write down all the foods you eat, the amounts, and how they affect your constipation. Pay close attention to how you feel after eating each new food and determine if it can be permanently reintroduced back into your diet. If any food bothers your stomach, stop eating it and add it to your list of problem foods. Move on to the next category. You can always retest a problem food at a later date.

At the end of this tough assignment, you will hopefully have identified all (or most all) foods that aggravate your IBS. Let's hope it's a short list. For the sake of good nutrition and food variety, here's my suggested order for reintroducing new foods:

1. Dairy (fat-free and reduced-fat milk, yogurt, cheese, etc.)
2. Wheat products (preferably whole wheat bread, pasta, cereal, and more)
3. Eggs
4. Increased portions of daily cooked vegetables (noncruciferous, no corn, no eggplant, no peppers)
5. More daily fruit (but avoid citrus varieties)
6. Shellfish
7. Soy foods
8. Nut butters

9. Whole nuts and seeds
10. Garlic and onion
11. Citrus fruits
12. Cooked cruciferous vegetables (plus cooked peppers and eggplant)
13. Beans and lentils
14. Raw vegetables
15. Corn
16. Ketchup, mustard, soy sauce, mayonnaise, and other condiments (test one at a time)
17. Dried fruit
18. Fruit juice, sugar, and honey
19. Alcohol
20. Coffee or tea
21. Chocolate

BREAKFAST OPTIONS

(Approximately 300 to 400 calories)

Oatmeal with Strawberries and Ground Flaxseed

½ cup dry *oatmeal prepared with water and topped with 1 cup sliced *strawberries and 2 tablespoons ground *flaxseed.

Cold Cereal with Raisins and Rice Milk

1½ cups puffed rice cereal with 1 cup plain or vanilla low-fat rice milk; with 3 tablespoons *raisins (or 1 sliced *banana) and 1 to 2 tablespoons ground *flaxseed.

Breakfast Potato with Cinnamon Applesauce

1 medium plain baked *white or *sweet potato. Serve with 1 cup natural unsweetened applesauce mixed with optional cinnamon.

LUNCH OPTIONS

(Approximately 400 to 500 calories)

Grilled Chicken with Cooked Carrots and Rice

5 ounces grilled chicken breast (or sliced turkey breast). Enjoy with ½ cup cooked *carrots and ¾ cup cooked brown rice or *barley.

Turkey and Avocado on Rice Cakes

5 ounces sliced turkey breast (or grilled chicken) divided over 2 to 3 brown rice cakes and each topped with 1 thin slice *avocado. Serve with 1 cup *raspberries.

Turkey Burger with Sweet Potato

5 ounces plain turkey burger topped with ½ cup mushrooms sautéed in nonstick cooking spray. Serve with 1 plain medium baked *sweet potato.

DINNER OPTIONS

(Approximately 500 to 600 calories)

Grilled Fish with Green Peas and Rice

Easy! 3-Step Microwave Salmon (page 345; omit the garlic) or 5 ounces grilled salmon, sole, trout, or tilapia with 1 teaspoon olive oil and other safe seasonings. Serve with ½ cup *green peas mixed with ½ cup cooked brown or wild rice.

Rosemary Chicken with Sautéed Spinach and Sweet Potato

5 ounces grilled Rosemary Chicken (page 347); 1 cup sautéed *spinach in 1 teaspoon olive oil with a pinch of salt and pepper; 1 plain medium baked *sweet potato (or *yam).

Roast Turkey with Cooked Carrots and Brown Rice

5 ounces roast turkey breast. Enjoy with 1 cup cooked *carrots and 1 cup cooked brown or wild rice (or 1 plain medium plain *white or *sweet potato topped with 1 tablespoon soft tub reduced-fat, trans fat–free margarine spread).

SNACK OPTIONS

100 calories or less

- *Fruit rich in soluble fiber:* 1 apple, pear, peach, or small banana; 1 cup berries (sliced strawberries, blackberries, raspberries); ½ cantaloupe; 4 apricots
- Other safe fruits: 1 cup watermelon; 1 nectarine; ½ mango
- ½ cup natural, unsweetened applesauce

100 to 200 calories

- 1 ounce baked potato chips (no olestra, check labels)
- ½ baked potato (*white or *sweet) with 1 teaspoon soft tub reduced fat, trans fat–free margarine spread
- *After you've tested eggs,* enjoy 1 of the following muffins as a snack or couple with 1 whole egg plus 2 to 3 egg whites for breakfast:
  - Banana Almond Muffin (page 414)
  - Berries and Jam Muffin (page 415)
  - Carrot 'n' Oat Muffin (page 416)

*Foods rich in soluble fiber that should be slowly introduced if you have severe diarrhea-predominant IBS

BANANA ALMOND MUFFINS

For only 180 calories per muffin, you'll get great taste, 4 grams of soluble fiber and 0 grams saturated fat. A muffin works well as an on-the-go snack . . . or enjoy one warm, out of the oven, with scrambled eggs for breakfast.

Makes 12

½	cup granulated white sugar or sugar substitute
½	cup soft tub reduced-fat, trans fat–free margarine spread
2	egg whites
3	bananas, mashed (about 1½ cups)
¼	cup water
1	teaspoon almond extract
1	teaspoon vanilla extract
½	cups barley flour
½	cup ground flaxseed
2	teaspoons baking powder
½	teaspoon baking soda
1	teaspoon ground cinnamon

1. Preheat the oven to 350°F. Line the cups of a 12-cup muffin pan with paper liners.
2. In a large bowl, mix the sugar or sugar substitute and margarine. Add the egg whites, one at a time, mixing well after each addition. Stir in the banana, water, almond extract, and vanilla. Add the flour, flaxseed, baking powder, baking soda, and cinnamon. Stir until the flour is just combined, but do not overmix.
3. Fill each muffin cup half full with the batter. Bake 13 to 16 minutes, until the tops of the muffins are lightly browned and a toothpick comes out clean when inserted in the center. Turn the muffins out on a wire rack to cool. Once cooled, the muffins can be stored in an airtight container at room temperature for up to 2 days, or frozen for up to 1 month.

PER MUFFIN
180 calories, 4 g protein, 30 g carbohydrate, 5 g fat, 0 mg cholesterol, 170 mg sodium, 4 g fiber

BERRIES AND JAM MUFFINS

Jam is one of those ingredients that everyone is automatically drawn to. It reminds us of our childhoods, breezy summer mornings, or cozy Sundays with the family. In this recipe, low-sugar jam sweetens and adds extra flavor possibilities. If you feel adventurous, substitute other berry flavors for the strawberry preserves.

Makes 12

½	cup granulated white sugar or sugar substitute
½	cup soft tub reduced-fat, trans fat–free margarine spread
2	egg whites
1	cup natural unsweetened applesauce
2	teaspoons vanilla extract
2	cups oat flour
2	teaspoons baking powder
½	teaspoon baking soda
½	cup strawberries, hulled and quartered
½	cup raspberries
¼	cup low-sugar strawberry preserves

1. Preheat the oven to 350°F. Line the cups of a 12-cup muffin pan with paper liners.
2. In a large bowl, mix the sugar or sugar substitute and margarine. Add the egg whites, one at a time, mixing well after each addition. Stir in the applesauce and vanilla. Add the oat flour, baking powder, and baking soda. Stir until the dry ingredients are just combined, but do not overmix. Fold in the strawberries and raspberries.
3. Fill each muffin cup half full with batter, and spoon a teaspoon of jam in the center of each. Bake 12 to 15 minutes, until the tops of the muffins are lightly browned and a toothpick comes out clean when inserted in the center.
4. Turn the muffins out on a wire rack to cool. Once cooled, the muffins can be stored in an airtight container at room temperature for up to 2 days, or frozen for up to 1 month.

PER MUFFIN
152 calories, 3 g protein, 24 g carbohydrate, 5 g fat (1 g saturated), 0 mg cholesterol, 167 mg sodium, 2 g fiber

CARROT 'N' OAT MUFFINS

Oat flour, raisins, carrots, and prunes provide four hits of soluble fiber! And because they taste so good, my 6-year-old daughter has no idea these muffins are good for her.

Makes 12

½	cup brown sugar or sugar substitute
½	cup soft tub, reduced-fat trans fat–free margarine spread
2	eggs whites
1	cup natural unsweetened applesauce
1	teaspoon vanilla extract
2	cups oat flour
2	teaspoons baking powder
½	teaspoon baking soda
1	teaspoon ground cinnamon
¼	teaspoon ground allspice
1	cup grated carrots
¼	cup raisins
¼	cup pureed prunes

1. Preheat the oven to 350°F. Line the cups of a 12-cup muffin pan with paper liners.
2. In a large bowl, mix the brown sugar or sugar substitute and margarine. Add the egg whites, one at a time, mixing well after each addition. Stir in the applesauce and vanilla. Add the oat flour, baking powder, baking soda, cinnamon, and allspice. Stir until the dry ingredients are just combined, but do not overmix. Fold in the carrots, raisins, and prunes.
3. Fill each muffin cup three-fourths full with batter. Bake 12 to 15 minutes, until the tops of the muffins are lightly browned and a toothpick comes out clean when inserted in the center. Turn the muffins out on a wire rack to cool. Once cooled, the muffins can be stored in an airtight container at room temperature for up to 2 days, or frozen for up to 1 month.

PER MUFFIN
151 calories, 3 g protein, 24 g carbohydrate, 5 g fat (1 g saturated), 0 mg cholesterol, 176 mg sodium, 2.5 g fiber

CHAPTER 18

CELIAC DISEASE

Celiac disease tends to take people by surprise—not just those who receive the diagnosis, but also family doctors, who are shocked when a physically robust patient's blood work comes back positive for the disease. That's because a couple of decades ago the stereotypical celiac patient was a pale, malnourished child, someone who wouldn't be out of place in a Charles Dickens novel eating gruel and wasting away in an orphanage. As screening tests became more sophisticated, we're learning that celiac disease is surprisingly common—affecting about one in every 100 people in the United States—and it can begin at any time in a person's life. There is no consistent set of symptoms—some people lose a tremendous amount of weight, others experience fatigue, joint pain, or seizures, but sometimes there are no symptoms at all and the disease is discovered quite by chance.

In my practice, clients often learn they have celiac disease when their doctors investigate possible causes for unexplained anemia. One minute you feel fine and you're having blood drawn for tests during a routine physical examination, the next you're facing nonnegotiable changes to your eating habits and the possibility of complications. If that scenario sounds familiar, you're lucky. If celiac disease remains undiagnosed or untreated, it can lead to osteoporosis, reproductive problems, skin rashes, epilepsy, and even some cancers. The good news is that celiac disease is treated entirely with dietary changes, so feeling better is as simple as knowing which foods are toxic to your gut.

WHAT AFFECTS CELIAC DISEASE?

Celiac disease (also called *celiac sprue, nontropical sprue,* and *gluten-sensitive enteropathy*) is genetic, which means that, in some people, the disease lies dormant until it is triggered. No one knows exactly what causes celiac disease to erupt, but experts believe that times of extreme emotional or physical stress—including surgery, a viral infection, pregnancy, or childbirth—can set the stage.

It's important to remember that celiac disease is NOT a food allergy. Some people call it an allergy as a short-hand way to explain why those with a diagnosis need to avoid certain foods, but that description is both misleading and dangerous. Celiac disease is an autoimmune disorder. The body's own immune system reacts to a protein called *gluten,* which is found in wheat. Related proteins are also found in rye and barley. When even the smallest amount of gluten enters the digestive system, it sets in motion a cascade of inflammatory processes, resulting in damage to the small intestine.

The small intestine is not merely a smooth tube connecting the stomach to the colon. The inner lining of the small intestine is jam-packed with protruding ridges called *villi,* which absorb nutrients as food passes through. In celiac disease, inflammation damages and sometimes destroys the villi, which means they can't do their job, and nutrients your body needs pass through your digestive system and are eliminated by waste. The outcome of this damage varies depending on the extent of the disease. In mild cases, there are no overt symptoms, but blood tests might reveal a deficiency in certain nutrients, especially folate, vitamin B_{12}, or iron (which can result in anemia). Over time, poor calcium absorption can lead to osteoporosis. In some people, celiac disease causes embarrassing and sometimes life-altering gastrointestinal symptoms, including gas, bloating, diarrhea or constipation, or weight loss. Other problems associated with celiac disease include nerve damage, migraines, seizures, infertility or miscarriages, joint pain, and even some cancers, including non-Hodgkin lymphoma and cancer of the esophagus or small intestine. The longer the disease goes untreated, the greater the risk of harm.

HOW FOOD AFFECTS CELIAC DISEASE

There is no cure for celiac disease, and the only treatment is to eliminate gluten from your diet. If you get a diagnosis early enough, your villi will eventually heal, and, with the right foods, you can replenish stores of the nutrients you've been missing. In terms of limiting damage, nutritional treatment for celiac disease is all about which foods to avoid. However, because the list of forbidden foods is so extensive, it is also critically important that you pay attention to the vitamins and minerals that most people normally get from gluten-containing foods, and be sure your diet is rich in other sources.

AVOIDING FOODS THAT CONTAIN GLUTEN

If you have an allergy to cats, or know other people who do, you've probably noticed that not every cat-allergy sufferer suffers in the same way. Some people start to sneeze if they are just in the same house with a cat, others remain sneeze-free until they bury their face in the animal's fur. That's not the case with celiac disease. Even the tiniest bit of gluten—the amount found in ⅛ teaspoon of wheat flour—can signal the body's immune system to respond with a full attack. The tricky part of celiac disease is that damage can occur without you noticing much in the way of symptoms. But the longer you eat foods containing gluten, the greater the damage until eventually, you become sick.

I wish the guidelines for avoiding gluten were as easy as telling you to stop eating wheat, barley, and rye bread. That's part of what you need to do——but it is much more complicated than that. There are many hidden sources of gluten, and beyond that, some common gluten-free products can be contaminated with gluten.

Here are lists of foods, ingredients, and additives to avoid. Photocopy the list—make more than one—and carry a copy in your wallet, and others your car and anywhere else you'll be able to refer to one easily when you're shopping for or eating a meal. Eventually, you'll have the foods memorized.

COMMON FOODS THAT CONTAIN GLUTEN

Barley (and anything with the word barley in it, such as barley malt)

Beer (all types)

Bleached flour

Bleu cheese (sometimes made with bread mold)

Bran (also called wheat bran)

Bread flour

Bulgur

Communion wafers

Couscous

Durum

Farina

Faro

Flour (this usually means wheat flour)

Graham flour

Groats

Kamut

Malt (and anything with the word malt in it, such as rice malt, malt extract or malt flavoring)

Malt beverages

Matzo

Oats and oat bran (see FAQ, page 421)

Orzo

Pasta (all varieties made with wheat, wheat starch, oats, barley, rye or any ingredients on this list)

Rye (and anything with the word rye in it)

Seitan

Semolina

Soy sauce (check ingredients, often made with wheat)

Spelt

Suet

Tabbouleh

Teriyaki sauce

Triticale

Triticum

Unbleached flour

Wheat (and anything with the word wheat in it, such as wheat grass, wheat starch; buckwheat is okay, and is the only exception)

Wheat germ

LESS COMMON FOODS THAT CONTAIN GLUTEN

Abyssinian hard (a wheat product)

Amp-isostearoyl hydrolyzed wheat
protein

Brewer's yeast

Cereal binding

Dextrimaltose

Disodium wheatgermamido Peg-2
sulfosuccinate

Edible starch

Einkorn

Emmer

Filler

Fu

Granary flour

Mir

Udon (wheat noodles)

Whole-meal flour

FOOD ADDITIVES THAT *MAY* CONTAIN GLUTEN

If a favorite food contains one of the following ingredients, contact the company and ask questions—depending on the manufacturing process, these suspect ingredients can sometimes be gluten-free.

Artificial color

Artificial flavoring

Bouillon cubes

Caramel color

Coloring

Dextrins

Dried fruit (may be dusted with wheat)

Flavored coffee

Flavored vinegar

Flavoring

Food starch

Glucose syrup

Gravy cubes

Ground spices (wheat is sometimes
added to prevent clumping)

Hydrolyzed plant protein (HPP)

Hydrolyzed vegetable protein (HVP)

Maltodextrin

Maltose

Miso

Modified food starch

Modified starch

Mono- and diglycerides

Monosodium glutamate (MSG)

Mustard powder (some brands contain
gluten, check ingredients)

Natural flavoring

Processed cheese (check ingredients)

Processed meats (cold cuts, hot dogs,
sausages, and canned meats which
contain wheat, barley, rye, oats,
gluten fillers, or stabilizers)

Shoyu

Smoke flavoring

Soba noodles

Starch

Stock/boullion cubes

Surimi (imitation seafood)

Textured vegetable protein (TVP)

Vegetable starch

Vitamins

MORE THINGS TO KNOW ABOUT HEALTHY EATING WITH CELIAC DISEASE

■ **Don't cheat.** I can't say this strongly enough. A miniscule amount of gluten can cause real damage to the small intestine. If you cheat, even a little, you can't help but get a toxic amount of gluten. A single cookie, half a slice a bread, even a single cracker is too much gluten for your system.

- **Don't cheat, part 2.** Unless you make every meal at home using absolutely no packaged products except those labeled "gluten-free," you will eat some gluten. If you ever eat in a restaurant or at a friend's house, or if you cook with any jarred, canned, or packaged foods, you will get some gluten in your food. There is really nothing you can do about it. In my office, we call this unintentional cheating because we know you don't mean to do it. But the bottom line is that you're getting some gluten even when you're doing your best to avoid it, so don't expose your intestines to more toxic gluten by consciously cheating.

- **Whenever possible, choose gluten-free (GF) packaged foods.** The best choices are foods that are specifically labeled gluten-free. Do not make the mistake of assuming that *wheat-free* or *yeast-free* means the same thing as *gluten-free*. Read the labels carefully, using the list of suspect ingredients as your guide. Also, check out the list of resources on page 429. You can order all sorts of gluten-free, safe products for delivery right to your door.

- **Go easy on gluten-free baked goods.** In order to make up for the lack of gluten and related proteins, many gluten-free baked goods contain unhealthy amounts of saturated fats or trans fats. Once your celiac disease is under control, your body will absorb more of these fats, leading to an increased risk of high cholesterol.

- **Be a gluten sleuth.** Everything that goes in your mouth or touches your tongue needs to be screened for gluten. Everything. Read labels on vitamin supplements, toothpaste, mouth rinses, cough medicine, and all over-the-counter medications. Talk with your pharmacist about avoiding gluten so that your prescription medications can be chosen with your special needs in mind (also, look up gluten-free medicines at www.celiac.com). Don't lick postage stamps or envelopes—the glue can contain gluten.

FAQS

I just found out I have celiac disease, and it seems as though I have to spend hours at the grocery store reading labels. Does it ever get any easier?

Yes, it does get easier. You have a lot of new information to assimilate, but it's knowledge that will serve you forever. Most of my clients with celiac disease only need to see me two or three times—after that, they understand exactly what they need to do to live a gluten-free life. I highly recommend consulting with a dietitian who specializes in celiac disease to get a handle on the details. Also, check out your local Whole Foods market—they offer a variety of gluten-free foods that are conveniently labeled. And certainly shop online at some of the gluten-free specialty stores. You'll find a helpful list of resources on page 429.

If you're struggling emotionally with the transition to a gluten-free lifestyle, you might find it helpful to talk with a psychologist or counselor. Some people need time to mourn the loss of favorite foods, or favorite family meals, or their vision of themselves as indestructible. One or two sessions with a professional can mean the difference between fighting the change and a journey of discovery. Read everything, join a celiac disease support group, befriend the health care professionals, and don't be afraid to ask questions. In addition, there are many wonderful resources to help you and those you love with celiac disease, regardless of whether the disease was diagnosed last week or ten years ago. Two of the best online sources of information are:

1. The Celiac Disease Center at Columbia University (www.CeliacDiseaseCenter.columbia.edu). Check out the online store and the specialized patient information provided by some of the country's best specialists.

2. www.Celiac.com. This celiac disease and gluten-free resource offers information, a message board for people to talk with each other, and links to additional resources and Web sites.

- **If you don't know, it's a no-go.** Foods that are sold from bins may contain gluten, no matter how they are marked. The problem is that you have no way of knowing what sort of food was in the bin before the food you are buying. You may think you're buying dried beans and dried beans alone, but you may also be getting dust from the bulgur wheat that was in the bin last week. The safest choice is to buy only packaged goods labeled *gluten-free* or with no suspect ingredients on the label. In restaurants, avoid fried foods. Even if your food doesn't contain gluten, the fry oil may have remnants of breading or other gluten-containing foods. Sauces, gravies, and many toppings also contain gluten. You are safest if you eat pure, fresh, whole foods from sources you can trust.

- **Beware of contamination in your own home.** In nearly every jar of jam or tub of margarine are bread crumbs left behind by the last person to dip a knife or spoon in them. You have two choices—either stock your own private pantry that other family members know is for your consumption alone, or make sure that everyone in the household uses only fresh, clean utensils to spoon out the products.

Foods that are generally considered safe for people with celiac disease are listed in the grocery list beginning on page 426.

BONUS POINTS

- **Get regular screenings.** Experts recommend that all adults with celiac disease get annual blood screenings for ferritin (a measure of the amount of iron stored in the body), folate, vitamin B_{12}, and thyroid-stimulating hormone (TSH, a measure of how well the thyroid is working). In addition, you will probably be tested for calcium absorption, which is measured by a test called a *24-hour urine catch*. This test is exactly what it sounds like—you urinate into a special container every time you use the bathroom during a 24-hour test period. These tests will allow you and your doctor to track how well your intestines have healed.

- **Ask your doctor if you should have a bone density scan.** Long-term malabsorption of calcium can lead to osteoporosis, thinning and weakening of bones. But osteoporosis often goes unnoticed. If a scan shows your bones are strong, it will be one less thing for you to worry about, and you'll have a good baseline measure for future reference. If your bones show signs of thinning, you and your doctor can begin a treatment plan.

- **Urge family members get tested.** Celiac disease is genetic, so first- and second-degree relatives should all be tested. People with autoimmune disorders, such as type 1 diabetes or Hashimoto's disease, also have an increased risk of celiac disease and should be tested.

- **If you are pregnant, or recently had a baby:** Remember that your child may have inherited celiac disease along with your soulful eyes. If it's still an option, consider breast-feeding, which seems to offer some protection from celiac disease. When it's time to start on solid food, the best time to introduce gluten-containing foods is when the child is between four and six months old. Research has shown that children who are at high risk of celiac disease have a greater risk of developing the disease if they are introduced to foods containing gluten *before* the fourth month, or *after* the seventh month.

■ **Take advantage of the Clan Thompson Company.** Clan Thompson LLC maintains numerous resources at www.ClanThompson.com, including a free email newsletter, lists of gluten-free foods and drugs, recipes, celiac news stories, travel information, and medical replies to more than 100 celiac disease-related questions. Free demos of their Celiac SmartList software (available for Windows, Mac, Palm handhelds, and Pocket PCs) are available for download. The SmartLists are a series of software programs which make it easy to find gluten information on thousands of items, including foods, prescription drugs, and over-the-counter products. Information is verified directly with each manufacturer, and a comments field provides additional details on issues like cross contamination. The SmartLists are updated quarterly, and the company will also research products at a subscriber's request. When they learn that product information has changed and an item is no longer gluten-free, the information is posted on their Gluten Alerts page and an email also goes out to each subscriber. This is a fabulous resource for anyone with celiac disease.

FAQS

I understand that it is important to read food labels so I know what foods to buy in the grocery store, but how do I make sure that foods I order in a restaurant don't contain gluten?

Most of the finer restaurants can prepare meals that are gluten-free—all you have to do is talk with the waiter about your options. This is the one time it is okay to use the word *allergy.* My clients with celiac disease find that most waiters don't understand the wide range of ingredients that could potentially contain *gluten* and may misguide you even if they don't mean to. If you tell the waiter that you have a severe allergy to even the smallest amounts of wheat, barley, and rye, you can usually count on respect for your food wishes. It can be helpful to become a "regular" at a favorite restaurant—if you develop a relationship with the chef and staff, you will be treated like family (or at least like a valued customer) and they will be more likely to cater to your needs. But it really is difficult to eat out with celiac disease. Most restaurants are a minefield of hidden gluten. You don't want to become a hermit, but you don't want to sacrifice your health for the sake of a fast food meal. Go for meals that are prepared simply, with no breading, no frying, and few added gravies or sauces. Choose from among fresh ingredients listed as safe on page 426.

SUPPLEMENTS

People with celiac disease should seriously consider taking supplements to help them get the nutrients they need but won't get in a gluten-free diet. I recommend:

1. **Multivitamin.** Because wheat products contain so many important nutrients, I like to recommend a good general multivitamin that provides plenty of the B vitamins, especially thiamin, riboflavin, vitamin B_6, and vitamin B_{12}. One of my favorites is Centrum Performance, which provides 300% DV of all those vitamins, plus 100% DV of folate.

What are your specific recommendations for staying gluten-free while dining out?

Appetizers: Vegetable salad with olive oil and balsamic vinegar requested on the side, or sliced tomatoes and mozzarella (again, request olive oil and balsamic vinegar on the side, and avoid prepared vinaigrette dressings).

Entrée: Grilled or broiled skinless chicken breast or fish (request seasoned with olive oil, salt, pepper, and lemon)

Unlimited Vegetables: Anything goes, steamed or sautéed in olive oil and garlic.

Starch: Plain baked white or sweet potato, plain brown or wild rice. Take advantage if a restaurant offers amaranth, millet, or quinoa on the menu.

Dessert: Fresh fruit

2. **Calcium, plus vitamin D.** Because so many people with celiac disease have osteoporosis, or have experienced malabsorption of calcium over the years, I always recommend women with celiac disease take a calcium supplement with vitamin D. Calcium can't be absorbed and used by the body without vitamin D, the most potent form. Because too much calcium may increase the risk of prostate cancer, if you're male and have celiac, speak with your physician before taking calcium supplements.

   For women: Take 500 to 600 milligrams of calcium twice a day—once in the morning and once in the evening—for a total of 1,000 to 1,200 milligrams per day. Choose a brand that also contains vitamin D_3 (also called *cholecalciferol*) at a dosage that will give you a total of 400 to 800 IU of vitamin D per day (the exact amount will depend on the dosage of vitamin D included in each calcium tablet—the daily total is the number to focus on).

3. **Others, as directed by a physician.** People with celiac disease can have multiple nutrient deficiencies before their disease gets under control. Once the disease is diagnosed, blood work will indicate which extra supplements you might need. All additional supplements should only be taken if recommended by a doctor, and only for as long as the doctor recommends—too much of a good thing can be harmful. For example, even though many people with newly diagnosed celiac disease have anemia, too much iron can be toxic. Also, folate supplements can mask a deficiency in vitamin B_{12}, so you might overlook a different problem if you start popping supplements on your own.

JOY'S 4-STEP PROGRAM
FOR CELIAC DISEASE

Follow this program if you have celiac disease.

STEP 1 ... START WITH THE BASICS

These are the first things you should do to take control of celiac disease.

- Make sure you thoroughly understand what foods and additives to avoid. If you have any questions or problems following a gluten-free diet, make an appointment with a dietitian who *specializes* in celiac disease. He or she will answer every question in as much detail as you need.

- Review all the products in your kitchen pantry, refrigerator, freezer, and bathroom medicine cabinet—including medications, toothpaste, and mouth rinses. Read the ingredients on all food labels. Find ways to separate safe products from those that contain gluten.

- Don't cheat!

- Talk with your doctor about the value of regular screenings for bone density, nutrient malnutrition, and celiac disease markers.

- Consider taking a multivitamin. If you're a woman, also consider a calcium supplement containing vitamin D_3.

STEP2 . . . YOUR ULTIMATE GROCERY LIST

Controlling celiac disease is not so much about foods you should eat as foods you shouldn't eat. The foods on this list are considered to be generally safe for people with celiac disease. You'll need to carefully check labels on all foods marked with an **asterisk (*)**—that's because ingredients can vary from brand to brand (for some categories, I provide gluten-free brands worth considering).

Because most of the popular grains contain gluten, it is important to try new, safe grains. You'll also need to eat a variety of fresh fruits and vegetables to make sure that you get a wide variety of naturally occurring vitamins, minerals, fiber, antioxidants, and other nutrients. Toward the end of the grocery list, I've listed additives and ingredients that are also thought to be safe. And to make your life even easier, I've provided a resource listing of companies (and their Web sites) that offer a variety of gluten-free food items. Take advantage and shop online!

FRUIT

ALL fresh fruits	Frozen whole fruits, with no additives	*Fruit juice	

VEGETABLES

ALL fresh vegetables	Artichokes	Beans, mung	Olives
ALL frozen vegetables with no additives, breading, or sauces	Avocado	Beans and peas, dried	Potatoes (all varieties)
	Beans, adzuki	Chickpeas (garbanzo beans)	*Pumpkin, canned, 100% pure puree
Alfalfa	*Beans, canned (no gluten additives)	Lentils	Seaweed

SEAFOOD

ALL fresh seafood	All frozen raw seafood with no additives or sauces

LEAN MEATS/EGGS/SOY FOODS

ALL fresh meats and poultry with no breading or additives	All frozen raw meats and poultry with no breading or additives	Eggs	Tofu
		Soybeans (including edamame)	

NUTS AND SEEDS (PREFERABLY UNSALTED)

ALL nuts	ALL seeds except rye and barley	Peanut butter and other nut butters

GRAINS, CEREALS, PASTA, AND MORE

Amaranth

Arrowroot starch

Buckwheat

*Cereals, cold: puffed and flake varieties made with amaranth, buckwheat, corn, millet, rice, or soy; good choices are Nature's Path Crispy Rice, Barbara's Bakery Brown Rice Crisps and Honey Rice Puffins, Health Valley's Organic Blue Corn Flakes

*Cereals, hot: cream and flake varieties

made with amaranth, cornmeal, buckwheat, hominy grits, rice, quinoa, or soy

Corn bran

Corn chips, plain (preferably baked)

Corn flour/corn meal products

Crackers, rice

Flour: buckwheat, carob, chickpea, lentil, potato, rice, sago, sorghum, soy

Grits (corn or soy)

Kasha (*not* the same as Kashi)

Masa

Millet

Pasta made from beans, rice, corn, peas, potato, quinoa, rice, or soy

Polenta

*Popcorn, gluten-free microwave varieties; good choices are Healthy Choice, Jolly Time Light, Newman's Light

Potato chips, plain (preferably baked)

Quinoa

Ragi

Rice (preferably brown or wild)

Rice cakes, plain

*Soba, 100% buckwheat

Sorghum and sorghum flour

Tacos shells made with corn, hard and soft

Teff

Tortillas made with corn, soy, or brown rice

DAIRY

*Cheese (preferably reduced-fat), *not* bleu cheese

Cheese, cottage, fat-free or 1% reduced-fat; good choices are from Cabot, Albertson's, Kemps, Axelrod, Friendship, Hood, Winn Dixie, Price Chopper

*Cheese, shredded fat-free Cheddar (for meal plan)

*Cream cheese (preferably reduced-fat)

*Ice cream (check labels, ingredients will vary from flavor to flavor)

Milk (preferably fat-

free, 1% reduced-fat, or enriched/fortified soy)

*Sour cream (preferably fat-free or reduced-fat), plain flavors *only;* good choices are from Cabot, Kemp, Albertson's, Winn Dixie, Hood, Friendship, Axelrod

*Yogurt, plain, unflavored (preferably fat-free or low-fat); good choices are from Stoneyfield Farms and Yoplait

MISCELLANEOUS

ALL pure herbs (*if herb mixes, check ingredients)

ALL pure spices (*if spice mixes, check ingredients)

*Alcohol: all distilled alcohols are gluten-free, but always check with manufacturer, or at www.celiac.com, to

be sure that there are no gluten-containing additives

Apple cider vinegar

Baking chocolate

Baking powder

Baking soda

*Beverages, some soy and rice beverages (check ingredients)

*Foods whose labels need to be carefully checked for gluten.

MISCELLANEOUS (cont.)

Cocoa powder

Coffee, instant and ground; check ingredients of *flavored coffee

Corn syrup

Cornstarch

Cream of tartar

Garlic

Gelatin

Herbs and spices (for meal plans): basil (dried), black pepper, Cajun spice, cinnamon, dill, garlic powder, nutmeg, parsley (fresh), rosemary, thyme (fresh)

Honey

*Hummus (check lablels; ingredients will vary from flavor to flavor); good choices are Trader Joe's garlic, original, kalamata, organic, roasted garlic, and roasted red pepper;

all flavors from Wildwood Harvest Foods except roasted red pepper; all flavors from Athenos

Jam and jelly

*Ketchup; good choices are Heinz, Del Monte, Price Chopper

Maple syrup

*Margarine spread, soft tub, trans fat–free; good choices are I Can't Believe It's Not Butter regular, light, and fat-free spray; Benecol regular and light; Promise soft tub, regular and light

*Mayonnaise (preferably reduced-fat); good choices are Hellman's and Best Foods' regular and reduced-fat, Cain's regular, light, and fat-free

Molasses

*Mustard; good choices

are French's Dijon, Laura Lynn, 365 Organic Every Day Dijon

Nonstick cooking spray; good choices are Pam Original and Butter flavor, however Pam Baking is NOT gluten-free)

Oil, canola

Oil, olive

Pickles

Relish

*Salad dressings; good choices are Newman's Own olive oil and vinegar, balsamic vinaigrette, light balsamic vinaigrette, light red wine and vinegar, light raspberry and walnut, light Italian, light Caesar

*Salsa; good choices are Amy's Kitchen, Albertson's, Newman's Own

*Snack bars; always check ingredients to be sure; good choice is Enjoy Life brand, Cocoa Loco or Caramel Apple flavors

*Soup, lentil or black bean (any gluten-free brand

*Soy crisps; good choice is Genisoy

*Soy sauce; good choices are La Choy, Hy-Vee soy sauce, Sav-A-Lot Jade Dragon, Bragg Liquid Aminos, Price Chopper

Sugar

Tapioca (not pudding)

Tea

Vanilla

Vinegar, balsamic, or red wine

Vinegar, white

Wine, red and white

SAFE (GLUTEN-FREE) ADDITIVES

Acacia gum

Adipic acid

Agar

Algae

Algin/alginate

Allicin

Annatto

Arabic gum

Arrowroot

Ascorbic acid

Aspartame

Aspic

Astragalus gummifer

Benzoic acid

BHA

BTA

Dextrose

Ester gum

Fructose

Guar gum

Locust bean gum

Malic acid

Methylcellulose

Microcrystallin cellulose

Pectin

Pepsin

Stearic acid

Sulfites

Tapioca starch/flour (not pudding)

Whey

Xanthan gum

*Foods whose labels need to be carefully checked for gluten.

FOOD COMPANIES THAT OFFER GLUTEN-FREE ITEMS

Adrienne's Gourmet Foods (www.adriennesgourmetfoods.com): Papadini Lentil Pasta

Amy's Kitchen (www.amys.com): Gluten-Free Chili, Pasta Sauce, Salsa, and Soup; look for the Gluten-Free symbol on product descriptions

Annie's Naturals (www.anniesnaturals.com): gluten-free dressings, sauces, and marinades: look for Special Dietary Needs on the Products page

Barbara's Bakery (www.barbarasbakery.com): look for the Special Diets section under the Product Line tab

Bell & Evans (www.bellandevans.com): look for Black Box packaging for its Gluten Free Chicken Breast Nuggets and Gluten Free Chicken Breast Tenders, both breaded with rice and corn flour

Eden Foods (www.edenfoods.com): large assortment of gluten-free products (condiments; Japanese)

Ener-G Foods (www.ener-g.com): gluten-free bread products

Enjoy Life (www.enjoylifefoods.com): breads, cereals, snack bars, and more

Fantastic World Foods (www.fantasticfoods.com): Gluten-Free Bean Dish Mixes, Soup, and Soup Mixes; see specific list under the FAQ tab

Food for Life Bread (www.foodforlife.com): gluten-free breads

Gluten-Free Mall (www.glutenfreemall.com)

Josefs Gluten-Free (www.josefsglutenfree.com)

Quinoa Corporation (www.quinoa.net): gluten-free grains and pasta

Thai Kitchen Asian (www.thaikitchen.com/allergyinfo.html): gluten-free noodle products and sauces

Westbrae (www.westbrae.com/products/condiments.php): condiments

Wild Oats Market (www.wildoats.com/u/health100305/): Gluten Free Shopping List

STEP3 ...GOING ABOVE AND BEYOND

There really is no "above and beyond" for people with celiac disease—the treatment is to stop eating gluten-containing foods and take supplements to make up for the shortfall in vitamins and minerals in this restricted diet. However, there are some things you can do to be helpful to others:

■ Recommend that first- and second-degree relatives get tested to make sure that they don't have undiagnosed celiac disease.

■ If you are pregnant or have a child, talk with the pediatrician about your celiac disease so that he/she can be aware of your child's increased risk.

THE OATMEAL QUESTION

Although oats are naturally gluten-free, they can be contaminated with wheat during the growing, milling, or packaging processes. If you want to add oats to your diet, here are some guidelines:

■ Add oats only after your health has stabilized on a gluten-free diet, and only with your doctor's okay.

■ Choose McCann's Irish Oatmeal, which is processed in a dedicated oats-only mill . . . or ask your doctor for a brand recommendation.

■ For the first few days, eat only a ¼ cup of oatmeal to see how your body reacts. Then move up to a ½ cup for another few days before eating a full portion.

■ Never order oats when you're out . . . and don't buy prepared or packaged food with oats.

STEP4 ...MEAL PLANS

These sample menus include foods that have been shown to be generally safe for people who have celiac disease. In addition, they provide plenty of vitamins and minerals that are often missing in a gluten-free diet.

Every day, choose *one* option for each of the three meals—breakfast, lunch, and dinner. Then, one or two times per day, choose from a variety of my suggested snacks. Approximate calories have been provided to help adjust for your personal weight management goals. If you find yourself hungry (and if weight is not an issue), feel free to increase the portion sizes for meals and snacks. Beverage calories are *not* included.

You can also prepare some of the delicious recipes in my other chapters by simply substituting gluten-free ingredients when necessary. And **always** remember to check *every* ingredient listed on condiments, spreads, and other prepared food. Enjoy!

BREAKFAST OPTIONS

(Approximately 300 to 400 calories)

Berry-Nut Yogurt Parfait

Spoon ⅓ cup fat-free yogurt in parfait glass. Top with 2 heaping tablespoons berries and 1 tablespoon chopped nuts or seeds (walnuts, pecans, peanuts, slivered almonds, sunflower seeds, or ground flaxseed). Repeat the three layers two times (yogurt, berries, and then nuts).

Cold Cereal with Milk and Fruit

1 cup gluten-free cereal (i.e., gluten-free brand of cornflakes, amaranth flakes, or puffed rice) mixed with 1 tablespoon ground flaxseed and 1 cup milk (fat-free, 1% reduced-fat, or calcium-enriched/fortified soy). Enjoy with ½ sliced banana (or ½ grapefruit or 1 orange).

Cantaloupe with Cottage Cheese and Sunflower Seeds

½ cantaloupe stuffed with 1 cup fat-free or 1% reduced-fat cottage cheese and sprinkled with 1 tablespoon sunflower seeds or chopped nuts (walnuts, pecans, almonds, peanuts, or cashews).

Mexican Breakfast Spud-let

1 medium baked potato split and stuffed with scrambled eggs: Beat 1 whole egg with 2 egg whites and cook in hot skillet coated with Pam Original nonstick cooking spray (*do not use* Pam Baking which contains gluten) or 1 teaspoon olive or canola oil). Season eggs with salt and pepper to taste and top with 2 heaping tablespoons salsa (check salsa ingredients).

Apple Slices with Peanut Butter

1 apple or banana, sliced and topped with 2½ tablespoons peanut butter. Or 1 slice gluten-free bread, toasted and topped with 1 level tablespoon peanut butter and served with 1 sliced banana or 1 apple.

Scrambled Eggs with Broccoli and Cheese

Beat 1 whole egg with 2 egg whites and cook in a hot skillet coated with Pam Original nonstick cooking spray (*not* Pam Baking). When eggs are almost cooked, add 1 cup cooked broccoli florets and 1 ounce shredded fat-free or reduced-fat cheese. Enjoy with ½ grapefruit (or ½ banana, ½ mango, or 1 orange).

Tropical Mango-Citrus Smoothie with Rice Cakes and Cottage Cheese

1 serving (2 cups) Tropical Mango-Citrus Smoothie (page 123). Enjoy with 2 plain rice cakes, each topped with sliced tomato and 1 heaping tablespoon fat-free or 1% reduced-fat cottage cheese.

Apple Cinnamon Pancakes with Lemon Yogurt Topping

1 serving Apple Cinnamon Pancakes with Lemon Yogurt Topping (page 437).

LUNCH OPTIONS

(Approximately 400 to 500 calories)

Turkey Sandwich with Avocado

4 ounces fresh turkey breast (or ham), 2 thin slices avocado, lettuce, tomato, and onion on 2 slices gluten-free bread (or 2 to 3 rice cakes, or wrap in gluten-free corn or brown rice tortilla). Spread with optional 1 level tablespoon reduced-fat mayo, mustard, or hummus (check condiment ingredients). Enjoy with sweet pepper and celery sticks.

Grilled Chicken Salad with Apple and Walnuts

2 to 4 cups romaine lettuce and baby spinach leaves mixed with unlimited preferred vegetables (chopped peppers, broccoli flowerets, sliced mushrooms, cherry tomatoes, cucumbers, carrots, or celery). Top with 4 ounces chopped skinless chicken breast and ½ chopped apple. Toss with 1 tablespoon chopped walnuts, plus 2 teaspoons olive oil and unlimited balsamic vinegar or fresh lemon juice (or 2 to 4 tablespoons gluten-free, reduced-calorie salad dressing). Season with a pinch of salt and pepper.

Turkey Burger with Baked Potato

1 (5-ounce) turkey burger (or extra-lean hamburger) topped with sliced tomato, onion, and 2 tablespoons gluten-free ketchup. Enjoy with ½ plain baked white or sweet potato and optional 1 to 2 tablespoons gluten-free reduced-fat sour cream.

Tomato-Cheese Omelet with Toast and Veggies

Beat 1 whole egg with 2 to 3 egg whites. Cook in heated skillet coated with Pam Original nonstick cooking spray (*not* Pam Baking). Add 3 tablespoons chopped tomatoes and optional dried basil. When bottom is cooked, gently flip over. Sprinkle with 1 ounce shredded reduced-fat or fat-free cheese, fold omelet in half and continue cooking until egg mixture firms and cheese melts. Enjoy with 1 slice gluten-free bread, toasted and topped with optional 1 teaspoon soft tub, trans fat–free margarine spread. Serve with 1 cup baby carrots or sugar snap peas.

Lentil Soup with Rice Cakes

2 cups lentil or black bean soup (any gluten-free brand, 350 calories or less). Enjoy with 2 rice cakes topped with sliced tomato and onion.

Chicken Tortilla with Tri-Colored Peppers

Sauté red, yellow, and green pepper sticks in 1 teaspoon olive or canola oil until soft; season with a pinch of salt and ground black pepper. Layer 1 corn, soy, or brown rice tortilla (any gluten-free brand 150 calories or less) with large lettuce leaves, the sautéed peppers, and 4 ounces grilled skinless chicken breast. Fold in ends and roll tightly. Enjoy with 1 cup preferred vegetables (sliced cucumbers, cherry tomatoes, celery, baby carrots, peppers, green beans, sugar snap peas).

Stuffed Baked Potato with Broccoli and Cheese

Split and stuff 1 medium baked potato with cooked chopped broccoli. Top with 1 ounce shredded reduced-fat or fat-free cheese (or ½ cup fat-free or 1% reduced-fat cottage cheese). Heat in 350°F oven or microwave on high until cheese is melted. Serve with mixed green vegetable salad tossed with 1 teaspoon olive oil and unlimited balsamic vinegar or fresh lemon juice (or 2 to 4 tablespoons gluten-free reduced-calorie salad dressing).

DINNER OPTIONS

(Approximately 500 to 600 calories)

Poached Red Snapper with Fresh Herbs and Vidalia Sweet Potatoes

6 ounces red snapper fillet poached in ⅔ cup of water with 2 tablespoons each fresh parsley, dill, thyme, and rosemary. (Or season any favorite fish with salt and ground black pepper and *lightly* brush with olive oil; grill or pan-roast on medium-high for about 3 minutes on each side, until golden brown; cooking times will vary depending on the fish.) Serve with 1 cup steamed Brussels sprouts, Swiss chard, asparagus, sugar snap peas, or green beans. Enjoy with 1 serving Vidalia Sweet Potatoes (page 438) or 1 medium baked sweet or white potato with optional 1 teaspoon soft tub reduced-fat trans fat–free margarine spread or 2 tablespoons reduced-fat sour cream (check ingredients).

Turkey Tacos

3 servings Turkey Tacos (page 250; use hard or soft corn taco shells and check ingredients on seasoning packet). Enjoy with optional salsa and hot sauce.

Sirloin Steak with Sautéed Spinach and Potato

5 ounces grilled sirloin steak (or pork tenderloin, veal, fish, or chicken breast) with unlimited sautéed spinach in 1 teaspoon olive oil and garlic. Enjoy with ½ baked potato with optional 1 teaspoon soft tub, reduced-fat, trans fat–free margarine spread or 2 tablespoons reduced-fat sour cream (check ingredients).

Rosemary Chicken with Swiss Chard and Brown Rice

5 ounces Rosemary Chicken (page 347), or coat skinless chicken breast with preferred safe seasonings and grill, lightly pan-fry, or bake. Enjoy with 1 cup Sautéed Swiss Chard (page 348) and 1 cup cooked brown or wild rice (or amaranth, quinoa, or millet).

Grilled Salmon with Edamame and Broccoli

1 cup boiled edamame (soybeans in the pod), lightly salted. Enjoy with 1 serving Easy 3-Step Microwave Salmon (page 345) or grill 5 ounces wild salmon with 1 teaspoon olive oil and preferred safe seasonings. Serve with 1 to 2 cups steamed broccoli or cauliflower.

Turkey Chili

2 cups (1 serving) Turkey Chili (page 367; when recipe calls for 2 teaspoons flour, use chickpea flour), topped with 1 ounce shredded fat-free Cheddar cheese. Serve with ½ cup cooked brown or wild rice (or amaranth or quinoa, or ½ plain baked potato). Optional side salad with lettuce, mushrooms, cucumbers, peppers, and onions tossed with 1 teaspoon olive oil and unlimited balsamic vinegar or fresh lemon juice.

Grilled Rockefeller Oysters with Cajun Fish and Asparagus

1 serving Grilled Rockefeller Oysters (page 180; when recipe calls for flour, use chickpea flour), with 6 ounces baked fish (tilapia, black cod, shrimp, wild salmon, or trout) rubbed with Cajun spice or preferred safe seasonings and baked or grilled. Enjoy with leafy green salad tossed with 1 teaspoon olive oil and fresh lemon juice or balsamic vinegar (or 2 tablespoons gluten-free reduced-calorie dressing). Serve with 1 cup steamed asparagus, broccoli, green beans, cauliflower, spinach, or other preferred vegetable.

SNACK OPTIONS

100 calories or less

- *Best Vegetables:* 1 cup raw or cooked bell peppers (red, green, yellow), bok choy, broccoli, broccoli raab, kale, Brussels sprouts, cabbage, sugar snap peas, tomatoes, okra, zucchini squash, carrots, lettuce and leafy greens, spinach, collard greens, Swiss chard, watercress, asparagus, kohlrabi, okra, artichokes, beets, cauliflower, or seaweed

- *Best Fruits:* 1 apple, small banana, orange, pear, peach, tangerine, persimmon, kiwi, or guava; 2 clementines or plums; ½ papaya, mango, grapefruit, or cantaloupe; 1 cup berries (all varieties), cherries, watermelon, honeydew, or pineapple; ½ cup lychee

- 1 cup fat-free milk

- 1 reduced-fat string cheese or 1 ounce fat-free or reduced-fat cheese

- 1 hard-boiled egg

- 1 rice cake with 1 level teaspoon peanut butter

- 1 level tablespoon peanut butter with celery sticks

- 10 raw almonds

100 to 200 calories

- 1 ounce plain baked potato chips, corn chips, or vegetable chips (check ingredients)

- 1 ounce Genisoy soy crisps (check ingredients on other brands of soy crisps)

- Enjoy Life snack bars (Cocoa Loco or Caramel Apple flavors)

- 8 ounces fat-free plain yogurt mixed with ½ cup canned 100% pure pumpkin and 1 teaspoon sugar or honey

- ½ cup low-fat or fat-free frozen yogurt or ice cream (any gluten-free brand 200 calories or less)

- 1 Gluten-Free Gingerbread Muffin (page 439)

- 2 cups Tropical Mango-Citrus Smoothie (page 123)

- 2 cups Strawberry-Kiwi Smoothie (page 122)

- 1 ounce nuts (about ¼ cup each): soy nuts, almonds, walnuts, pecans, cashews, or peanuts

- ¼ cup sunflower seeds or pistachio nuts in the shell

- 1 cup boiled edamame (soybeans in the pod), lightly salted

- 1 cup baby carrots and/or pepper sticks with ¼ cup hummus (check ingredients)

- ½ cup fat-free or 1% reduced-fat cottage cheese mixed with 2 tablespoons ground flax-seed (or 1 tablespoon chopped nuts)

- Sliced apple with 1 level tablespoon peanut butter

- 10 almonds plus 1 serving of fruit

APPLE-CINNAMON PANCAKES WITH LEMON YOGURT TOPPING

Nobody should have to live without pancakes! While testing this gluten-free version, ten "non-celiac" breakfast guests confirmed that scrumptious flapjacks do not need all-purpose wheat flour. Enjoy the pancakes, which include extra calcium and fiber!

Makes 4 servings, 3 pancakes and ¼ cup topping each

TOPPING

1	cup fat-free, plain unflavored yogurt
1	tablespoon grated lemon zest
1	tablespoon honey
1	teaspoon vanilla extract
1	teaspoon ground cinnamon

PANCAKES

1	cup buckwheat flour
1	cup fat-free milk
1	egg white
¼	cup fat-free yogurt
1	tablespoon honey
2	teaspoons vanilla extract
1	teaspoon ground cinnamon
⅛	teaspoon freshly grated nutmeg
½	teaspoon baking soda
1	cup diced apple, preferably Golden Delicious
1	tablespoon canola oil

1. To make the topping: Whisk together the yogurt, lemon zest, honey, vanilla, and cinnamon in a small bowl. Set aside.
2. To make the pancakes: In a blender, combine the flour, milk, egg white, yogurt, honey, vanilla, cinnamon, nutmeg, and baking soda. Blend until smooth. Stir in the apple.
3. Spray a griddle or large frying pan with nonstick cooking spray. Add the oil and heat over medium-high heat. When the oil is hot (but not smoking), ladle about 2 tablespoons batter onto the griddle for each pancake. Cook until small bubbles form around the edges, 2 to 3 minutes. Flip the pancakes, and cook 2 to 3 minutes longer, until the centers are cooked through. Serve immediately with the topping, or allow to cool and freeze in an air-tight container.

PER SERVING
261 calories, 11 g protein, 45 g carbohydrate, 5 g fat (0 g saturated), 0 mg cholesterol, 260 mg sodium, 4.5 g fiber; plus 259 mg calcium (26% of DV)

VIDALIA SWEET POTATOES

When my producer at the *Today* show, Rainy Farrell, mentioned her delicious sweet potato dish, my mouth was watering! I knew it had to be included in the book. Her version was meant for the grill but the weekend I got my hands on the recipe, it stormed non-stop and I was forced to create an indoor version. I hope you love it as much as I do!

Makes 2 servings

2	medium sweet potatoes (about 7 ounces each)
1	teaspoon garlic powder
	Salt
1	Vidalia onion, thinly sliced
4	teaspoons soft tub, reduced-fat, trans fat–free margarine spread

1. Preheat the oven or toaster oven to 400°F. Line a baking sheet with aluminum foil or parchment paper; set aside.
2. With the tines of a fork, prick the potatoes several times. Microwave the potatoes on high for 5 to 6 minutes.
3. Make a large, lengthwise slit down the center of the potatoes. Sprinkle each potato with ½ teaspoon garlic powder and season with salt. Press the onion slices inside, and top with the margarine. Season with additional salt to taste.
4. Bake on the top rack of the oven for 9 to 10 minutes, until the onion begins to brown and the potato is tender when pierced with a fork. Serve immediately.

PER SERVING
264 calories, 4 g protein, 56 g carbohydrate, 3 g fat (0 g saturated), 0 mg cholesterol, 171 mg sodium, 9 g fiber

GLUTEN-FREE GINGERBREAD MUFFINS

Enjoy warm gingerbread muffins as a late afternoon snack, or serve for a relaxed Sunday-morning breakfast with low-fat cottage cheese or scrambled eggs. Muffins can be stored in an airtight container at room temperature for up to 2 days, or frozen for up to 1 month.

Makes 12

½	cup honey (or sugar substitute)
½	cup soft tub reduced-fat, trans fat–free margarine spread
2	eggs whites
1	cup plain fat-free yogurt
1	tablespoon grated lemon zest
1	teaspoon vanilla extract
2	cups teff flour
2	teaspoons baking powder
½	teaspoon baking soda
½	teaspoon dried ginger
½	teaspoon ground cinnamon
½	teaspoon ground nutmeg
¼	teaspoon ground cloves
1	tablespoon crystallized ginger, chopped

1. Preheat the oven to 350°F. Line the cups of a 12-cup muffin pan with paper liners.
2. In a large bowl, mix the honey or sugar substitute with the margarine. Stir in the egg whites, yogurt, lemon zest, and vanilla. Add the teff flour, baking powder, baking soda, dried ginger, cinnamon, nutmeg, and cloves. Stir until the flour is just incorporated, but do not overmix. Fold in the crystallized ginger.
3. Fill each muffin liner three-fourths full with batter. Bake 12 to 15 minutes, until the tops of the muffins are lightly browned and a toothpick comes out clean when inserted in the center. Turn the muffins out on a cooling rack.

Tip: If you have trouble finding teff flour in your local health food store, order it online ; or you can buy teff seeds and grind your own flour using a clean, electric coffee grinder.

PER MUFFIN
200 calories, 5 g protein, 35 g carbohydrate, 4 g fat (0 g saturated), 0 mg cholesterol, 186 mg sodium, 4 g fiber

PART SIX

SMOOTH SAILING

DECODING A NUTRITION LABEL

Once you become comfortable with the layout and information provided on food labels, you won't be able to resist checking out the stats on every package you buy. Before long, you'll be one of those people you see lingering in the grocery store aisles with reading glasses and a shopping cart full of healthy choices. Here's how to decode a nutrition label (see sample label on page 445):

1. **Serving Size and Servings Per Container.** Look here first. All the other information on the label is based on a single serving, so you need to know the size of a single serving, and how many servings are contained in the package. You may be surprised. Some packages look small, but they could contain two or more servings. Serving sizes are standardized, so you can compare similar foods and choose the one with the best nutrient profile.

2. **Calories.** If you are watching your weight (as most of us are), calories are key. This number is the total number of calories in a single serving. If you eat two servings, multiply the number of calories by two; if you eat three servings, multiply the number of calories by three, and so on.

3. **Calories from Fat.** This tells you the number of calories in a single serving that come from fat. Some foods—such as margarines and oils—are all fat, so this number will be the same as the total number of calories.

4. **Total Fat.** This section specifies the amount of total fat, plus the amounts of the two most dangerous types of fats—saturated fats and trans fats. (These are displayed in grams. To convert to calories from fat, multiply by 9.) You'll notice there is a second number for both total fat and saturated fat—**% Daily Value**. This shows what percent of your total daily calories (based on a 2,000-calorie diet) is contained in one serving. As a general rule, I recommend aiming for no more than 35 percent of your total daily calories coming from total fat, and no more than 10 percent from saturated fat. There is no safe amount of trans fats, so aim to get as few grams per day as possible.

5. **Cholesterol.** Only animal products contain cholesterol, so don't get too excited if your breakfast cereal doesn't have any. Aim for a daily total of 300 milligrams or less per day. (To keep track of your daily totals, you can add the milligrams of cholesterol for

all foods you eat, or add the numbers specified by **% Daily Value,** being careful not to eat more than 100 percent during the day.)

6. **Sodium.** This tells you the amount of salt in a single serving. Aim for a daily total of 2300 milligrams or less per day. (To keep track of your daily total, you can add the milligrams of sodium for all foods you eat, or add the numbers specified by **% Daily Value,** being careful not to eat more than 100 percent during the day.) If you are salt-sensitive or have high blood pressure, your doctor may recommend that you restrict your sodium intake even more.

7. **Carbohydrates.** I divide carbohydrates into two broad categories—high-quality and low-quality. The goal is to eat more high-quality carbs and fewer low-quality carbs. Food labels tell you the amount of **Total Carbohydrates** in one serving. The label also gives you a few clues to the general quality of the carbohydrate via two categories: **Dietary Fiber** and **Sugars.** Sugars are typically low-quality carbohydrates, and they should be eaten only in small quantities. (If you subtract grams of Sugars from Total Carbohydrates, you can often get an estimate of the amount of healthy high-quality carbs.) Dietary fiber typically accompanies high-quality carbohydrate. Experts recommend that you consume 25 to 35 grams of total fiber daily. The label will also sometimes specify the amount of Soluble Fiber and Insoluble Fiber, which may be of interest to people fighting diabetes or cardiovascular disease.

   The **% Daily Values** for total carbohydrate and dietary fiber help you to gauge how much a serving will contribute to your personal goals. The standard is based on a 2,000-calorie diet containing 60 percent of its calories from total carbohydrates and 25 grams of total dietary fiber.

8. **Protein.** Take your weight in pounds, and divide it in half. That's approximately how many grams of protein you should eat per day. This listing will help you figure out how much protein is contained in packaged foods.

9. **Vitamins and minerals.** Below the thick dividing line under Protein is the space for listing significant vitamins and minerals and the percent of the Recommended Daily Value contained in one serving. This can be helpful if you want to boost your intake of particular nutrients.

10. **Goals for certain calorie diets.** Some of the larger food labels also contain a small chart that lists recommended goals for various nutrients based on both a 2,000-calorie diet and a 2,500-calorie diet. These are simply reminders, and they do not provide additional information about the food.

11. **Calorie guide.** Some larger food labels also contain an informational section that lists the Calories per gram for Fat (9 calories per gram), Carbohydrate (4 calories per gram), Protein (4 calories per gram), and Alcohol (7 calories per gram). This is informational; it does not describe the specific food.

12. **Ingredients.** Somewhere outside the Nutrition Facts box is a list of ingredients, in descending order of predominance according to weight. That means that the first food listed is the most abundant (by weight).

13. **Special notations.** Look for special notations that might tell you more about the product, such as "enriched" or "fortified" (which tells you that extra vitamins or minerals have been added, or replaced after processing), or "contains wheat ingredients" (which tells you it isn't safe for people with celiac disease or wheat sensitivities), or "may contain peanuts" (as a warning to people with peanut allergies).

14. **Contact information.** All labels must include a way for you to contact the company, such as the company name, address, telephone number, and/or Web site address. Don't hesitate to contact the company if you have questions about its products.

Nutrition Facts

Serving Size
Servings Per Container

Amount Per Serving

Calories 0	Calories from Fat 0

	% Daily Value*
Total Fat 0g	0%
Saturated Fat 0g	0%
Trans Fat 0g	
Cholesterol 0mg	0%
Sodium 0mg	0%
Total Carbohydrate 0g	0%
Dietary Fiber 0g	0%
Soluble Fiber 0g	0%
Insoluble Fiber 0g	0%
Sugars 0g	
Protein 0g	

Vitamin A 0%	•	Vitamin C 0%
Calcium 0%	•	Iron 0%
Phosphorus 0%	•	Magnesium 0%

* Percent Daily Values are based on a 2,000 calorie diet. Your daily values may be higher or lower depending on your calorie needs:

	Calories:	2,000	2,500
Total Fat	Less than	0g	0g
Sat Fat	Less than	0g	0g
Cholesterol	Less than	0mg	0mg
Sodium	Less than	0mg	0mg
Potassium		0mg	0mg
Total Carbohydrate		0g	0g
Dietary Fiber		0g	0g

Calories per gram:

Fat 0 • Carbohydrate 0 • Protein 0

INGREDIENTS: Whole Wheat Flour, (Stone Ground Whole Oats, Hard Red Winter Wheat, Rye, Long Grain Brown Rice, Triticale, Buckwheat, Barley, Sesame Seeds), Malted Barley, Salt, Yeast, Mixed Tocopherols (Natural Vitamin E) for Freshness.

CONTAINS WHEAT INGREDIENTS

DISTRIBUTED BY
COMPANY NAME
ADDRESS
CITY, STATE, ZIP
WEB ADDRESS

JOY'S FOOD PICKS

It can be difficult to choose from among all the available brands of packaged foods. That's why I have created this list of my personal picks. These are some of the "best of the best"—brands that I've evaluated and love. They are healthy, tasty, and fit perfectly in all of my meal plans. Most of these brands should be available in your local supermarket, although you may need to visit a health food store for some. I encourage you to be a little adventurous, to step outside of your food comfort zone and discover how wonderful these healthful products really are.

BREAD, PITA, WHOLE WHEAT

When shopping for whole wheat pita bread, choose those that have at least 2 grams of fiber. There are two sizes of pita—regular (which has 140 to 170 calories per pita) and mini (which have an **asterisk** (*) and typically provide about 70 to 80 calories per pita). The first ingredient on the label should always be whole grain or whole wheat flour.

*Aladdin's Whole Wheat Pocket Pita Pocket, regular size
*Aladdin's Whole Wheat Pocket Pita Pocket, small size
*Kangaroo Whole Grain Sandwich Pocket
Khoubiz Whole Wheat Pita
*Khoubiz Whole Wheat Pita, small
Thomas' Sahara Mini 100% Whole Wheat Pita Bread
*Thomas' Sahara 100% Whole Wheat Pita Bread
Toufayan Wheat Pita Bread
Trader Joe's Whole Wheat Pita Bread

BREAD, WHOLE WHEAT

When shopping for whole wheat bread, choose those that have at least 2 grams of fiber and 80 calories or less per slice. The first ingredient on the label should always be whole grain or whole wheat flour.

Arnold Carb Counting 100% Wheat
Arnold Stoneground 100% Whole Wheat

Healthy Choice Hearty 100% Whole Grain
Home Pride 100% Whole Wheat
Home Pride Honey Whole Wheat
Nature's Own 100% Whole Wheat
Pepperidge Farm 100% Whole Wheat Stoneground
Pepperidge Farm Carb Style 100% Whole Wheat
Sara Lee Heart Healthy 100% Plus Whole Wheat
Sara Lee Heart Healthy 100% Whole Wheat Classic
Sara Lee Soft & Smooth 100% Whole Wheat
Stroehmann Family Grains Heart Healthy 100% Whole Wheat

BREAD, WHOLE WHEAT, REDUCED-CALORIE

Choose brands that list the first ingredient as whole grain or whole wheat flour and have 45 calories or less per slice. Most brands listed provide at least 2 grams fiber.

Arnold Bakery Light Wheat
Healthy Life Natural All Whole Grain 100% Whole Wheat
Nature's Own Double Fiber Wheat
Weight Watchers 100% Whole Wheat

CEREAL, WHOLE GRAIN

When choosing breakfast cereal, look for those with at least 3 grams of fiber and no more than 120 calories and 6 grams of sugar per ¾ to 1 cup serving. Check the nutrition label to make sure.

Barbara's Multigrain Shredded Spoonfuls
Barbara's Puffins, Original and Cinnamon
General Mills Cheerios, Plain and MultiGrain
General Mills Fiber One
General Mills Wheaties
General Mills Total, Whole Grain
Kashi GoLean
Kashi Heart to Heart
Kellogg's All Bran, original
Kellogg's Complete All Bran Oat Bran Flakes
Kellogg's Complete All Bran Wheat Bran Flakes
Kellogg's Special K, Protein Plus
Post Bran Flakes
Post Grape-Nut Flakes
South Beach Diet Whole Grain Crunch
Weetabix Organic Crispy Flakes

CRACKERS, WHOLE GRAIN

When choosing crackers, the first ingredient should be whole grain and one serving should provide at least 2 grams fiber and no more than 130 calories. The number of crackers per 1-ounce serving will vary, so be sure to check the label on the box before indulging.

Ak-Mak 100% Whole Wheat Stone Ground Sesame Crackers
Kashi TLC Original 7 Grain
Kashi TLC Natural Ranch
Kashi TLC Honey Sesame
Kavli 5 Grain Crisp Bread
Kavli Crispy Thin Crisp Bread
Kavli Hearty Thick Crisp Bread
Manischewitz Whole Wheat Matzo
Nabisco Triscuit, Deli-Style Rye
Nabisco Triscuit, Reduced Fat
Ry Krisp Natural
Ry Krisp Seasoned
Ry Krisp Sesame
Ryvita Fruit Crunch
Wasa Fiber Rye
Wasa Hearty Rye
Wasa Light Rye
Whole Food 365 Crackers Woven Wheats

BURGERS, LEAN TURKEY

When purchasing burgers, look for brands that are 250 calories or less per 4-ounce serving and provide no more than 3 grams saturated fat.

Jennie-O Turkey Store—fresh: Lean and Seasame Lean
Jennie-O Turkey Store—frozen: Original ¼ Pound, and Savory Seasonal
Perdue Fresh Ground Turkey Patties
Shady Brook Farms 93% Lean Ground Turkey Patties

BURGERS, VEGGIE AND SOY

These meatless burgers are great choices for lean protein. Each of them contains no more than 150 calories and 2 grams of saturated fat and provides at least 10 grams of protein.

Amy's All American Veggie Burger
Amy's Texas Veggie
Boca Burgers All American Flame Grilled
Boca Burgers Cheeseburger
Boca Burgers Grilled Vegetable

Boca Burgers Original

Boca Burgers Roasted Onion

Gardenburger GardenVegan

Morningstar Farms Grillers Vegan

Morningstar Farms Okara Pattie

Morningstar Farms Veggie Medley Burger

Morningstar Farms Zesty Tomato Basil Burger

Veggie Patch Meatless Garlic Portabella Burger

Yves the Good Burger Veggie Chick'n Burger

Yves the Good Burger Veggie Original

Yves the Good Burger Veggie Authentic

CHEESE, COTTAGE

All of the products listed below are great sources of fat-free and low-fat protein (as well as calcium). If you're watching your sodium intake, be sure to go for the no-salt-added options, as the other can have between 350 and 470 milligrams of sodium per ½-cup serving.

Axelrod's 1% low-fat, no-salt

Axelrod's nonfat

Hood, low-fat

Hood, fat-free

Hood, no salt added, 1% low-fat

Friendship 1% low-fat

Friendship 1% low-fat, no salt added

Friendship nonfat

Light n' Lively, low-fat

Trader Joe's 1% organic low-fat

Trader Joe's fat-free

CHEESE, LOW-FAT

Check cheese labels carefully, and choose the brands that meet your personal health needs. Although all of the brands listed are lower in calories, total fat, and saturated fat than regular whole-milk cheese, some are far leaner than others. For example, 1 ounce of reduced-fat cheese typically provides about 4.5 grams saturated fat, but 1-ounce of fat-free cheese provides 0 grams of saturated fat.

Alpine Lace Reduced-Fat Cheddar

Alpine Lace Reduced-Fat Low Moisture Mozzarella

Alpine Lace Yellow Reduced-Fat and Reduced-Sodium American

CHEESE, LOW-FAT *(cont.)*

Alpine Lace Reduced-Fat Swiss
Borden Singles, all fat-free varieties
Cabot Vermont 75% Reduced-Fat Sharp
Cracker Barrel 2% Milk Reduced Fat Natural Extra Sharp Cheddar,
Cracker Barrel 2% Milk Reduced Fat Natural Sharp Cheddar
Cracker Barrel 2% Milk Reduced Fat Natural Vermont's Sharp-White
Kraft 2% Milk Singles, American
Kraft Fat Free Shredded, Cheddar
Kraft Fat Free Singles, American, Sharp Cheddar, Mozzarella, and Swiss
Kraft Natural Low-Moisture, Part-Skim Shredded, Mozzarella
Laughing Cow Mini Babybel Original, Light
Laughing Cow Wedges, Original Swiss, LightPolly-O String Reduced-Fat
Mozzarella, 2% Milk
Polly0O—Ums String cheese mozzarella, Reduced-fat
Sargento Fat-Free Ricotta
Sargento Light Ricotta
Sargento Reduced Fat Deli-Style Sliced Provolone
Sargento Reduced Fat Deli-Style Sliced Swiss
Sargento Reduced Fat Mild Cheddar, Shredded
Sargento Reduced Fat Mozzarella, Shredded

CHILI, CANNED AND FROZEN

The following brands of chili are no more than 250 calories and 550 milligrams of sodium per 1-cup serving. Plus, they each provide at least 7 grams of fiber.

Amy's Organic (light in sodium), Medium or Spicy
Health Valley Organic Chunky Chile—all varieties
Westbrae Natural, vegetarian

EGG SUBSTITUTE

For each of the egg substitutes listed below, a serving size of ¼ cup contains only 30 calories and 0 grams of fat—making these products a great source of lean protein!

Better'n Eggs
Eggbeaters Egg White
Eggbeaters Original
Eggology 100% Egg Whites
Horizon Organic Liquid Egg Whites
Just Whites Egg Substitute
Organic Valley Egg Whites

HUMMUS

These hummus options are delicious and contain approximately 100 calories per ¼ cup.

Athenos Original Hummus
Guiltless Gourmet Original Hummus
Tribe of Two Sheiks

MAYONNAISE, REDUCED FAT

My picks for reduced-fat mayonnaise have 25 calories or less per 1-tablespoon serving.

Best Foods Light
Hellman's, reduced fat
Wish-Bone, reduced fat

PASTA

Two ounces of dry pasta comes out to 1 cup of cooked (about 200 calories). The pastas I've listed below are all good sources of fiber, with 4 or more grams per 1-cup serving.

Barilla Plus
Catelli Healthy Harvest Whole Wheat Pasta
DeBoles Organic Whole Wheat—Spaghetti style and Angel Hair
De Cecco Whole Wheat
Golden Grain Mission MultiGrain Penne Rigate
Heartland MultiGrain Spaghetti
Hodgson Mill Organic Whole Wheat
Mueller's MultiGrain Penne
Ronzoni Healthy Harvest Whole Wheat Blend—all varieties
Wild Oats, Whole Wheat

SALAD DRESSING

My picks for salad dressings have 50 calories or less per 2-tablespoon serving. Some of these options can be quite high in sodium, so check the label to find the best fit for your eating program.

Kraft Free Catalina Dressing
Kraft Free Fat Free Honey Dijon
Kraft Free Italian Dressing
Kraft Free Fat Free Ranch Dressing
Kraft Free Fat Free Thousand Island
Newman's Own Lighten Up! Balsamic Vinaigrette
Newman's Own Lighten Up! Low Fat Sesame Ginger
Wishbone Just 2 Good! Blue Cheese
Wish-Bone Just 2 Good! Creamy Caesar
Wish-Bone Just 2 Good! Deluxe French-style

SALAD DRESSING *(cont.)*

Wish-Bone Just 2 Good! Parmesan Peppercorn Ranch

Wish-Bone Just 2 Good! Sweet 'n' Spicy French

Wish-Bone Just 2 Good! Thousand Island

SALSA

I love adding salsa to many foods for a low-calorie, low-fat flavor boost. All of the brands listed below have less than 20 calories per 2-tablespoon serving.

Amy's Organic Salsa, Medium and Mild

Bravos Salsa Mild, Medium Hot

Chi-Chi's Salsa, Original Recipe, Mild or Medium, Fiesta, Mild, Medium, or Hot, and All Natural

Desert Pepper Trading Company Salsa Divino, Mild; Salsa Del Rio, Medium; Salsa Diablo, Hot!

Doritos Dippas, Hot Salsa

Drew's All Natural Organic Salsa, Hot—all varieties

Mrs. Renfros's Gourmet Salsa—Jalapeño Green Salsa—Hot

Muir Glen Organic Salsa, all variety of flavors

Newman's Own All-Natural Bandito Salsa, Mild, Medium, and Hot

Tostitos All Natural Salsa Mild, Medium, and Hot

SAUCE, BARBECUE

The following brands provide no fat and are less than 25 calories per 2-tablespoon serving. Watch the sodium, if salt is an issue in your eating plan.

Stubb's BBQ Sauce—Spicy, Original, and Mild

Stubb's Smokey Mesquite Bar-B-Q Sauce

Walden Farm Calorie Free Original Barbeque Sauce

Walden Farms Calorie Free Thick N Spicy Barbeque Sauce

SAUCE, PASTA

All of my picks for pasta sauce have no saturated fat and have 60 calories or less per ½-cup serving. Some can pack a big sodium punch, however, with up to 400 milligrams per serving. Check the nutrition label to find the best option for you.

Amy's Organic Low Sodium Marinara

Classico Carbernet Marinara with Herbs

Classico Fire Roasted Tomato & Garlic

Classico Spicy Red Pepper

Classico Tomato & Basil

Enrico's—All Natural Fat-Free—all varieties

Enrico's Original—Traditional

Healthy Choice Garlic & Herb

Healthy Choice Super Chunky Tomato Mushroom & Garlic

Muir Glen Organic Chunky Tomato & Herb

Muir Glen Organic Italian Herb

Muir Glen Organic Portabello Mushroom

Progresso Red Clam

Walnut Acres Garlic-Garlic

Walnut Acres Organic Low Sodium Tomato & Basil

Walnut Acres Organic Tomato & Mushroom

Walnut Acres Zesty Basil

SAUSAGES, SOY

The following vegetarian brands have no more than 160 calories and 1 gram of saturated fat per serving—a terrific alternative to high fat sausage.

Boca Meatless Breakfast Links

Boca Meatless Sausages, Italian

Gardenburger Veggie Breakfast Sausage

Lightlife Gimme Lean Sausage Style

Morningstar Farms Veggie Breakfast Sausage Links

Morningstar Farms Veggie Breakfast Sausage Patties

SAUSAGES, TURKEY AND CHICKEN

The following brands of lean poultry sausage provide no more than 150 calories and 2.5 grams of saturated fat per link. Sodium content ranges between 340 and 660 milligrams, so be sure to check the labels if salt is an issue.

al fresco All Natural Fully Cooked Chicken Sausages

Applegate Farms—Organic Chick and Apple, Organic Andouille Poultry Sausage, and Organic Sweet Italian Poultry Sausage

Casual Gourmet Chicken Sausage

Coleman Organic Chicken Sausages—Mild Italian Chicken Sausage and Spicy Italian Chicken Sausage

Hans Cooked Chicken Sausages—Green Onion Bermuda; Roast Red Pepper and Garlic Sante Fe

Shady Brook Farms, Lean Italian Turkey Sausages—Hot and Sweet

Trader Joe's Chicken Sausages

SOUP, CANNED

I'm a big fan of all of the varieties of the following brands. They're all lower in sodium and great for a fast and healthy meal.

Amy's Organic Light in Sodium

Campbell's Low Sodium Soup

Health Valley, all varieties

Healthy Choice
Progresso 50% Less Sodium

SOY MILK

When choosing soy milk, go for those that contain at least 30% of your daily value for calcium and 130 calories or less.

Silk Light Soymilk, Chocolate
Silk Light Soymilk, Plain
Silk Light Soymilk, Vanilla
Silk Soymilk, Unsweetened
Silk Soymilk, Vanilla
Vitasoy Complete Original
Vitasoy Creamy Original
Vitasoy Smooth Vanilla
Vitasoy Light Original
Vitasoy Unsweetened Original
WestSoy Plus Soymilk, Plain

SPREAD, SOFT TUB, REDUCED FAT

Go for the spreads that have no more than 1 gram of saturated fat and 0 trans fats per 1-tablespoon serving. All of the following brands fit the bill and provide no more than 50 calories.

Benecol Light Spread
Blue Bonnet Light Soft Spread
Fleischmann's Light
I Can't Believe It's Not Butter! Fat Free
I Can't Believe It's Not Butter! Light
Promise Fat-Free Buttery Spread
Smart Beat Trans Fat Free Super Light
Take Control Light

TOFU

The following brands of tofu contain 60 calories or less and provide between 4 and 8 grams of protein for every 3-ounce serving.

House Organic Firm Tofu, Medium
Mori-Nu Silken Extra Firm Tofu
Mori-Nu Silken Firm Tofu
Mori-Nu Silken Lite Extra Firm Tofu
Mori-Nu Silken Lite Firm Tofu
Mori-Nu Silken Soft Tofu

TORTILLAS

All of the following brands provide at least 2 grams of fiber and between 50 and 170 calories per tortilla (wraps that are 100 calories or less have an asterisk).

Aladdin Low-Carb Wheat Wrap

*La Tortilla Factory Low-Carb, Low Fat Original Tortillas

La Tortilla Factory Whole Grain Wraps

*Mission Carb Balance Whole Wheat Tortillas

Mission Multigrain Tortillas

Thomas' Sahara Wraps, 100% Whole Wheat

YOGURT

In the list below, I've noted which brands contain artificial sweeteners. Also, the serving sizes for yogurt can vary from 6 ounces to 8 ounces, so keep an eye on the number of calories per serving.

Dannon All Natural

*Dannon Light & Fit, Non Fat with artificial sweeteners—all varieties

*Dannon Light & Fit, Crave Control with artificial sweeteners—all varieties

Dannon Fruit on the Bottom, all varieties

FAGE Total 0%

FAGE Total Light

Horizon Organic Fat Free

Horizon Organic Lowfat Blended, all flavors

Stonyfield Farm All Natural Fat Free, all flavors

Stonyfield Farm Organic Lowfat, all flavors

Trader Joe's Organic 1% Low Fat Vanilla

REFERENCES

WEIGHT LOSS, Chapter 3

Andrade A, Minaker T, Melanson K. Eating rate and satiation. Presentation at the 2006 Annual Scientific Meeting of NAASO: The Obesity Society. Boston, MA: October 20-24, 2006.

Czernichow S, Bertrais S, Preziosi P, et al. Indicators of abdominal obesity in middle-aged participants of the SU.VI.MAX study: relationships with educational level, smoking status and physical inactivity. *Diabetes Metabolism*. 2004;30(2):153-159.

Davis JN, Hodges VA, Gillham MB. Normal-weight adults consume more fiber and fruit than their age-and height-matched overweight/obese counterparts. *Journal of the American Dietetic Association*. 2006;106(6):833-840.

Gillum RF, Sempos CT. Ethnic variation in validity of classification of overweight and obesity using self-reported weight and height in American women and men: the Third National Health and Nutrition Examination Survey. *Nutrition Journal* [serial online]. 2005;4:27.

Gray DS, Fujioka K. Use of relative weight and body mass index for the determination of adiposity. *Journal of Clinical Epidemiology*. 1991;44(6):545-550.

Harrison GG. Height-weight tables. *Annals of Internal Medicine*. 1985;103(6 part 2):989–994.

Howard BV, Manson JE, Stefanick, ML, et al. Low-fat dietary pattern and weight change over 7 years: the Women's Health Initiative dietary modification trial. *Journal of the American Medical Association*. 2006;295(1):39-49.

Howarth NC, Huang TT, Roberts SB, McCrory MA. Dietary fiber and fat are associated with excess weight in young and middle-aged US adults. *Journal of the American Dietetic Association*. 2005;105(9):1365-1372.

Howarth NC, Saltzman E, Roberts SB. Dietary fiber and weight regulation. *Nutrition Reviews*. 2001;59(5): 129-139.

Littman AJ, Kristal AR, White E. Effects of physical activity intensity, frequency, and activity type on 10-y weight change in middle-aged men and women. *International Journal of Obesity*. 2005;29(5):524–533.

Monti V, Carlson JJ, Hunt SC, Adams TD. Relationship of ghrelin and leptin hormones with body mass index and waist circumference in a random sample of adults. *Journal of the American Dietetic Association*. 2006;106(6):822-828.

Nelson LH, Tucker LA. Diet composition related to body fat in a multivariate study of 203 men. *Journal of the American Dietetic Association*. 1996;96(8):771-777.

Price GM, Uauy R, Breeze E, et al. Weight, shape, and mortality risk in older persons: elevated waist-hip ratio, not high body mass index, is associated with a greater risk of death. *American Journal of Clinical Nutrition*. 2005;84(2):449-460.

Schoeller DA, Buchholz AC. Energetics of obesity and weight control: does diet composition matter? *Journal of the American Dietetic Association*. 2005;105(5 Suppl 1);S24-S28.

St Jeor ST, Howard BV, Prewitt TE, et al. Dietary protein and weight reduction: a statement for healthcare professionals from the Nutrition Committee of the Council on Nutrition, Physical Activity, and Metabolism of the American Heart Association. *Circulation*. 2001;104(15):1869-1874.

Weigley ES. Average? Ideal? Desirable? A brief overview of height-weight tables in the United States. *Journal of the American Dietetic Association*. 1984;84(4):417-423.

Willett WC. The Mediterranean diet: science and practice. *Public Health Nutrition*. 2006;9(1A):105-110.

Williams PT, Pate RR. Cross-sectional relationships of exercise and age to adiposity in 60,617 male runners. *Medicine and Science in Sports and Exercise*. 2005;37(8):1329-1337.

Williams PT, Satariano WA. Relationships of age and weekly running distance to BMI and circumferences in 41,582 physically active women. *Obesity Research*. 2005;13(8):1370-1380.

Williams PT, Wood PD. The effects of changing exercise levels on weight and age-related weight gain. *International Journal of Obesity*. 2006;30(3):543-551.

Yao M, Roberts SB. Dietary energy density and weight regulation. *Nutrition Reviews*. 2001;59(8 Pt 1):247-258.

Zemel MB. The role of dairy foods in weight management. *Journal of the American College of Nutrition*. 2005;24(6 Suppl):537S-546S.

BEAUTIFUL SKIN, Chapter 4

Adebamowo CA, Spiegelman D, Danby FW, et al. High school dietary dairy intake and teenage acne. *Journal of the American Academy of Dermatology*. 2005; 52 (2): 207-214.

Duffield-Lillico AJ, Slate EH, Reid ME, et al. Selenium supplementation and secondary prevention of non-melanoma skin cancer in a randomized trial. *Journal of the National Cancer Institute*. 2003;95(19):1477-1481.

Hakim IA, Harris RB, Ritenbaugh C. Fat intake and risk of squamous cell carcinoma of the skin. *Nutrition and Cancer*. 2000;36(2):155-162.

Schwartz JR, Marsh RG, Draelos ZD. Zinc and skin health: overview of physiology and pharmacology. *Dermatologic Surgery*. 2005;31(7 Pt 2):837-847.

Sies HO, Stahl W. Nutritional protection against skin damage from sunlight. *Annual Review of Nutrition*. 2004;24:173-200.

Skolnik P, Eaglstein WH, Ziboh VA. Human essential fatty acid deficiency: treatment by topical application of linoleic acid. *Archives of Dermatology*. 1977;113(7):939-941.

Steele VE, Kelloff GJ, Balentine D, et al. Comparative chemopreventive mechanisms of green tea, black tea and selected polyphenol extracts measured by *in vitro* bioassays. *Carcinogenesis*. 2000;21(1):63-67.

Wilson D, Varigos G, Ackland ML. Apoptosis may underlie the pathology of zinc-deficient skin. *Immunology and Cell Biology*. 2006;84(1):28-37.

HEALTHY HAIR, Chapter 5

Birch MP, Lalla SC, Messenger AG. Female pattern hair loss. *Clinical and Experimental Dermatology*. 2002;27(5):383-388.

Corazza GR, Andreani ML, Venturo N, et al. Celiac disease and alopecia areata: report of a new association. *Gastroenterology*. 1995;109(4):1333-1337.

Harkey MR. Anatomy and physiology of hair. *Forensic Science International*. 1993;63(1-3):9-18.

Rushton DH. Nutritional factors and hair loss. *Clinical and Experimental Dermatology*. 2002;27(5):396-404.

Springer K, Brown M, Stulberg DL. Common hair loss disorders. *American Family Physician*. 2003;68(1): 93-102.

Trost LB, Bergfeld WF, Calogeras E. The diagnosis and treatment of iron deficiency and its potential relationship to hair loss. *Journal of the American Academy of Dermatology*. 2006;54(5):824-844.

Wiedemeyeer K, Schill WB, Loser C. Diseases on hair follicles leading to hair loss part: nonscarring alopecias. *Skinmed*. 2004;3(4):209-214.

FEEDING A BEAUTIFUL SMILE, Chapter 6

Bergstrom J. Cigarette smoking as a risk factor in chronic periodontal disease. *Community Dentistry and Oral Epidemiology*. 1989;17(5):245-247.

Briggs JE, McKeown PP, Crawford VL, et al. Angiographically confirmed coronary heart disease and periodontal disease in middle-aged males. *Journal of Periodontology.* 2006;77(1):95-102.

Bsoul SA, Terezhalmy GT. Vitamin C in health and disease. *Journal of Contemporary Dental Practice.* 2004;5(2):1-13.

Hamilton-Miller JMT. Anti-cariogenic properties of tea (*Camellia sinensis*). *Journal of Medical Microbiology.* 2001;50(4):299-302.

Nishida M, Grossi SG, Dunford RG, et al. Calcium and the risk for periodontal disease. *Journal of Periodontology.* 2000;71(7):1057-1066.

Nishida M, Grossi SG, Dunford RG, et al. Dietary vitamin C and the risk for periodontal disease. *Journal of Periodontology.* 2000;71(8):1215-1223.

Wang PL, Shirasu S, Shinohara M, et al. Salivary amylase activity of rats fed a low calcium diet. *Japanese Journal of Pharmacology.* 1998;78(3):279-283.

CARDIOVASCULAR DISEASE, Chapter 7

Andersen LF, Jacobs Jr DR, Carlsen MH, Blomhoff R. Consumption of coffee is associated with reduced risk of death attributed to inflammatory and cardiovascular diseases in the Iowa Women's Health Study. *American Journal of Clinical Nutrition.* 2006;82(5):1039-1046.

Austin MA, Hokanson JE, Edwards KL. Hypertriglyceridemia as a cardiovascular risk factor. *American Journal of Cardiology.* 1998;81(4A):7B-12B.

Blache D, Devaux S, Joubert O, et al. Long-term moderate magnesium-deficient diet shows relationships between blood pressure, inflammation and oxidant stress defense in aging rats. *Free Radical Biology & Medicine.* 2006;41(2):277-284.

Borek C. Garlic reduces dementia and heart-disease risk. *Journal of Nutrition.* 2006;136(3 Suppl):810S-812S.

Brown CD, Higgins M, Donato KA, et al. Body mass index and the prevalence of hypertension and dyslipidemia. *Obesity Research.* 2000;8(9):605-619.

Brown L, Rosner B, Willett WW, Sacks FM. Cholesterol-lowering effects of dietary fiber: a meta-analysis. *American Journal of Clinical Nutrition.* 1999;69(1):30-42.

Chrysohoou C, Panagiotakos DB, Pitsavos C, et al. The association between pre-hypertension status and oxidative stress markers related to atherosclerotic disease: The ATTICA study. *Atherosclerosis.* 2006;May 25. (Epub)

Davidson MH, Maki KC, Umporowicz DM, et al. Safety and tolerability of esterified phytosterols administered in reduced-fat spread and salad dressing to healthy adult men and women. *Journal of the American College of Nutrition.* 2001;20(4):307-319.

Ding EL, Hutfless SM, Ding X, Girotra S. Chocolate and prevention of cardiovascular disease: a systematic review. *Nutrition and Metabolism* (London) [online]. 2006;3:2.

Gill JM, Mees GP, Frayn KN, Hardman AE. Moderate exercise, postprandial lipaemia and triacylglycerol clearance. *European Journal of Clinical Investigation.* 2001;31(3):201-207.

Gonen A, Harats D, Rabinkov A, et al. The antiatherogenic effect of allicin: possible mode of action. *Pathobiology.* 2005;72(6):325-334.

Grubben MJ, Boers GH, Blom HJ, et al. Unfiltered coffee increases plasma homocysteine concentrations in healthy volunteers: a randomized trial. *American Journal of Clinical Nutrition.* 2000;71(2):480-484.

Guyton JR. Extended-release niacin for modifying the lipoprotein profile. *Expert Opinion on Pharmacotherapy.* 2004;5(6):1385-1398.

Halperin RO, Sesso HD, Ma J, et al. Dyslipidemia and the risk of incident hypertension in men. *Hypertension.* 2006;47(1):45-50.

He K, Liu K, Daviglus ML, et al. Magnesium intake and incidence of metabolic syndrome among young adults. *Circulation.* 2006;113(13):1675-1682.

Hendriks HF, Brink EJ, Meijer GW, et al. Safety of long-term consumption of plant sterol esters-enriched spread. *European Journal of Clinical Nutrition.* 2003;57(5):681-692.

Hokanson JE, Austin MA. Plasma triglyceride level is a risk factor for cardiovascular disease independent of high-density lipoprotein cholesterol level: a meta-analysis of population-based prospective studies. *Journal of Cardiovascular Risk.* 1996;3(2):213-219.

Hu FB, Manson JE, Willett WC. Types of dietary fat and risk of coronary heart disease: a critical review. *Journal of the American College of Nutrition*. 2001;20(1):5-19.

Hu FB, Rimm EB, Stampfer MJ, et al. Prospective Study of major dietary patterns and risk of coronary heart disease in men. *American Journal of Clinical Nutrition*. 2000;72(4):912-921.

Jakubowski M, McAllister PJ, Bajwa ZH, et al. Exploding vs. imploding headache in migraine prophylaxis with Botulinum Toxin A. Pain 2006;125(3):286-295.

Jorde R, Bonaa KH. Calcium from dairy products, vitamin D intake, and blood pressure: the Tromso Study. *American Journal of Clinical Nutrition*. 2000;71(6):1530-1535.

Katsanos CS. Prescribing aerobic exercise for the regulation of postprandial lipid metabolism: current research and recommendations. *Sports Medicine*. 2006;36(7):547-560.

Kolovou GD, Salpea KD, Anagnostopoulou KK, Mikhailidis DP. Alcohol use, vascular disease, and lipid-lowering drugs. *Journal of Pharmacology and Experimental Therapeutics*. 2006;318(1):1-7.

Lee KW, Lip GYH. The role of omega-3 fatty acids in the secondary prevention of cardiovascular disease. *Quarterly Journal of Medicine*. 2003;96;465-480.

Lichtenstein A, Appel LJ, Brands M, et al. Diet and lifestyle recommendations revision 2006: a scientific statement from the American Heart Association Nutrition Committee. *Circulation*. 2006;114(1):82-96.

Lonn E, Yusuf S, Arnold MJ, et al. Homocysteine lowering with folic acid and B vitamins in vascular disease. *New England Journal of Medicine*. 2006;354(15):1567-1577.

Lopez-Garcia E, van Dam RM, Willett WC, et al. Coffee consumption and coronary heart disease in men and women: a prospective cohort study. *Circulation*. 2006;113(17):2045-2053.

Makela P, Valkonen T, Martelin T. Contribution of deaths related to alcohol use of socioeconomic variation in mortality: register based follow up study. *British Medical Journal*. 1997;315(7102):211-216.

Maki KC, Davidson MH, Umporowicz DM, et al. Lipid responses to plant-sterol-enriched reduced-fat spreads incorporated into a National Cholesterol Education Program Step I diet. *American Journal of Clinical Nutrition*. 2001;74(1):33-43.

McTigue K, Larson JC, Valoski A, et al. Mortality and cardiac and vascular outcomes in extremely obese women. *Journal of the American Medical Association*. 2006;296(1):79-86.

Nam BH, Kannel WB, D'Agostino RB. Search for an optimal atherogenic lipid risk profile: from the Framingham Study. *American Journal of Cardiology*. 2006;97(3):372-375.

Oh K, Hu FB, Manson JE, et al. Dietary fat intake and risk of coronary heart disease in women: 20 years of follow-up of the nurses' health study. *American Journal of Epidemiology*. 2005;161(7):672-679.

Reilly MP, Wolfe ML, Localoi AR, Rader, DJ. C-reactive protein and coronary artery calcification: the study of inherited risk of coronary atherosclerosis (SIRCA). *Arteriosclerosis, Thrombosis, and Vascular Biology*. 2003;23:1851-1856.

Ridker PM, Stampfer MJ, Rifai N. Novel risk factors for systemic atherosclerosis: a comparison of C-reactive protein, fibrinogen, homocysteine, lipoprotein(a), and standard cholesterol screening as predictors of peripheral arterial disease. *Journal of the American Medical Association*. 2001;285(19):2481-2485.

Rimm EB, Williams P, Fosher K, et al. Moderate alcohol intake and lower risk of coronary heart disease: meta-analysis of effects on lipids and haemostatic factors. *British Medical Journal*. 1999;319(7224):1523-1528.

Rossi GP, Maiolino G, Seccia TM, et al. Hyperhomocysteinemia predicts total and cardiovascular mortality in high-risk women. *Journal of Hypertension*. 2006;24(5):851-859.

Sacks FM, Lichtenstein A, Van Horn L, et al. Soy protein, isoflavones, and cardiovascular health: an American Heart Association Science Advisory for Professionals from the Nutrition Committee. *Circulation*. 2006;113(7):1034-1044.

Salonen JT, Lakka TA, Lakka HM, et al. Hyperinsulinemia is associated with the incidence of hypertension and dyslipidemia in middle-aged men. *Diabetes*. 1998;47(2):270-275.

Sesso HD, Buring JE, Chown MJ, et al. A prospective study of plasma lipid levels and hypertension in women. *Archives of Internal Medicine*. 2005;165(20):2420-2427.

Sesso HD, Buring JE, Rifai N, et al. C-reactive protein and the risk of developing hypertension. *Journal of the American Medical Association*. 2003;290(22):2945-2951.

Shai I, Rimm EB, Hankinson SE, et al. Multivariate assessment of lipid parameters as predictors of coronary heart disease among postmenopausal women: potential implications for clinical guidelines. *Circulation*. 2004;110(18):2824-2830.

Tanne D, Koren-Morag N, Graff E, Goldbourt U. Blood lipids and first-ever ischemic stroke/transient ischemic attack in the bezafibrate infarction prevention (BIP) registry: high triglycerides constitute an independent risk factor. *Circulation.* 2001;104:2892-2897.

Thomson M, Al-Qattan KK, Bordia T, Ali M. Including garlic in the diet may help lower blood glucose, cholesterol, and triglycerides. *Journal of Nutrition.* 2006:136(3 Suppl):800S-802S.

Tobias K, Moore SC, Gaziano M, et al. Healthy lifestyle and the risk of stroke in women. *Archives of Internal Medicine.* 2006;166(13):1403-1409.

Troughton JA, Woodside JV, Young IS, et al. Homocysteine and coronary heart disease risk in the PRIME study. *Atherosclerosis.* 2006;Jun13; [Epub]

Weststrate JA, Meijer GW. Plant sterol-enriched margarines and reduction of plasma total-and LDL-cholesterol concentrations in normocholesterolaemic and mildly hypercholesterolaemic subjects. *European Journal of Clinical Nutrition.* 1998;52(5):334-343.

Wexler R, Aukerman G. Nonpharmacologic strategies for managing hypertension. *American Family Physician.* 2006;73(11):1953-1956.

Wilburn AJ, King DS, Glisson J, et al. The natural treatment of hypertension. *Journal of Clinical Hypertension* (Greenwich). 2004;6(5):219-221.

Wildman RP, Sutton-Tyrrell K, Newman AB, et al. Lipoprotein levels are associated with incident hypertension in older adults. *Journal of the American Geriatric Society.* 2004;52(6):916-921.

Yan LL, Daviglus ML, Liu K, et al. Midlife body mass index and hospitalization and mortality in older age. *Journal of the American Medical Association.* 2006;295(2):190-198.

ARTHRITIS, Chapter 8

Ahmed S, Wang N, Lalonde M, et al. Green tea polyphenol epigallocatechin-3-gallate (EGCG) differentially inhibits interleukin-1 beta-induced expression of matrix metalloproteinase-1 and -13 in human chondrocytes. *Journal of Pharmacology and Experimental Therapeutics.* 2004;308(2):767-773.

Altman RD, Marcussen KC. Effects of a ginger extract on knee pain in patients with osteoarthritis. *Arthritis and Rheumatism.* 2001;44(11):2531-2538.

Belch J, Hill A. Evening primrose oil and borage oil in rheumatologic conditions. *American Journal of Clinical Nutrition.* 2000;71(Suppl):352S-356S.

Chainani-Wu N. Safety and anti-inflammatory activity of curcumin: a component of turmeric (Curcuma longa). *Journal of Alternative and Complementary Medicine.* 2003;9(1):161-168.

Choi HK. Dietary risk factors for rheumatic diseases. *Current Opinion in Rheumatology.* 2005;17(2):141-146.

Choi HK, Atkinson K, Karlson EW, et al. Alcohol intake and risk of incident gout in men: a prospective study. *Lancet.* 2004;363:1277-1281.

Choi HK, Atkinson K, Karlson EW, et al. Purine-rich foods, dairy and protein intake, and the risk of gout in men. *New England Journal of Medicine.* 2004;350(11):1093-1103.

Choi HK, Atkinson K, Karlson EW. Alcohol intake and risk of incident gout in men: a prospective study. *Lancet.* 2004;363(9417):1251-1252.

Choi HK, Curhan G. Gout: epidemiology and lifestyle choices. *Current Opinion in Rheumatology.* 2005;17(3): 341-345.

Clegg DO, Reda DJ, Harris CL, et al. Glucosamine, chondroitin sulfate, and the two in combination for painful knee osteoarthritis. *New England Journal of Medicine.* 2006;354(8):795-808.

Cleland LG, James MJ, Proudman SM. Fish oil: what the prescriber needs to know. *Arthritis Research & Therapy.* 2005;8(1):202.

Cleland LG, James MJ, Proudman SM. The role of fish oils in the treatment of rheumatoid arthritis. *Drugs.* 2003;63(9):845-853.

Ding C, Cicuttini F, Scott F, et al. Natural history of knee cartilage defects and factors affecting change. *Archives of Internal Medicine.* 2006;166(6):651-658.

Funk JL, Oyarzo JN, Frye JB, et al. Turmeric extracts containing curcuminoids prevent experimental rheumatoid arthritis. *Journal of Natural Products.* 2006;69(3):351-355.

Grant WB. Epidemiology of disease risks in relation to vitamin D insufficiency. *Progress in Biophysics and Molecular Biology.* 2006;92(1):65-79.

Hochberg M, Lixing L, Barker B, et al. Traditional Chinese acupuncture is effective as adjunctive therapy in patients with osteoarthritis of the knee. *Arthritis and Rheumatism.* 2001;44:819-825.

Hooper MM, Stellato TA, Hallowell PT, et al. Musculoskeletal findings in obese subjects before and after weight loss following bariatric surgery. *International Journal of Obesity* (Lond) [serial online]. 2006;Apr 25.

Ishikawa Y, Kitamura M. Bioflavonoid quercetin inhibits mitosis and apoptosis of glomerular cells in vitro and in vivo. *Biochemical and Biophysical Research Communications.* 2000;279(2):629-634.

Kopp W. The atherogenic potential of dietary carbohydrate. *Preventive Medicine.* 2006;42(5):336-342.

Kraus VB, Huebner JL, Stabler T, et al. Ascorbic acid increases severity of spontaneous knee osteoarthritis in a guinea pig model. *Arthritis and Rheumatism.* 2004;50(6):1822-1831.

Lee SJ, Terkeltaub RA, Kavanaugh A. Recent developments in diet and gout. *Current Opinion in Rheumatology.* 2006;18(2):193-198.

Luk AJ, Simkin PA. Epidemiology of hyperuricemia and gout. *American Journal of Managed Care.* 2005;11(15 Suppl):S435-S442.

Martinez-Dominguez E, de la Puerta R, Ruiz-Gutierrez V. Protective effects upon experimental inflammation models of a polyphenol-supplemented virgin olive oil diet. *Inflammation Research.* 2001;50(2):102-106.

Messier SP, Gutekunst DJ, Davis C, DeVita P. Weight loss reduces knee-joint loads in overweight and obese older adults with knee osteoarthritis. *Arthritis and Rheumatism.* 2005;52(7):2026-2032.

Messier SP, Loeser RF, Miller GD, et al. Exercise and dietary weight loss in overweight and obese older adults with knee osteoarthritis: the arthritis, diet, and activity promotion trial. *Arthritis and Rheumatism.* 2004;50(5):1501-1510.

Morelli V, Naquin C, Weaver, V. Alternative therapies for traditional disease states: osteoarthritis. *American Family Physician.* 2003;67(2):339-344.

Najm WI, Reinsch S, Hoehler F, et al. S-Adenosyl methionine (SAMe) versus celecoxib for the treatment of osteoarthritis symptoms: a double-blind cross-over trial. *BMC Musculoskeletal Disorders* [serial online]. 2004;5:6.[Epub]

Padyukov L, Silva C, Stolt P, et al. A gene-environment interaction between smoking and shared epitope genes in HLA-DR provides a high risk of seropositive rheumatoid arthritis. *Arthritis and Rheumatism.* 2004;50(10): 3085-3092.

Pattison DJ, Silman AJ, Goodson NJ, et al. Vitamin C and the risk of developing inflammatory polyarthritis: prospective nested case-control study. *Annals of the Rheumatic Diseases.* 2004;63(7):843-847.

Pattison DJ, Symmons DP, Lunt M, et al. Dietary beta-cryptoxanthin and inflammatory polyarthritis: results from a population-based prospective study. *Journal of Clinical Nutrition.* 2005;82(2):451-455.

Pattison DJ, Symmons DPM, Lunt M, et al. Dietary risk factors for the development of inflammatory poly-arthritis: evidence for a role of high level of red meat consumption. *Arthritis and Rheumatism.* 2004;50(12): 3804-3812.

Piscoya J, Rodriguez Z, Bustamante SA, et al. Efficacy and safety of freeze-dried cat's claw in osteoarthritis of the knee: mechanisms of action of the species Uncaria guianensis. *Inflammation Research.* 2001;50(9):442-448.

Sato M, Miyazaki T, Kambe F. Quercetin, a bioflavonoid, inhibits the induction of interleukin 8 and mono-cyte chemoattractant protein-1 expression by tumor necrosis factor-alpha in cultured human synovial cells. *Journal of Rheumatology.* 1997;24(9):1680-1684.

Schlesinger N. Dietary factors and hyperuricaemia. *Current Pharmaceutical Design.* 2005;11(32):4133-4138.

Shishodia S, Sethi G, Aggarwal BB. Curcumin: getting back to the roots. *Annals of the New York Academy of Sciences.* 2005;1056:206-217.

Teixeira S. Bioflavonoids: proanthocyanidins and quercetin and their potential roles in treating musculosk-eletal conditions. *Journal of Orthopaedic and Sports Physical Therapy.* 2002;32(7):357-363.

Yoon JH, Baek SJ. Molecular targets of dietary polyphenols with anti-inflammatory properties. *Yonsei Medical Journal.* 2005;46(5):585-596.

TYPE 2 DIABETES, Chapter 9

Agardh EE, Carlsson S, Ahlbom A, et al. Coffee consumption, type 2 diabetes and impaired glucose tolerance in Swedish men and women. *Journal of Internal Medicine.* 2004;255(6):645-652.

Althuis MD, Jordan NE, Ludington EA, Wittes JT. Glucose and insulin responses to dietary chromium supplements: a meta-analysis. *American Journal of Clinical Nutrition*. 2002;76(1):148-155.

Carlsson S, Hammar N, Grill V, Kaprio J. Alcohol consumption and the incidence of type 2 diabetes: a 20-year follow-up of the Finnish Twin Cohort Study. *Diabetes Care*. 2003;26(10):2785-2790.

Davies M, Brophy S, Williams R, Taylor A. The prevalence, severity, and impact of painful diabetic peripheral neuropathy in type 2 diabetes. *Diabetes Care*. 2006;29(7):1518-1522.

Delarue J, LeFoll C, Corporeau C, Lucas D. N-3 long chain polyunsaturated fatty acids: a nutritional tool to prevent insulin resistance associated to type 2 diabetes and obesity? *Reproduction, Nutrition, Development*. 2004;44(3):289-299.

Fung TT, Hu FB, Pereira MA, et al. Whole-grain intake and the risk of type 2 diabetes: a prospective study in men. *American Journal of Clinical Nutrition*. 2002;76(3):535-540.

Gerhard GT, Ahmann A, Meeuws K, et al. Effects of a low-fat diet compared with those of a high-monounsaturated fat diet on body weight, plasma lipids and lipoproteins, and glycemic control in type 2 diabetes. *American Journal of Clinical Nutrition*. 2004;80(3):668-673.

Gillen LJ, Tapsell LC, Patch CS, et al. Structured dietary advice incorporating walnuts achieves optimal fat and energy balance in patients with type 2 diabetes mellitus. *Journal of the American Dietetic Association*. 2005;105(7):1087-1096.

Gumbiner B, Low CC, Reaven PD. Effects of a monounsaturated fatty acid-enriched hypocaloric diet on cardiovascular risk factors in obese patients with type 2 diabetes. *Diabetes Care*. 1998;21(1):9-15.

Haag M, Dippenaar NG. Dietary fats, fatty acids and insulin resistance: short review of a multifaceted connection. *Medical Science Monitor*. 2005;11(12):RA359-367.

Harsch IA, Schahin SP, Bruckner K, et al. The effect of continuous positive airway pressure treatment on insulin sensitivity in patients with obstructive sleep apnoea syndrome and type 2 diabetes. *Respiration*. 2004;71(3):252-259.

Hasanain B, Mooradian AD. Antioxidant vitamins and their influence in diabetes mellitus. *Current Diabetes Reports*. 2002;2(5):448-456.

Howard AA, Arnsten JH, Gourevitch MN. Effect of alcohol consumption on diabetes mellitus: a systematic review. *Annals of Internal Medicine*. 2004;140(3):211-219.

Hu FB, Manson JE, Stampfer MJ, et al. Diet, lifestyle, and the risk of type 2 diabetes mellitus in women. *New England Journal of Medicine*. 2001;345(11):790-797.

Ip MSM, Lam B, Ng MMT, et al. Obstructive sleep apnea is independently associated with insulin resistance. *American Journal of Respiratory and Critical Care Medicine*. 2002;165(5):670-676.

Khader YS, Dauod AS, El-Qaderi SS, et al. Periodontal status of diabetics compared with nondiabetics: a meta-analysis. *Journal of Diabetes Complications*. 2006;20(1):59-68.

Khan A, Safdar M, Ali Khan MM, et al. Cinnamon improves glucose and lipids of people with type 2 diabetes. *Diabetes Care*. 2003;26(12):3215-3218.

Kiran M, Arpak N, Unsal E, Erdogan MF. The effect of improved periodontal health on metabolic control in type 2 diabetes mellitus. *Journal of Clinical Periodontology*. 2005;32(3):266-272.

Kleefstra N, Houweling ST, Jansman FG, et al. Chromium treatment has no effect in patients with poorly controlled, insulin-treated type 2 diabetes in an obese Western population: a randomized, double-blind, placebo-controlled trial. *Diabetes Care*. 2006;29(3):521-525.

Knowler WC, Barrett-Connor E, Fowler SE, et al. Diabetes Prevention Program Research Group. Reduction in the incidence of type 2 diabetes with lifestyle intervention or metformin. *New England Journal of Medicine*. 2002;346(6):393-403.

Liese AD, Schulz M, Fang F, et al. Dietary glycemic index and glycemic load, carbohydrate and fiber intake, and measures of insulin sensitivity, secretion, and adiposity in the Insulin Resistance Atherosclerosis Study. *Diabetes Care*. 2005;28(12):2832-2838.

Lombardo YB, Chicco AG. Effects of dietary polyunsaturated n-3 fatty acids on dyslipidemia and insulin resistance in rodents and humans. A review. *Journal of Nutritional Biochemistry*. 2006;17(1):1-13.

Lopez-Garcia E, van Dam RM, Willett WC, et al. Coffee consumption and coronary heart disease in men and women: a prospective cohort study. *Circulation*. 2006;113(17):2045-2053.

Lopez-Ridaura R, Willett WC, Rimm EB, et al. Magnesium intake and risk of type 2 diabetes in men and women. *Diabetes Care*. 2004;27(1):134-140.

Mang B, Wolters M, Schmitt B, et al. Effects of a cinnamon extract on plasma glucose, HbA, and serum lipids in diabetes mellitus type 2. *European Journal of Clinical Investigation*. 2006;36(5):340-344.

Meyer KA, Kushi LH, Jacobs Jr DR, Folsom AR. Dietary fat and incidence of type 2 diabetes in older Iowa women. *Diabetes Care*. 2001;24(9):1528-1535.

Montonen J, Knekt P, Jarvinen R, et al. Whole-grain and fiber intake and the incidence of type 2 diabetes. *American Journal of Clinical Nutrition*. 2003;77(3):622-629.

Ostman E, Granfeldt, Y, Persson L, Bjorck I. Vinegar supplementation lowers glucose and insulin responses and increases satiety after a bread meal in healthy subjects. *European Journal of Clinical Nutrition*. 2005;59(9):983-988.

Partanen J, Niskanen L, Lehtinen J, et al. Natural history of peripheral neuropathy in patients with non-insulin-dependent diabetes mellitus. *New England Journal of Medicine*. 1995;333(2):89-94.

Pereira MA, Parker ED, Folsom AR. Coffee consumption and risk of type 2 diabetes mellitus: an 11-year prospective study of 28,812 postmenopausal women. *Archives of Internal Medicine*. 2006;166(12):1311-1316.

Pittas AG, Dawson-Hughes B, Li T, et al. Vitamin D and calcium intake in relation to type 2 diabetes in women. *Diabetes Care*. 2006;29(3):650-656.

Rasmussen OW, Thomsen C, Hansen KW, et al. Effects on blood pressure, glucose, and lipid levels of a high-monounsaturated fat diet compared with a high-carbohydrate diet in NIDDM subjects. *Diabetes Care*. 1993;16(12):1565-1571.

Rodrigues DC, Taba MJ, Novaes AB, et al. Effect of non-surgical periodontal therapy on glycemic control in patients with type 2 diabetes mellitus. *Journal of Periodontology*. 2003;74(9):1361-1367.

Salmeron J, Hu FB, Manson JE, et al. Dietary fat intake and risk of type 2 diabetes in women. *American Journal of Clinical Nutrition*. 2001;73(6):1019-1026.

Thomas DE, Elliott EJ, Naughton GA. Exercise for type 2 diabetes mellitus (review). *Cochrane Review* [serial online]. 2006;3.

Tuomilehto J, Lindstrom J, Eriksson JG, et al. Prevention of type 2 diabetes mellitus by changes in lifestyle among subjects with impaired glucose tolerance. *New England Journal of Medicine*. 2001;334(18):1343-1350.

van Dam RM, Willett WC, Manson JE, Hu FB. Coffee, caffeine, and risk of type 2 diabetes. *Diabetes Care*. 2006;29(2):308-403.

Wannamethee SG, Camargo Jr CA, Manson JE, et al. Alcohol drinking patterns and risk of type 2 diabetes mellitus among younger women. *Archives of Internal Medicine*. 2003;163(11):1329-1336.

Wiernsperger N, Nivoit P, Bouskela E. Obstructive sleep apnea and insulin resistance: a role for microcirculation? *Clinics*. 2006;61(3):253-266.

Wing RR, Venditti E, Jakicic JM, et al. Lifestyle intervention in overweight individuals with a family history of diabetes. *Diabetes Care*. 1998;21(3):350-359.

Yeh GY, Eisenberg DM, Kaptchuk TJ, Phillips RS. Systematic review of herbs and dietary supplements for glycemic control in diabetes. *Diabetes Care*. 2003;26(4):1277-1294.

OSTEOPOROSIS, Chapter 10

Bacon L, Stern JS, Keim, NL, Van Loan MD. Low bone mass in premenopausal chronic dieting women. *European Journal of Clinical Nutrition*. 2004;58(6):966-971.

Bonjour JP. Dietary protein: an essential nutrient for bone health. *Journal of the American College of Nutrition*. 2005;24(6 Suppl):526S-536S.

Booth SL, Tucker KL, Chen H, et al. Dietary vitamin K intakes are associated with hip fracture but not with bone mineral density in elderly men and women. *American Journal of Clinical Nutrition*. 2000;71(5):1201-1208.

Feskanich D, Weber P, Willett WC, et al. Vitamin K intake and hip fractures in women: A prospective study. *American Journal of Clinical Nutrition*. 1999;69(1):74-79.

Gjesdal CG, Vollset SE, Ueland PM, et al. Plasma total homocysteine level and bone mineral density: the Hordaland Homocysteine Study. *Archives of Internal Medicine*. 2006;166(1):88-94.

Ikeda Y, Iki M, Morita A, et al. Intake of fermented soybeans, natto, is associated with reduced bone loss in postmenopausal women: Japanese Population-Based Osteoporosis Study (JPOS). *Journal of Nutrition*. 2006;136(5):1323-1328.

Ilich JZ, Brownbill RA, Tamorini L, Crncevic-Orlic Z. To drink or not to drink: how are alcohol, caffeine and past smoking related to bone mineral density in elderly women? *Journal of the American College of Nutrition*. 2002;21(6):526-544.

Ilich JZ, Kerstetter JE. Nutrition in bone health revisited: A story beyond calcium. *Journal of the American College of Nutrition*. 2000;19(6):715-737.

Jacka FN, Pasco JA, Henry MJ, et al. Depression and bone mineral density in a community sample of peri-menopausal women: Geelong Osteoporosis Study. *Menopause*. 2005;12(1):88-91.

Judge JO, Kleppinger A, Kenny A, et al. Home-based resistance training improves femoral bone mineral density in women on hormone therapy. *Osteoporosis International*. 2005;16(9):1096-1108.

Kamer AR, El-Ghorab N, Marzec N, et al. Nicotine induced proliferation and cytokine release in osteoblastic cells. *International Journal of Molecular Medicine*. 2006;17(1):121-127.

Kerstetter JE, O'Brien KO, Caseria DM, et al. The impact of dietary protein on calcium absorption and kinetic measures of bone turnover in women. *Journal of Clinical Endocrinology and Metabolism*. 2005;90(1):26-31.

Kerstetter JE, O'Brien KO, Insogna KL. Dietary protein, calcium metabolism, and skeletal homeostasis revisited. *American Journal of Clinical Nutrition*. 2003;78(3 suppl):584S-592S.

Kerstetter JE, O'Brien KO, Insogna KL. Low protein intake: the impact on calcium and bone homeostasis in humans. *Journal of Nutrition*. 2003;133(3):855S-861S.

Macdonald HM, New SA, Fraser, et al. Low dietary potassium intakes and high dietary estimates of net endogenous acid production are associated with low bone mineral density in premenopausal women and increased markers of bone resorption in postmenopausal women. *American Journal of Clinical Nutrition*. 2005;81(4):923-933.

Macdonald HM, New SA, Golden MHN, et al. Nutritional associations with bone loss during the menopausal transition: evidence of a beneficial effect of calcium, alcohol, and fruit and vegetable nutrients and of a detrimental effect of fatty acids. *American Journal of Clinical Nutrition*. 2004;79(1):155-165.

Mussolino ME. Depression and hip fracture risk: the NHANES I epidemiologic follow-up study. *Public Health Reports*. 2005;120(1):71-75.

National Institutes of Health. Osteoporosis Prevention, Diagnosis, and Therapy. *NIH Consensus Statement*. [Online]. 2000; March 27-29;17(1):1-36.

New SA, Robins SP, Campbell MK, et al. Dietary influences on bone mass and bone metabolism: Further evidence of a positive link between fruit and vegetable consumption and bone health? *American Journal of Clinical Nutrition*. 2000;71(1):142-151.

Nieves JW. Osteoporosis: The role of micronutrients. *American Journal of Clinical Nutrition*. 2005;81(5):1232S-1239S.

Rapuri PB, Gallagher JC, Balhorn KE, Ryschon KL. Alcohol intake and bone metabolism in elderly women. *American Journal of Clinical Nutrition*. 2000;72(5):1206-1213.

Reinwald S, Weaver CM. Soy isoflavones and bone health: a double-edged sword? *Journal of Natural Products*. 2006;69(3):450-459.

Ryder KM, Shorr RI, Bush AJ, et al. Magnesium intake from food and supplements is associated with bone mineral density in healthy older white subjects. *Journal of the American Geriatric Society*. 2005;53(11):1875-1880.

Setchell KD, Lydeking-Olsen E. Dietary phytoestrogens and their effect on bone: evidence from in vitro and in vivo, human observational, and dietary intervention studies. *American Journal of Clinical Nutrition*. 2003;78(3 suppl):593S-609S.

Suominen H. Muscle training for bone strength. *Aging Clinical and Experimental Research*. 2006;18(2):85-93.

Tucker KL, Hannan MT, Chen H, et al. Potassium, magnesium, and fruit and vegetable intakes are associated with greater bone mineral density in elderly men and women. *American Journal of Clinical Nutrition*. 1999;69(4):727-736.

van Meurs JB, Dhonukshe-Rutten RA, Pluijm SM, et al. Homocysteine levels and the risk of osteoporotic fracture. *New England Journal of Medicine*. 2004; 350(20):2033-2041.

Weaver CM, Cheong JM. Soy isoflavones and bone health: the relationship is still unclear. *Journal of Nutrition*. 2005;135(5):1243-1247.

Weber P. Vitamin K and bone health. *Nutrition*. 2001;17(10):880-887.

Zhang X, Shu XO, Li H, et al. Prospective cohort study of soy food consumption and risk of bone fracture among postmenopausal women. *Archives of Internal Medicine*. 2005;165(16):1890-1895.

CATARACTS AND MACULAR DEGENERATION, Chapter 11

Ferrigno L, Aldigeri R, Rosmini F, et al. Associations between plasma levels of vitamins and cataract in the Italian-American Clinical Trial of Nutritional Supplements and Age-Related Cataract (CTNS):CTNS Report #2. *Ophthalmic Epidemiology.* 2005;12(2):71-80.

Gale CR, Hall NF, Phillips DIW, Martyn CN. Lutein and zeaxanthin status and risk of age-related macular degeneration. *Investigative Ophthalmology & Visual Science.* 2003;44(6):2461-2465.

Jacques PF, Taylor A, Moeller S, et al. Long-term nutrient intake and 5-year change in nuclear lens opacities. *Archives of Ophthalmology.* 2005;123(4):517-526.

Kuzniarz M, Mitchell P, Cumming RG, Flood VM. Use of vitamin supplements and cataract: the Blue Mountains Eye Study. *American Journal of Ophthalmology.* 2001;132(1):19-26.

Leske MC, Chylack LT Jr, Wu SY. The Lens Opacities Case-Control Study. Risk factors for cataract. *Archives of Ophthalmology.* 1991;109(2):244-251.

Moeller SM, Taylor A, Tucker KL, et al. Overall adherence to the Dietary Guidelines for Americans is associated with reduced prevalence of early age-related nuclear lens opacities in women. *Journal of Nutrition.* 2004;134(7):1812-1819.

Newsome DA, Rothman RJ. Zinc uptake in vitro by human retinal pigment epithelium. *Investigative Ophthalmology & Visual Science.* 1987;28(11):1795-1799.

Richer S, Stiles W, Statkute L, et al. Double-masked, placebo-controlled, randomized trial of lutein and antioxidant supplementation in the intervention of atrophic age-related macular degeneration: the Veterans LAST study (Lutein Antioxidant Supplementation Trial). *Optometry.* 2004;76(4):216-230.

Robertson JM, Donner AP, Trevithick JR. A possible role for vitamins C and E in cataract prevention. *American Journal of Clinical Nutrition.* 1991;53(1 Suppl):346S-351S.

Santosa S, Jones PJH. Oxidative stress in ocular disease: does lutein play a protective role? *Canadian Medical Association Journal.* 2005;173(8):861-862.

Sperduto RD, Hu TS, Milton RC, et al. The Linxian cataract studies. Two nutrition intervention trials. *Archives of Ophthalmology.* 1993;111(9):1246-1253.

Tavani A, Negri E, La Vecchia C. Food and nutrient intake and risk of cataract. *Annals of Epidemiology.* 1996;6(1):41-46.

Thiagarajan G, Chandani S, Sundari CS, et al. Antioxidant properties of green and black tea, and their potential ability to retard the progression of eye lens cataract. *Experimental Eye Research.* 2001;73(3):393-401.

van Leeuwen R, Boekhoorn S, Vingerling JR, et al. Dietary intake of antioxidants and risk of age-related macular degeneration. *Journal of the American Medical Association.* 2005;294(24):3101-3107.

Vinson JA, Zhang J. Black and green teas equally inhibit diabetic cataracts in a streptozotocin-induced rat model of diabetes. *Journal of Agricultural and Food Chemistry.* 2005;53(9):3710-3713.

Yang CS, Landau JM. Effects of tea consumption on nutrition and health. *Journal of Nutrition.* 2000;130(10):2409-2412.

MEMORY, Chapter 12

Andres-Lacueva C, Shukitt-Hale B, Galli RL, et al. Anthocyanins in aged blueberry-fed rats are found centrally and may enhance memory. *Nutritional Neuroscience.* 2005;8(2):111-120.

Bryan J, Calvaresi E, Hughes D. Short-term folate, vitamin B-12 or vitamin B-6 supplementation slightly affects memory performance but not mood in women of various ages. *Journal of Nutrition.* 2002;132(6):1345-1356.

Casadesus G, Shukitt-Hale B, Stellwagen HM, et al. Modulation of hippocampal plasticity and cognitive behavior by short-term blueberry supplementation in aged rats. *Nutritional Neuroscience.* 2004;7(5-6):309-316.

Dang-Vu TT, Desseilles M, Peigneux P, Maquet P. A role for sleep in brain plasticity. *Pediatric Rehabilitation.* 2006;9(2):98-118.

Jennings JR, Muldoon MF, Ryan C, et al. Reduced cerebral blood flow response and compensation among patients with untreated hypertension. *Neurology.* 2005;64(8):1358-1365.

Jones N, Rogers PJ. Preoccupation, food, and failure: an investigation of cognitive performance deficits in dieters. *International Journal of Eating Disorders.* 2003;33(2):185-192.

Kang JH, Ascherio A, Grodstein F. Fruit and vegetable consumption and cognitive decline in aging women. *Annals of Neurology.* 2005;57(5):713-720.

Mahoney CR, Taylor HA, Kanarek RB, Samuel P. Effect of breakfast composition on cognitive processes in elementary school children. *Physiology and Behavior.* 2005;85(5):635-645.

Maquet P. The role of sleep in learning and memory. *Science.* 2001;294(5544):1048-1052.

Morris MC, Evans DA, Tangney CC, et al. Fish consumption and cognitive decline with age in a large community study. *Archives of Neurology.* 2005;62(12):1849-1853.

Mosavi Jazayeri SM, Amani R, Mugahi NK. Effects of breakfast on memory in healthy young adults. *Asia Pacific Journal of Clinical Nutrition.* 2004;13(Suppl):S130.

O'Brien LT, Hummert ML. Memory performance of late middle-aged adults: contrasting self-stereotyping and stereotype threat accounts of assimilation to age stereotypes. *Social Cognition.* 2006;24(3):338-358.

Rovio S, Karebolt I, Helkala EL, et al. Leisure-time physical activity at midlife and the risk of dementia and Alzheimer's disease. *Lancet Neurology.* 2005;4(11):705-711.

Singh A, Naidu PS, Kulkarni SK. Reversal of aging and chronic ethanol-induced cognitive dysfunction by quercetin a bioflavonoid. *Free Radical Research.* 2003;37(11):1245-1252.

Solfrizzi V, Panza F, Capurso A. The role of diet in cognitive decline. *Journal of Neural Transmission.* 2003;110(1):95-110.

Tucker KL, Qiao N, Acott T, et al. High homocysteine and low B vitamins predict cognitive decline in aging men: the Veterans Affairs Normative Aging Study. *American Journal of Clinical Nutrition.* 2005;82(3):627-635.

Wesnes KA, Pincock C, Richardson D, et al. Breakfast reduces declines in attention and memory over the morning in schoolchildren. *Appetite.* 2003;41(3):329-331.

Winocur G, Greenwood CF. The effects of high fat diets and environmental influences on cognitive performance in rats. *Behavioural Brain Research.* 1999;101(2):153-161.

Zimmerman FJ, Christakis DA. Children's television viewing and cognitive outcomes: a longitudinal analysis of national data. *Archives of Pediatric and Adolescent Medicine.* 2005;159(7):619-625.

MOOD, Chapter 13

Bottiglieri T. Homocysteine and folate metabolism in depression. *Progress in Neuropsychopharmacology & Biological Psychiatry.* 2005;29(7):1103-1112.

Coppen A, Bolander-Gouaille C. Treatment of depression: time to consider folic acid and vitamin B12. *Journal of Psychopharmacology.* 2005;19(1):59-65.

Diehl DJ, Gershon S. The role of dopamine in mood disorders. *Comprehensive Psychiatry.* 1992;33(2):115-120.

Gloth FM 3rd, Alam W, Hollis B. Vitamin D vs broad spectrum phototherapy in the treatment of seasonal affective disorder. *Journal of Nutrition, Health, & Aging.* 1999;3(1):5-7.

Haskell CF, Kennedy DO, Wesnes KA, Scholey AB. Cognitive and mood improvements of caffeine in habitual consumers and habitual non-consumers of caffeine. *Psychopharmacology* (Berl). 2005;179(4):813-825.

Hypericum Depression Trial Study Group. Effect of Hypericum perforatum (St John's wort) in major depressive disorder: a randomized controlled trial. *Journal of the American Medical Association.* 2002;287(14):1807-1814.

James JE, Rogers PJ. Effects of caffeine on performance and mood: withdrawal reversal is the most plausible explanation. *Psychopharmacology* (Berl). 2005;182(1):1-8.

Lansdowne AT, Provost SC. Vitamin D3 enhances mood in healthy subjects during winter. *Psychopharmacology* (Berl). 1998;135(4):319-323.

Lee S, Gura KM, Kim S, et al. Current clinical applications of omega-6 and omega-3 fatty acids. *Nutrition in Clinical Practice.* 2006;21(4):323-341.

Parker G, Gibson NA, Brotchie H, et al. Omega-3 fatty acids and mood disorders. *American Journal of Psychiatry.* 2006;163(6):969-978.

Shelton RC, Keller MB, Gelenberg A, et al. Effectiveness of St John's wort in major depression: a randomized controlled trial. *Journal of the American Medical Association.* 2001;285(15):1978-1986.

Smith A, Sutherland D, Christopher G. Effects of repeated doses of caffeine on mood and performance of alert and fatigued volunteers. *Journal of Psychopharmacology*. 2005;19(6):620-626.

Sontrop J, Campbell MK. Omega-3 polyunsaturated fatty acids and depression: a review of the evidence and a methodological critique. *Preventive Medicine*. 2006;42(1):4-13.

Szegedi A, Kohnen R, Dienel A, Kieser M. Acute treatment of moderate to severe depression with hypericum extract WS 5570 (St John's wort): randomized controlled double blind non-inferiority trial versus paroxetine. *British Medical Journal* [serial online]. 2005;330(7490):503.

Trivedi MH, Greer TL, Grannemann BD, et al. Exercise as an augmentation strategy for treatment of major depression. *Journal of Psychiatric Practice*. 2006;12(4):205-213.

Vieth R, Kimball S, Hu A, Walfish PG. Randomized comparison of the effects of the vitamin D3 adequate intake versus 100 mcg (4000 IU) per day on biochemical responses and the wellbeing of patients. *Nutrition Journal* [serial online]. 2004;3:8.

MIGRAINE HEADACHES, Chapter 14

Allais G, Bussone G, De Lorenzo C, et al. Advanced strategies of short-term prophylaxis in menstrual migraine: state of the art and prospects. *Neurological Science*. 2005: 26(Suppl2):S125-S129.

Bic Z, Blix GG, Hopp HP, et al. The influence of a low-fat diet on incidence and severity of migraine headaches. *Journal of Women's Health & Gender-Based Medicine*. 1999;8(5):623-630.

Bigal ME, Liberman JN, Lipton RB. Obesity and migraine: a population study. *Neurology*. 2006;66:545-550.

Biondi DM. Physical treatments for headache: a structured review. *Headache*. 2005;45(6):738-746.

Boardman HF, Thomas E, Millson DS, Croft PR. Psychological, sleep, lifestyle and comorbid associations with headache. *Headache*. 2005;45(6):657-669.

Crawford P, Simmons M. What dietary modifications are indicated for migraines? *Journal of Family Practice*. 2006;55(1):62-64.

Diener HC, Pfaffenrath V, Pageler L, et al. The fixed combination of acetylsalicylic acid, paracetamol and caffeine is more effective than single substances and dual combination for the treatment of headache: a multicentre, randomized, double-blind, singe-dose, placebo-controlled parallel group study. *Cephalalgia*. 2005;25(10):776-787.

Goldstein J, Silberstein SD, Saper JR, et al. Acetaminophen, aspirin, and caffeine versus sumatriptan succinate in the early treatment of migraine: results from the ASSET trial. *Headache*. 2005;45(8):973-982.

Harel Z, Gascon G, Riggs S, et al. Supplementation with omega-3 polyunsaturated fatty acids in the management of recurrent migraines in adolescents. *Journal of Adolescent Health*. 2002;31(2):154-161.

Jakubowski M, McAllister PJ, Bajwa ZH, et al. Exploding vs. imploding headache in migraine prophylaxis with Botulinum Toxin A. *Pain* 2006: 125(3):286-295

Modi S, Lowder DM. Medications for migraine prophylaxis. *American Family Physician*. 2006;73(1):72-78.

Nadelson C. Sport and exercise-induced migraines. *Current Sports Medicine Reports*. 2006;5(1):29-33.

Rasura M, Spalloni A, Ferrari M, et al. A case series of young stroke in Rome. *European Journal of Neurology*. 2006;13(2):146-152.

Sándor PS, Di Clemente L, Coppola G, et al. Efficacy of coenzyme Q10 in migraine prophylaxis: a randomized controlled trial. *Neurology*. 2005;64(4):713-715.

Wagner W, Nootbaar-Wagner U. Prophylactic treatment of migraine with gamma-linolenic and alpha-linolenic acids. *Cephalalgia*. 1997;17(2):127-130.

PREMENSTRUAL SYNDROME, Chapter 15

Bendich A. The potential for dietary supplements to reduce premenstrual syndrome (PMS) symptoms. *Journal of the American College of Nutrition*. 2000;19(1):3-12.

Bertone-Johnson ER, Hankinson SE, Bendich A, et al. Calcium and vitamin D intake and risk of incident premenstrual syndrome. *Archives of Internal Medicine*. 2005;165(11):1246-1252.

Bianchi-Demicheli F, Ludicke F, Lucas H, Chardonnens D. Premenstrual dysphoric disorder: current status of treatment. *Swiss Medical Weekly.* 2002;132(39-40):574-578.

Case AM, Reid RL. Menstrual cycle effects on common medical conditions. *Comprehensive Therapy.* 2001;27(1):65-71.

Daugherty JE. Treatment strategies for premenstrual syndrome. *American Family Physician.* 1998;58(1):183-192,197-198.

Frackiewicz EJ, Shiovitz TM. Evaluation and management of premenstrual syndrome and premenstrual dysphoric disorder. *Journal of the American Pharmaceutical Association.* 2001;41(3):437-447.

Kljakovic M, Pullon S. Allergy and the premenstrual syndrome (PMS). *Allergy.* 1997;52(6):681-683.

Shamberger RJ. Calcium, magnesium, and other elements in the red blood cells and hair of normals and patients with premenstrual syndrome. *Biological Trace Element Research.* 2003;94(2):123-129.

Thys-Jacobs S. Micronutrients and the premenstrual syndrome: the case for calcium. *Journal of the American College of Nutrition.* 2000;19(2):220-227.

INSOMNIA, Chapter 16

Bootzin RR, Perlis ML. Nonpharmacologic treatments of insomnia. *Journal of Clinical Psychiatry.* 1992;53(suppl):37-41.

Buscemi N, Vandermeer B, Pandya R, et al. Melatonin for treatment of sleep disorders. *Evidence Report Technology Assessment.* 2004;108:1-7.

Eddy M, Walbroehl GS. Insomnia. *American Family Physician.* 1999;59(7):1911-1916,1918.

Hadley S, Petry JJ. Valerian. *American Family Physician.* 2003;67(8):1755-1758.

Hudson C, Hudson SP, Hecht T, MacKenzie J. Protein source tryptophan versus pharmaceutical grade tryptophan as an efficacious treatment for chronic insomnia. *Nutritional Neuroscience.* 2005;8(2):121-127.

Lewith GT, Godfrey AD, Prescott P. A single-blinded, randomized pilot study evaluating the aroma of Lavandula augustifolia as a treatment for mild insomnia. *Journal of Alternative and Complementary Medicine* 2005;11(4):631-637.

Morin CM, Hauri PJ, Espie CA, et al. Nonpharmacologic treatment of chronic insomnia. An *American Academy of Sleep Medicine* review. *Sleep.* 1999;22(8):1134-1156.

Rajput V, Bromley SM. Chronic insomnia: a practical review. *American Family Physician.* 1999;60(5):1431-1438.

Tworoger SS, Yasui Y, Vitiello MV, et al. Effects of a yearlong moderate-intensity exercise and a stretching intervention on sleep quality in postmenopausal women. *Sleep.* 2003;26(7):830-836.

Youngstedt SD. Effects of exercise on sleep. *Clinics in Sports Medicine.* 2005;24(2):355-365.

IRRITABLE BOWEL SYNDROME, Chapter 17

Bach DR, Erdmann G, Schmidtmann M, Monnikes H. Emotional stress reactivity in irritable bowel syndrome. *European Journal of Gastroenterology and Hepatology.* 2006;18(6):629-636.

Bundy R, Walker AF, Middleton RW, et al. Artichoke leaf extract reduces symptoms of irritable bowel syndrome and improves quality of life in otherwise healthy volunteers suffering from concomitant dyspepsia: a subset analysis. *Journal of Alternative and Complementary Medicine.* 2004;10(4):667-669.

Creed F. How do SSRIs help patients with irritable bowel syndrome? *Gut.* 2006;55(8):1065-1067.

Dapoigny M, Stockbrugger RW, Azpiroz F, et al. Role of alimentation in irritable bowel syndrome. *Digestion.* 2003;67(4):225-233.

Floch MH. Use of diet and probiotic therapy in the irritable bowel syndrome: analysis of the literature. *Journal of Clinical Gastroenterology.* 2005;39(4 Suppl 3):S243-246.

Friedman G. Diet and the irritable bowel syndrome. *Gastroenterology Clinics of North America.* 1991;20(2):313-324.

Gerson CD, Gerson MJ. A collaborative health care model for the treatment of irritable bowel syndrome. *Clinical Gastroenterology and Hepatology.* 2003;1(6):446-452.

Grigoleit HG, Grigoleit P. Peppermint oil in irritable bowel syndrome. *Phytomedicine.* 2005;12(8):601-606.

Kennedy T, Jones R, Darnley S, et al. Cognitive behaviour therapy in addition to antispasmodic treatment for irritable bowel syndrome in primary care: randomized controlled trial. *British Medical Journal.* 2005;331(7514):435-440.

Levy RL, Linde JA, Feld KA, et al. The association of gastrointestinal symptoms with weight, diet, and exercise in weight-loss program participants. *Clinical Gastroenterology and Hepatology.* 2005;3(10):992-996.

Lindfors P, Unge P, Bjornsson S, et al. Effects of hypnotherapy on IBS in different clinical settings—results from two randomized, controlled trials. Presentation at Digestive Disease Week 2006 conference. Los Angeles, CA: May 20-25, 2006.

Liu JH, Chen GH, Yeh HZ, et al. Enteric-coated peppermint-oil capsules in the treatment of irritable bowel syndrome: a prospective, randomized trial. *Journal of Gastroenterology.* 1997;32(6):765-768.

Logan AC, Beaulne TM. The treatment of small intestinal bacterial overgrowth with enteric-coated peppermint oil: a case report. *Alternative Medicine Review.* 2002;7(5):410-417.

McKay DL, Blumberg JB. A review of the bioactivity and potential health benefits of peppermint tea (Mentha piperita L.). *Phytotherapy Research* [serial online]. 2006; Jun 12.

Morgan T, Robson KM. Irritable bowel syndrome: diagnosis is based on clinical criteria. *Postgraduate Medicine.* 2002;112(5):30-32,35-36,39-41.

Nobaek S, Johansson ML, Molin G, et al. Alteration of intestinal microflora is associated with reduction in abdominal bloating and pain in patients with irritable bowel syndrome. *American Journal of Gastroenterology.* 2000;95(5):1231-1238.

O'Mahony L, McCarthy J, Kelly P, et al. Lactobacillus and bifidobacterium in irritable bowel syndrome: symptom responses and relationship to cytokine profiles. *Gastroenterology.* 2005;128(3):541-551.

Pittler MH, Ernst E. Peppermint oil for irritable bowel syndrome: a critical review and metaanalysis. *American Journal of Gastroenterology.* 1998;93(7):1131-1135.

Posserud I, Agerforz P, Ekman R, et al. Altered visceral perceptual and neuroendocrine response in patients with irritable bowel syndrome during mental stress. *Gut.* 2004;53(8):1102-1108.

Posserud I, Ersryd A, Simren M. Functional findings in irritable bowel syndrome. *World Journal of Gastroenterology.* 2005;12(18):2830-2838.

Roberts L, Wilson S, Singh S, et al. Gut-directed hypnotherapy for irritable bowel syndrome: piloting a primary care-based randomized controlled trial. *British Journal of General Practice.* 2006;56(523):115-121.

Santosa S, Farnworth E, Jones PJ. Probiotics and their potential health claims. *Nutrition Reviews.* 2006;64(6):265-274.

CELIAC DISEASE, Chapter 18

Akobeng AK, Ramanan AV, Buchan I, Heller RF. Effect of breast feeding on risk of celiac disease: a systematic review and meta-analysis of observational studies. *Archives of Disease in Childhood.* 2006;91(1): 39-43.

Alaedini A, Green PHR. Narrative review: celiac disease: understanding a complex autoimmune disorder. *Annals of Internal Medicine.* 2005;142(4):289-298.

Biagi F, Campanella J, Martucci S, et al. A milligram of gluten a day keeps the mucosal recovery away: a case report. *Nutrition Reviews.* 2004;62(9):360-363.

Dahele A, Ghosh S. Vitamin B12 deficiency in untreated celiac disease. *American Journal of Gastroenterology.* 2001;96(3):745-750.

Helms S. Celiac disease and gluten-associated diseases. *Alternative Medicine Review.* 2005;10(3):172-192.

Hischenhuber C, Crevel R, Jarry B, et al. Review article: safe amounts of gluten for patients with wheat allergy or coeliac disease. *Alimentary Pharmacology & Therapeutics.* 2006;23(5):559-575.

Kupper C. Dietary guidelines and implementation for celiac disease. *Gastroenterology.* 2005;128(4 Suppl 1): S121-127.

Lee SK, Green PH. Celiac sprue (the great modern-day imposter). *Current Opinions in Rheumatology.* 2006;18(1):101-107.

Norris JM, Barriga K, Hoffenberg EJ. Risk of celiac disease autoimmunity and timing of gluten introduction in the diet of infants at increased risk of disease. *Journal of the American Medical Association.* 2005;293(19):2343-2351.

Srinivasan U, Jones E, Carolan J, Feighery C. Immunohistochemical analysis of coeliac mucosa following ingestion of oats. *Clinical and Experimental Immunology.* 2006;144(2):197-203.

Storsrud S, Olsson M, Arvidsson Lenner R, et al. Adult coeliac patients do tolerate large amounts of oats. *European Journal of Clinical Nutrition.* 2003;57(1):163-169.

Thompson T. Oats and the gluten-free diet. *Journal of the American Dietetic Association.* 2003;103(3):376-379.

Thompson T, Dennis M, Higgins LA, et al. Gluten-free diet survey: are Americans with coeliac disease consuming recommended amounts of fibre, iron, calcium and grain foods? *Journal of Human Nutrition and Dietetics.* 2005;18(3):163-169.

INDEX

Underscored page references indicate boxed text and tables. **Boldface** references indicate illustrations.